T0348634

Ambulatory Anesthesia

Editor

MICHAEL T. WALSH

ANESTHESIOLOGY CLINICS

www.anesthesiology.theclinics.com

Consulting Editor
LEE A. FLEISHER

June 2019 • Volume 37 • Number 2

ELSEVIER

1600 John F. Kennedy Boulevard • Suite 1800 • Philadelphia, Pennsylvania, 19103-2899

http://www.theclinics.com

ANESTHESIOLOGY CLINICS Volume 37, Number 2
June 2019 ISSN 1932-2275, ISBN-13: 978-0-323-68222-0

Editor: Colleen Dietzler
Developmental Editor: Kristen Helm

Photocopying

Single photocopies of single articles may be made for personal use as allowed by national copyright laws. Permission of the Publisher and payment of a fee is required for all other photocopying, including multiple or systematic copying, copying for advertising or promotional purposes, resale, and all forms of document delivery. Special rates are available for educational institutions that wish to make photocopies for non-profit educational classroom use. For information on how to seek permission visit www.elsevier.com/permissions or call: (+44) 1865 843830 (UK)/(+1) 215 239 3804 (USA).

Derivative Works

Subscribers may reproduce tables of contents or prepare lists of articles including abstracts for internal circulation within their institutions. Permission of the Publisher is required for resale or distribution outside the institution. Permission of the Publisher is required for all other derivative works, including compilations and translations (please consult www.elsevier. com/permissions).

Electronic Storage or Usage

Permission of the Publisher is required to store or use electronically any material contained in this periodical, including any article or part of an article (please consult www.elsevier.com/permissions). Except as outlined above, no part of this publication may be reproduced, stored in a retrieval system or transmitted in any form or by any means, electronic, mechanical, photocopying, recording or otherwise, without prior written permission of the Publisher.

Notice

No responsibility is assumed by the Publisher for any injury and/or damage to persons or property as a matter of products liability, negligence or otherwise, or from any use or operation of any methods, products, instructions or ideas contained in the material herein. Because of rapid advances in the medical sciences, in particular, independent verification of diagnoses and drug dosages should be made.

Although all advertising material is expected to conform to ethical (medical) standards, inclusion in this publication does not constitute a guarantee or endorsement of the quality or value of such product or of the claims made of it by its manufacturer.

Anesthesiology Clinics (ISSN 1932-2275) is published quarterly by Elsevier Inc., 360 Park Avenue South, New York, NY 10010-1710. Months of issue are March, June, September, and December. Periodicals postage paid at New York, NY and at additional mailing offices. Subscription prices are $100.00 per year (US student/resident), $360.00 per year (US individuals), $446.00 per year (Canadian individuals), $693.00 per year (US institutions), $876.00 per year (Canadian institutions), $225.00 per year (Canadian and foreign student/resident), $469.00 per year (foreign individuals), and $876.00 per year (foreign institutions). To receive student and resident rate, orders must be accompanied by name of affiliated institution, date of term, and the *signature* of program/residency coordinator on institutions letterhead. Orders will be billed at individual rate until proof of status is received. Foreign air speed delivery is included in all *Clinics'* subscription prices. All prices are subject to change without notice. POSTMASTER: Send address changes to *Anesthesiology Clinics,* Elsevier Health Sciences Division, Subscription Customer Service, 3251 Riverport Lane, Maryland Heights, MO 63043. Customer Service (orders, claims, online, change of address): Elsevier Health Sciences Division, Subscription Customer Service, 3251 Riverport Lane, Maryland Heights, MO 63043. **Tel:1-800-654-2452 (U.S. and Canada); 314-447-8871 (outside U.S. and Canada). Fax: 314-447-8029. E-mail: journalscustomerservice-usa@elsevier. com (for print support); journalsonlinesupport-usa@elsevier.com (for online support).**

Reprints. For copies of 100 or more of articles in this publication, please contact the Commercial Reprints Department, Elsevier Inc., 360 Park Avenue South, New York, NY 10010-1710. Tel.: 212-633-3874; Fax: 212-633-3820; E-mail: reprints@elsevier.com.

Anesthesiology Clinics, is also published in Spanish by McGraw-Hill Inter-americana Editores S. A., P.O. Box 5-237, 06500 Mexico D. F., Mexico.

Anesthesiology Clinics, is covered in *MEDLINE/PubMed (Index Medicus), Current Contents/Clinical Medicine, Excerpta Medica, ISI/BIOMED,* and *Chemical Abstracts.*

Contributors

CONSULTING EDITOR

LEE A. FLEISHER, MD
Robert D. Dripps Professor and Chair of Anesthesiology and Critical Care, Professor of Medicine, Perelman School of Medicine, University of Pennsylvania, Philadelphia, Pennsylvania, USA

EDITOR

MICHAEL T. WALSH, MD
Assistant Professor, Department of Anesthesiology and Perioperative Medicine, Mayo Clinic College of Medicine and Science, Mayo Clinic, Rochester, Minnesota, USA

AUTHORS

BASEM ABDELMALAK, MD, FASA
Professor of Anesthesiology, Departments of General Anesthesiology and Outcomes Research, Director, Anesthesia for Bronchoscopic Surgery, Director, Center for Sedation, Cleveland Clinic, Cleveland, Ohio, USA

ANOUSHKA M. AFONSO, MD, FASA
Director, Enhanced Recovery Programs (ERP), Assistant Attending, Department of Anesthesiology and Critical Care Medicine, Josie Robertson Surgery Center, Memorial Sloan Kettering Cancer Center, New York, New York, USA

ADAM W. AMUNDSON, MD
Assistant Professor of Anesthesiology, Department of Anesthesiology and Perioperative Medicine, Mayo Clinic, Rochester, Minnesota, USA

ALBERTO E. ARDON, MD, MPH
Assistant Professor, Department of Anesthesiology, University of Florida Jacksonville, Jacksonville, Florida, USA

VIKRAM K. BANSAL, MD
Assistant Professor of Clinical Anesthesiology, Department of Anesthesiology, Division of Ambulatory Anesthesiology, Vanderbilt University Medical Center, Nashville, Tennessee, USA

SEKAR S. BHAVANI, MD
Staff Anesthesiologist, Section Head NORA, Associate Residency Program Director, Department of General Anesthesiology, Cleveland Clinic, Cleveland, Ohio, USA

JOSHUA A. BLOOMSTONE, MD, MSc, FASA
Associate Professor, Division of Surgery and Interventional Sciences, University College London, London, United Kingdom; Clinical Professor of Anesthesiology, The University of Arizona College of Medicine Phoenix, Senior Vice President for Clinical Innovation, Envision Physician Services, Plantation, Florida, USA

EVELYN JANE BROCK, DO
Associate Professor of Clinical Anesthesiology, Department of Anesthesiology, Division of Ambulatory Anesthesiology, Vanderbilt University Medical Center, Nashville, Tennessee, USA

STEVEN F. BUTZ, MD
Associate Professor of Anesthesiology, Medical College of Wisconsin, Medical Director, Children's Hospital of Wisconsin Surgicenter, Milwaukee, Wisconsin, USA

TIMOTHY DEL ROSARIO, MD
Fellow, Business and Leadership Ambulatory Anesthesia Fellowship, Department of Anesthesiology, The Ohio State University Wexner Medical Center, Columbus, Ohio, USA

KATHERINE H. DOBIE, MD
Associate Professor of Clinical Anesthesiology, Department of Anesthesiology, Vanderbilt University Medical Center, Nashville, Tennessee, USA

REBECCA M. GERLACH, MD
Assistant Professor, Department of Anesthesia and Critical Care, The University of Chicago, Chicago, Illinois, USA

ROY GREENGRASS, MD, FRCP
Professor, Department of Anesthesiology and Perioperative Medicine, Mayo Clinic, Jacksonville, Florida, USA

GAGANPREET GREWAL, MD
Assistant Professor of Anesthesiology and Pain Management, The University of Texas Southwestern Medical Center, Dallas, Texas, USA

MICHAEL GUERTIN, MD, MBA, CPE, FASA
Associate Professor, Department of Anesthesiology, The Ohio State University Wexner Medical Center, Jameson Crane Sports Medicine Institute, Columbus, Ohio, USA

JARRETT HEARD, MD, MBA
Assistant Professor, Department of Anesthesiology, The Ohio State University Wexner Medical Center, Columbus, Ohio, USA

ADAM K. JACOB, MD
Associate Professor of Anesthesiology, Department of Anesthesiology and Perioperative Medicine, Mayo Clinic, Rochester, Minnesota, USA

CHRISTOPHER J. JANKOWSKI, MD, MBOE
Assistant Professor of Anesthesiology, Mayo Clinic College of Medicine and Science, Rochester, Minnesota, USA

GIRISH P. JOSHI, MBBS, MD, FFARCSI
Professor of Anesthesiology and Pain Management, The University of Texas Southwestern Medical Center, Dallas, Texas, USA

GERALD A. MACCIOLI, MD, MBA, FCCM, FASA
Chief Quality Officer, Medical Director, Clinical Research and Scientific Intelligence, The Envision Healthcare Center for Quality and Patient Safety, The Physicians Quality Registry, Envision Healthcare, Plantation, Florida, USA

KEIRA P. MASON, MD
Senior Associate in Perioperative Anesthesia, Department of Anesthesiology, Critical Care and Pain Medicine, Bader 3, Boston Children's Hospital, Associate Professor of Anaesthesia, Harvard Medical School, Boston, Massachusetts, USA

ROBERT LEWIS McCLAIN, MD
Senior Associate Consultant, Department of Anesthesiology and Perioperative Medicine, Mayo Clinic, Jacksonville, Florida, USA

PATRICK J. McCORMICK, MD, MEng
Vice Chair for Informatics, Assistant Attending, Department of Anesthesiology and Critical Care Medicine, Memorial Sloan Kettering Cancer Center, New York, New York, USA

M. STEPHEN MELTON, MD
Assistant Professor, Department of Anesthesiology, Duke University Medical Center, Durham, North Carolina, USA

DOUGLAS G. MERRILL, MD, MBA, MA, FASA
Merrill Healthcare, Reno, Nevada, USA

KAREN C. NIELSEN, MD
Assistant Professor, Department of Anesthesiology, Duke University Medical Center, Durham, North Carolina, USA

OBIANUJU OKOCHA, MD
Assistant Professor, Department of Anesthesiology, Northwestern University, Chicago, Illinois, USA

BRIAN M. OSMAN, MD
Assistant Professor, Department of Anesthesiology, Perioperative Medicine and Pain Management, University Health Tower, University of Miami Miller School of Medicine, Miami, Florida, USA

JASON K. PANCHAMIA, DO
Assistant Professor of Anesthesiology, Department of Anesthesiology and Perioperative Medicine, Mayo Clinic, Rochester, Minnesota, USA

ARUN PRASAD, MBBS, FRCA, FRCPC
Assistant Professor, Department of Anesthesiology, University of Toronto, Women's College Hospital, Toronto, Ontario, Canada

LEOPOLDO V. RODRIGUEZ, MD, FAAP, FASA
Vice-President, Society for Ambulatory Anesthesiology (SAMBA), Member, ASA Committee on Performance and Outcome Measures, Medical Director, Surgery Center of Aventura, Assistant National Medical Director for Ambulatory Anesthesiology, South Florida Director of Clinical Quality and Performance Improvement for Ambulatory Anesthesiology, Envision Physician Services, Plantation, Florida, USA

MARK A. SAXEN, DDS, PhD
Volunteer Clinical Associate Professor, Anesthesia, Oral Surgery and Hospital Dentistry, Indiana University School of Dentistry, Private Practice, Indiana Office-Based Anesthesia, Indianapolis, Indiana, USA

FRED E. SHAPIRO, DO, FASA
Associate Professor, Department of Anesthesia, Critical Care and Pain Medicine, Beth Israel Deaconess Medical Center, Harvard Medical School, Boston, Massachusetts, USA

BOBBIEJEAN SWEITZER, MD, FACP
Professor, Department of Anesthesiology, Northwestern University, Chicago, Illinois, USA

HANAE K. TOKITA, MD, FASA
Assistant Attending, Department of Anesthesiology and Critical Care, Director of Regional Anesthesia, Josie Robertson Surgery Center, Memorial Sloan Kettering Cancer Center, New York, New York, USA

JAMES W. TOM, DDS, MS
Associate Clinical Professor, Section on Dental Anesthesiology, Herman Ostrow School of Dentistry, University of Southern California, Dentist Anesthesiologist, Divisions 1 & 3, Herman Ostrow School of Dentistry, University of Southern California, Los Angeles, California, USA

REBECCA S. TWERSKY, MD, MPH, FASA
Professor of Anesthesiology, Department of Anesthesiology and Critical Care Medicine, Chief of Anesthesia, Josie Robertson Surgery Center, Memorial Sloan Kettering Cancer Center, New York, New York, USA

MICHAEL T. WALSH, MD
Assistant Professor, Department of Anesthesiology and Perioperative Medicine, Mayo Clinic College of Medicine and Science, Mayo Clinic, Rochester, Minnesota, USA

Contents

Most surgery in the United States occurs in offices, free-standing surgicenters, and hospital-based outpatient facilities. Patients are frequently elderly with comorbidities, and procedures are increasingly complex. Traditionally, patients have been evaluated on the day of surgery by anesthesia providers. Obtaining information on patients' health histories, establishing criteria for appropriateness, and communicating medication instructions streamline throughput, lower cancellations and delays, and improve provider and patient satisfaction. Routine testing does not lower risk or improve outcomes. Evaluating and optimizing patients with significant diseases, especially those with suboptimal management, has positive impact on ambulatory surgery and anesthesia.

Obesity and obstructive sleep apnea (OSA) are often associated with increased perioperative risks and challenges for the anesthesiologist. This article addresses the current controversies surrounding perioperative care of morbidly obese patients with or without OSA scheduled for ambulatory surgery, particularly in a free-standing ambulatory center. Topics discussed include preoperative selection of obese and OSA patients for ambulatory surgeries, intraoperative methods to reduce perioperative risk, and appropriate postoperative care.

Although enhanced recovery pathways were initially implemented in inpatients, their principles are relevant in the ambulatory setting. Opioid minimization and addressing pain and nausea through multimodal analgesia, regional anesthesia, and robust preoperative education programs are integral to the success of ambulatory enhanced recovery programs. Rather than measurements of length of stay as in traditional inpatient programs, the focus of enhanced recovery programs in ambulatory surgery should be on improved quality of recovery, pain management, and early ambulation.

As more surgeries are moving out of the hospital setting, effective emergency response in freestanding ambulatory surgery centers requires organized preparedness. Rapid, consistent emergency response can be challenged by their rarity of occurrence, fast-paced environment, and relative lack of resources. Anesthesiologists who practice in these settings must be aware of the differences between the management of an anesthetic emergency in the hospital with virtually unlimited resources and staff, versus an ambulatory surgery center with limited resources and slightly different goal: stabilization and transfer of care. Regular simulation-based training schedules are effective for ambulatory surgery center preparedness for emergency response.

Demand for low-cost, high-quality health care has forced the total joint replacement (TJR) industry to evaluate and mitigate high variable costs. Minimizing hospital stay can significantly reduce total cost of care. A shortened hospital stay does not compromise patient safety or satisfaction, and may reduce perioperative complications compared with multiple-day hospitalizations. Through the use of enhanced recovery clinical pathways, outpatient TJRs have progressively shortened hospitalizations. Successful ambulatory TJR can be accomplished through advances in surgical technique, presurgical patient education, opioid-sparing multimodal analgesia, anesthetic techniques that facilitate rapid recovery, and progressive rehabilitation.

Proper pain control is critical for ambulatory surgery. Regional anesthesia can decrease postoperative pain, improve patient satisfaction, and expedite patient discharge. This article discusses the techniques, clinical pearls, and potential pitfalls associated with those blocks, which are most useful in an ambulatory perioperative setting. Interscalene, supraclavicular, infraclavicular, axillary, paravertebral, erector spinae, pectoralis, serratus anterior, transversus abdominis plane, femoral, adductor canal, popliteal, interspace between the popliteal artery and capsule of the knee, and ankle blocks are described.

Ambulatory surgery in the pediatric population can be similar to adult ambulatory with a few different challenges. Success is best determined by appropriate preoperative screening. Issues common in pediatrics are the respiratory infection, asthma, congenital heart disease and syndromes, as well as sleep apnea. Risk factors for adverse respiratory events and patient transfer differ from adults as do data for rapid discharge.

and other health care workers to manage and continuously improve their work. This article reviews some of the steps necessary to successfully adopt lean in an ambulatory surgical setting.

Health care professionals see measurement through their own eyes and biases. This article makes the patient central to what is measured. Patient-reported experience measures and patient-reported outcome measures are of the utmost importance. In addition, as clinicians continue to evolve how they measure what really matters, they need to be mindful of the time taken from direct patient care to achieve these activities. In addition, and most important, clinicians must ensure that all measures are designed to ensure that population health is improved, that patient experience and outcomes are enhanced, and that the cost of care is reduced.

Congress passed the Medicare Access and Chip Reauthorization Act of 2015 to replace the flawed sustainable growth rate system and it consolidates all pay-for-performance programs. These programs are intended to reduce health care costs but do not address the lack of funding for the social networks that (in all other developed countries) support better health and lower health care use and cost. These programs require reporting by providers about performance on quality, cost, and other metrics, leading to bonuses for those who exceed Centers for Medicare & Medicaid Services–determined metrics and financial penalties for those who do not.

The ambulatory surgery center medical director is a physician leader who recognizes the need to develop a culture that encourages communication and empowerment of employees and professional staff, leading to engagement that optimize care through patient selection, safety and satisfaction requires vision and guidance from the medical director and is central to success of the ASC. Innovative thinking further improves patient care and long-term success by leveraging advances in technology and sustainable practices.

ANESTHESIOLOGY CLINICS

ISSUE OF RELATED INTEREST

Orthopedic Clinics of North America, January 2018 (Vol. 49, No. 1)
Outpatient Surgery
Michael J. Beebe, Clayton C. Bettin, James H. Calandruccio,
Benjamin J. Grear, Benjamin M. Mauck, William M. Mihalko,
Jeffrey R. Sawyer, Thomas (Quin) Throckmorton, Patrick C. Toy,
and John C. Weinlein, *Editors*
Available at: http://www.orthopedic.theclinics.com/

THE CLINICS ARE AVAILABLE ONLINE!
Access your subscription at:
www.theclinics.com

Foreword

Ambulatory Anesthesia: The Innovating Edge of Perioperative Medicine?

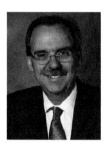

Lee A. Fleisher, MD
Consulting Editor

The origin of ambulatory anesthesia can be traced all the way back to 1898 when James Hendson Nicoll performed almost 9000 ambulatory surgical procedures. It took almost 7 decades later before free-standing ambulatory surgery centers were developed. During the past half century, there has been amazing progress in this. These include advances in the preoperative evaluation and preparation of the ambulatory surgery patient and a marked expansion of both the conditions of the patient having surgery as an outpatient and the types of surgery being performed. The advancement of regional and Enhanced Recovery After Surgery techniques has pushed this expansion. Finally, outcomes and metrics for ambulatory surgery and anesthesia are finally being developed. In this issue of the *Anesthesiology Clinics*, innovations in safely allowing more patients to undergo ambulatory are discussed.

Michael T. Walsh, MD is Assistant Professor of Anesthesiology and a consultant in the Department of Anesthesiology and Perioperative Medicine at the Mayo Clinic. He is the immediate past president of the Society for Ambulatory Anesthesia and the Vice Chair of the Standards Committee of the American Association for

Anesthesiology Clin 37 (2019) xiii–xiv
https://doi.org/10.1016/j.anclin.2019.03.002
1932-2275/19/© 2019 Published by Elsevier Inc.

anesthesiology.theclinics.com

Accreditation of Ambulatory Surgery Facilities. He is, therefore, well qualified to edit this issue of ambulatory anesthesia.

Lee A. Fleisher, MD
Perelman School of Medicine at
University of Pennsylvania
3400 Spruce Street, Dulles 680
Philadelphia, PA 19104, USA

E-mail address:
Lee.Fleisher@uphs.upenn.edu

Preface
Ambulatory Anesthesia

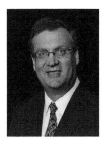

Michael T. Walsh, MD
Editor

We're all ambulatory anesthesiologists now!

This quote originated with Keynesian economic theory in the 1970s and has a couple of meanings: solidarity, to be sure, but also a sense of inevitable dominance. I think both meanings help illustrate my point when it comes to ambulatory anesthesia. First, the percentage of ambulatory surgical procedures and anesthetics continues to grow with greater than 60% of all surgeries in the United States classified as ambulatory. Office-based procedures have grown even faster. As of 2014, 11% of the estimated 885 million office visits in the United States were for a surgical procedure. Of course, not everyone is literally practicing ambulatory anesthesia every day, but many subspecialties and procedures once thought to be confined to the inpatient realm are beginning to shift to same-day surgery and 23-hour stay. Outpatient minimally invasive cardiac and vascular procedures, total joint arthroplasty, spine surgery, and minimally invasive neurosurgery are seeing a growing migration toward ambulatory surgery. The nonoperating room procedural practice is seeing explosive growth, and ambulatory patients make up the lion's share.

The dominance of ambulatory surgery and anesthesia is not just about the numbers. More importantly, it's about the mindset; the idea that all anesthetics should return patients to their preoperative functional status as quickly as possible and with minimal pain or side effects. Ambulatory anesthesia was an early proponent of minimizing opioids and utilizing multimodal therapy for pain control and PONV treatment. The enhanced recovery protocols currently popular for inpatient procedures that emphasize early discharge and same-day ambulation and oral intake are a perfect example of the ambulatory philosophy taken to the next level. We can't discharge all our patients in the first day (yet!), but our anesthetic approach continually strives to reach that lofty goal, and as minimally invasive surgical techniques and pain control continue

Anesthesiology Clin 37 (2019) xv–xvi
https://doi.org/10.1016/j.anclin.2019.03.001
1932-2275/19/© 2019 Published by Elsevier Inc.

to improve, someday, the promise of nearly all anesthesiologists being ambulatory anesthesiologists may come to fruition.

This issue of *Anesthesiology Clinics* focuses on the present state of ambulatory anesthesia; however, because of ambulatory's broad reach, I think the topics will be of interest to all anesthesiologists. Clinical topics begin with an article on preoperative evaluation, with special emphasis on cardiac conditions and chronic pain patients. A separate article on obesity and obstructive sleep apnea explores the current data and latest guidelines for these commonly encountered conditions. Other important clinical articles include an ambulatory-based focus on enhanced recovery and emergency response. Specific patient groups are discussed in articles on total joint arthroplasty, regional anesthesia, pediatrics, and GI/NORA. Finally, safety in office-based anesthesia and the special concerns of pediatric dental anesthesia rounds out the clinical section.

In 1970, anesthesiologists John Ford and Wallace Reed opened the first free-standing ASC, and ambulatory anesthesiologists have been involved in the practice management side of same-day surgery ever since. While not every ambulatory anesthesiologist holds the actual title of medical director, most of us practice with that mindset: always looking for ways to improve quality, efficiency, and patient satisfaction. It is hoped that the practice management articles focusing on quality, outcomes, and payment will make that job easier. The article on medical director issues offers a nice synopsis and invaluable thoughts on leadership.

I want to thank all of the authors for their time and talents in contributing to this issue. Their dedication and expertise really shine through and it is hoped will offer valuable tips and strategies to help you improve the care of your patients, no matter where you practice.

Michael T. Walsh, MD
Department of Anesthesiology &
Perioperative Medicine
Mayo Clinic
100 1st Street SW
Rochester, MN 55901, USA

E-mail address:
walsh.michael1@mayo.edu

Preoperative Evaluation for Ambulatory Anesthesia
What, When, and How?

Obianuju Okocha, MD[a], Rebecca M. Gerlach, MD[b],
BobbieJean Sweitzer, MD[a],*

KEYWORDS

- Ambulatory surgery • Preoperative assessment • Risk assessment • Cardiac testing
- Cataract surgery • Ischemic heart disease • Heart failure • Hypertension

KEY POINTS

- Preoperative evaluation of patients anticipating ambulatory surgery can improve care and reduce risk.
- Advanced age and comorbidities increase adverse outcomes in patients having outpatient procedures.
- Patients with ischemic heart disease, heart failure, valvular disease, hypertension, or diabetes mellitus and those requiring dialysis commonly may benefit from evaluation before the day of surgery.
- Routine testing does not improve outcomes for patients having ambulatory surgery.
- Cataract surgery is very low risk despite patients typically being elderly with multiple comorbidities.

INTRODUCTION

With increasing volumes of ambulatory procedures, appropriate preoperative assessment is critical to provide efficient, cost-effective, and safe care. With appropriate patient selection and optimization, ambulatory surgery is safe for most patients. Many low-risk patients are efficiently evaluated immediately before surgery. More complex patients benefit from assessment in advance of surgery. The American Society of Anesthesiologists physical status (ASA-PS) classification provides a starting point for triaging patients. Ambulatory surgery can be safe in patients with elevated ASA-PS classification. In a European multicenter study investigating 57,709 procedures, including ASA-PS III patients, major complications, such as stroke, myocardial infarction (MI), and pulmonary embolism, were low, and no deaths were definitively related to surgery.[1]

[a] Department of Anesthesiology, Northwestern University, NMH/Feinberg 5-704, 251 East Huron Street, Chicago, IL 60611, USA; [b] Department of Anesthesia & Critical Care, University of Chicago, 5841 South Maryland Avenue, MC 4028, Chicago, IL 60637, USA
* Corresponding author.
E-mail address: Bobbie.sweitzer@nm.org

Anesthesiology Clin 37 (2019) 195–213
https://doi.org/10.1016/j.anclin.2019.01.014   anesthesiology.theclinics.com

The preoperative assessment serves to screen, evaluate, and intervene to decrease morbidity and mortality and predict perioperative outcomes.[2] Preoperative evaluation determines if patients are candidates for ambulatory surgery. Risk assessment may lead to changes in venue, medical management, alternatives to the planned surgery, selection of specialized anesthetic techniques, or planning for appropriate care. Inadequate evaluation and optimization are associated with perioperative mortality[3] and increases complications, costs, delays, and cancellation of surgeries.[4,5]

Appropriately triaging patients allows for efficient screening of low-risk ASA-PS I and II patients. ASA-PS III and IV patients may benefit from more intensive assessment and optimization before the day of surgery (DOS). Patients with severe systemic diseases (eg, ASA-PS III and above) or risk factors (eg, frailty, poor functional status, limited medical care) may require testing, coordination of care, and initiation of therapies. A health history surveys for conditions (bolded, asterisked items in **Fig. 1**) requiring further in-person (ideally in a preoperative clinic) evaluation before surgery or directs healthier patients to telephone screening or assessment on the DOS. Ideally, the survey is completed as soon as surgery is contemplated, which can be before referral to a surgeon.

Regardless of when assessment occurs, anesthesia providers in the ambulatory setting are tasked with evaluating patients and deciding on both fitness for ambulatory surgery and the appropriate venue (eg, office-based, free-standing surgicenter, hospital-based ambulatory center). Particularly challenging conditions, cardiac or neurologic diseases (eg, ischemic heart disease, heart failure [HF], undiagnosed murmurs, valvular disease, stroke or neuromuscular disorders), hypertension, or diabetes mellitus (DM) are not uncommon. Elderly patients present particular challenges with increased postoperative complications and hospital readmissions. Reducing testing provides an opportunity to streamline care and save costs. Care coordination for complex patients, such as those with cardiac implantable electronic devices (CIED), those undergoing dialysis, or those with chronic pain, improves care. This review highlights important challenges in the preoperative evaluation of ambulatory surgery patients.

COMMON MEDICAL CONDITIONS OR PATIENT GROUPS
Ischemic Heart Disease

Cardiac risk assessment and optimization are necessary in preoperative evaluation. The 2014 American College of Cardiology/American Heart Association (ACC/AHA) guidelines on perioperative cardiovascular evaluation for noncardiac surgery include a stepwise algorithm for patients 55 years and older, or those with risk factors for, or diagnosis of, coronary artery disease (CAD) (**Fig. 2**).[6] Step 3 in the algorithm considers patient and surgical factors to estimate the risk of major adverse cardiac events (MACE). Various risk assessment tools exist, including the Myocardial Infarction or Cardiac Arrest (MICA),[7] the National Surgical Quality Improvement Project (NSQIP) database risk model,[8] and the Revised Cardiac Risk Index (RCRI).[9] MICA is available at www.surgicalriskcalculator.com/miorcardiacarrest. NSQIP is also a free online resource (www.riskcalculator.facs.org). **Table 1** summarizes the RCRI. Of note, for low-risk surgeries, there is wide variability among the risk assessment tools when predicting cardiac complications. Using more than one risk assessment tool can lead to differences in decision making.[10] Assessment tools inform discussions of appropriateness of surgery, and direct testing. Cardiac testing is indicated only if the results will impact management.[6,11] Excessive testing increases cost and leads to harm if results prompt further testing, particularly in patients at low risk of MACE who are unlikely to benefit from preoperative interventions. Cataract and minor plastic surgery are

Name _____ DOB _____

Preferred Daytime Phone #_____Preferred Language _____

Planned surgery _____ Today's Date _____

Surgeon _____Primary Care Physician _____PCP Phone #_____

Please list all previous surgeries (and approximate dates)

Please list any allergies to medications, latex, food or other (and your reactions to them)

List all medications (include over-the-counter drugs, inhalers, herbals, supplements and aspirin)

Drug Name	Dose and How Often?	Drug Name	Dose and How Often?
1.		7.	
2.		8.	
3.		9.	
4.		10.	
5.		11.	
6.		12.	

Weight: (lbs or kg) _____ Height: (inches or cm) _____ (Circle the measurement units you use)

Please check any of the following that apply to your health:

☐ Heart attack at any time*	☐ Heart stent at any time*	☐ LVAD*
☐ Heart attack within past 60 days*	☐ Atrial fibrillation*	☐ Heart device*
☐ Chest pain or pressure with activity*	☐ Arrhythmia*	☐ Pacemaker*
☐ Angina*	☐ Congenital heart disease*	☐ Defibrillator*
☐ Heart failure*	☐ Hypertension	☐ Fainted in the last year*
☐ Heart surgery*	☐ Murmur*	☐ Pain in legs while walking
☐ Heart stent in the last 6 months*	☐ Valve disorder*	☐ None of these
☐ Unable to climb 2 flights of stairs or walking 2 blocks because of chest pain or trouble breathing*		

☐ Oxygen at home*	☐ Asthma*	☐ Pneumonia in last 2 months*	☐ None of these
☐ Pulmonary hypertension*	☐ COPD*	☐ Any problems with your lungs*	
☐ Trouble breathing at rest or with minimal exertions*	☐ Severe cough*		

Fig. 1. Preoperative health history survey. Bolded, asterisked conditions are associated with elevated perioperative risks. Patients with these conditions may benefit from being seen ahead of the day of surgery. AVM, arteriovenous malformation; COPD, chronic obstructive pulmonary disease; CPAP, continuous positive airway pressure; DOB, date of birth; excl., excluding; HIV, human immunodeficiency virus; LVAD, left ventricular assist device.

considered very low risk, and preoperative cardiac testing is not indicated.[6] The NSQIP calculator, which allows specification of the planned surgery and was derived from populations that included ambulatory surgical patients, likely best determines overall surgical risk.

Procedures are delayed if possible for 60 days after an MI because of the high risk of MACE.[6] Surgery requiring interruption of dual-antiplatelet therapy (DAPT) is delayed for a minimum of 1 month following bare-metal stent placement and 6 months after drug-eluting stent (DES) placement.[12] If a DES was placed for an acute coronary syndrome (ACS), 12 months of DAPT is indicated before interruption. Stopping DAPT after 3 to 6 months following DES placement is considered for urgent surgery, when the harm of delaying outweighs the risk of stent thrombosis.[12]

Name _____

☐ Face, arm or leg weakness	☐ **Dementia***	☐ **Spinal cord injury***
☐ **Stroke/TIA within past 3 months***	☐ **Parkinson's**	☐ **Brain tumor***
☐ Stroke or TIA at any time	☐ **Myasthenia gravis***	☐ **Brain aneurysm or AVM***
☐ Paralysis	☐ **Muscular dystrophy***	☐ **Epilepsy, blackouts or seizures***
☐ Difficulty speaking	☐ **Multiple Sclerosis***	☐ None of these

☐ **Hospitalized in last 30 days***	☐ Hepatitis B/C	☐ **Rheumatoid arthritis***
☐ Diabetes	☐ **Jaundice***	☐ Sjogren's
☐ **Cancer: What type?_____***	☐ **Hyperthyroidism***	☐ **HIV***
☐ **Chemo or radiation last 3 months***	☐ Hypothyroidism	☐ **Use illegal drugs (excl. marijuana)***
☐ **Kidney disease other than stones***	☐ **Adrenal disorder***	☐ **Kidney failure***
☐ **Liver disease***	☐ **Pituitary disorder***	☐ Taking antibiotics for any reason
☐ **Cirrhosis***	☐ **Dialysis***	☐ None of these
☐ **Lupus***	☐ **Scleroderma***	

☐ **Blood thinners or anticoagulants other than aspirin***	☐ **Hemophilia***	☐ **Sickle cell disease***
☐ **Bleeding with surgery or tooth extractions***	☐ **Von Willebrands***	☐ **Anemia***
☐ **Blood transfusion in last 3 months***	☐ **Known bleeding disorder***	☐ Severe nose bleeds
☐ **Blood clots/ Pulmonary embolus***	☐ **Jehovah's Witness / Refusal of blood products***	☐ None of these

☐ **Malignant hyperthermia (in blood relatives or self) with anesthesia***	☐ Dentures
	☐ Problems opening your mouth
☐ **Severe nausea or vomiting from anesthesia***	☐ Loose teeth
☐ Difficult airway with anesthesia	☐ None of the these

☐ **Unintentional weight loss > 10 lbs***	☐ Feel that everything you did was an effort: ____ days in the last week
☐ Difficulty getting out of bed/chair by yourself	
☐ Difficulty making your own meals	☐ **Need assistance with eating or bathing or dressing***
☐ Your physical abilities limit your daily activities	☐ Fallen in the last 6 months (___ times)
☐ Difficulty doing your own shopping	☐ None of the these

☐ Very loud snoring	☐ High blood pressure/ Hypertension	☐ Sleep apnea; Uses CPAP
☐ Tired/fall asleep frequently during the day		☐ None of these
☐ **Observed to stop breathing during sleep***	☐ **Sleep apnea; NO CPAP***	

☐ Cannot speak and/or understand English	☐ Deaf	☐ None of these
☐ Cannot lie flat for 45 min	☐ Blind	
☐ Currently pregnant. Last menstrual period began:_____		
☐ Smoker (current or past) _____ packs/day for _____ years. Quit date_____		
☐ Drink alcohol. How much each day? _____ beers _____ glasses of wine _____ shots of hard alcohol		

Fig. 1. (*continued*).

Guideline-directed medical therapy, with statins, aspirin, and in certain instances, β-blockers, lowers perioperative risk.[6]

Heart Failure

HF is an independent risk factor for adverse outcomes after surgery and doubles the mortality after major noncardiac surgery over CAD alone.[13] Systolic HF, reduced ejection fraction, and decompensated HF increase risk. Decompensated HF presents as a major risk for MACE. Elective surgery is delayed for coordinated treatment with a cardiologist. Transthoracic echocardiography (TTE) is reasonable (class IIa recommendation) in patients with HF and worsening dyspnea or clinical changes or may be considered (class IIb recommendation) if there has been no reassessment within the last year.[6]

B-type natriuretic peptide (BNP) or N-terminal pro-BNP is used to assess HF or suspected HF. BNP is a plasma biomarker synthesized by cardiac myocytes and fibroblasts in response to ventricular-filling pressures and wall stress. Many cardiac and

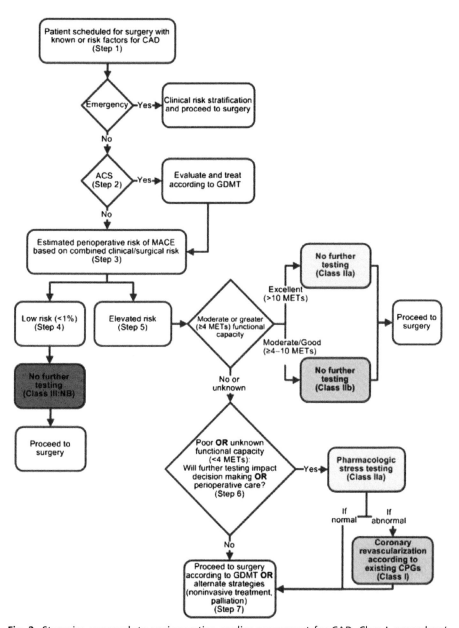

Fig. 2. Stepwise approach to perioperative cardiac assessment for CAD. Class I, procedure/treatment should be performed/administered; Class IIa, it is reasonable to perform procedure/administer treatment; Class IIb, procedure/treatment may be considered; Class III, procedure not helpful/treatment not proven benefit; CPG, clinical practice guideline; GDMT, guideline-directed medical therapy; MET, metabolic equivalent; NB, no benefit. (*Adapted from* Fleisher LA, Fleischmann KE, Auerbach AD, et al. 2014 ACC/AHA guideline on perioperative cardiovascular evaluation and management of patients undergoing noncardiac surgery: a report of the American College of Cardiology/American Heart Association Task Force on practice guidelines. J Am Coll Cardiol 2014;64(22):e94; with permission.)

Table 1
Risk assessment using the revised cardiac risk index

Risk Factor	Definition of Risk Factor
High-risk surgical procedures	• Intraperitoneal • Intrathoracic • Suprainguinal vascular
Ischemic heart disease	• History of MI • History of positive exercise test • Current complaint of chest pain presumed due to myocardial ischemia • Use of nitrate therapy • ECG with pathologic Q waves
Congestive HF	• History of congestive HF • Pulmonary edema • Paroxysmal nocturnal dyspnea • Bilateral rales or S3 gallop • Chest radiograph showing pulmonary vascular redistribution
History of transient ischemic attack (TIA) or cerebrovascular accident (CVA)	—
Insulin therapy for diabetes	—
Creatinine >2.0 mg/dL	—

Each risk factor is assigned 1 point: 0 to 1 point predicts low risk of MACE at less than 1%; 2 points predict elevated risk of MACE at 6.6% and 3 or more points predict elevated risk of MACE at 11%.

Modified from Lee TH, Marcantonio ER, Mangione CM, et al. Derivation and prospective validation of a simple index for prediction of cardiac risk of major noncardiac surgery. Circulation 1999;100(10):1047.

noncardiac conditions (eg, HF, ACS, valvular heart disease [VHD], atrial fibrillation, advanced age, renal failure, anemia, pulmonary hypertension) elevate BNP, but a low BNP effectively rules out *significant* heart disease.[14] Patients with HF may have an elevated BNP, and serial monitoring guides optimization and timing of surgery. Surgery is best delayed until the BNP is at baseline.

Undiagnosed Murmurs

The differential diagnosis of a systolic murmur includes aortic stenosis (AS) or sclerosis, mitral or tricuspid regurgitation, pulmonic stenosis, ventricular septal defect, hypertrophic cardiomyopathy, and hyperdynamic states. A diastolic murmur always has significant implications, and may be caused by mitral stenosis (MS). A TTE is warranted before surgery to investigate a new murmur. If a new pathologic condition is discovered, follow-up with a primary care provider or cardiologist should be arranged. Symptoms of dyspnea, chest pain, or syncope with an undiagnosed murmur warrant postponement of surgery pending an echocardiogram.

Valvular Heart Disease

Providers need to be aware of the indications for interventions, the valvular pathologic condition, symptoms, anticoagulation, and results of TTE in patients with VHD. Patients with asymptomatic or mild disease are at low risk perioperatively, whereas patients with symptoms or severe disease benefit from possible valve replacement or valvuloplasty before surgery and are not candidates for ambulatory surgery. VHD progresses over time, and periodic monitoring with TTE is indicated (**Table 2**). Symptoms

Table 2
Frequency of echocardiograms in patients with valvular heart disease (asymptomatic and normal left ventricular function)

	Valve Lesion			
Severity	Aortic Stenosis (Normal SV)	Aortic Regurgitation	Mitral Stenosis	Mitral Regurgitation
Mild	Every 3–5 y (V_{max} 2.0–2.9 m/s)	Every 3–5 y	Every 3–5 y (MVA >1.5 cm^2)	Every 3–5 y
Moderate	Every 1–2 y (V_{max} 3.0–3.9 m/s)	Every 1–2 y		Every 1–2 y
Severe	Every 6–12 mo (V_{max} ≥4 m/s)	Every 6–12 mo Dilating LV: more frequently	Every 1–2 y (MVA 1.0–1.5 cm^2) Once every year (MVA <1.0 cm^2)	Every 6–12 mo Dilating LV: more frequently

Patients with mixed valve disease may require more frequent evaluations than is recommended for single valve lesions.

TTE is recommended in patients with known VHD with any change in symptoms or physical examination findings. This table refers to only patients with asymptomatic VHD and normal left ventricular function. Patients with symptomatic severe VHD and decompensated ventricular function will usually undergo valvular intervention.

Abbreviations: LV, left ventricle; MVA, mitral valve area; SV, stroke volume; V_{max}, maximum velocity.

Adapted from Nishimura RA, Otto CM, Bonow RO, et al. 2014 AHA/ACC guideline for the management of patients with valvular heart disease: a report of the American College of Cardiology/American Heart Association Task Force on practice guidelines. J Am Coll Cardiol 2014;63(22):e66; with permission.

(eg, dyspnea, syncope, exercise limitation, angina) predict disease severity. Patients with severe AS may not exercise sufficiently to elicit symptoms.[15] Patients with severe AS (valve area ≤1.0 cm^2, V_{max} >4 m/s, or mean pressure gradient >40 mm Hg) can proceed with minor procedures if asymptomatic with normal ventricular function. **Fig. 3** details staging of AS and indications for valve replacement.[16] MS is less common than AS. Severe MS is a valve area ≤1.5 cm^2 and elevated pulmonary artery systolic pressure greater than 30 mm Hg. Percutaneous balloon valvuloplasty may be indicated preoperatively in severe symptomatic rheumatic valvular stenosis.[16] The severity of VHD guides the use of invasive monitoring, surgical venue, or suitability for discharge home. Discontinuation of anticoagulation and bridging is coordinated with prescribing physicians.

Hypertension

Elevated blood pressure (BP) is challenging to manage. A BP value that is too high to proceed with surgery is not well defined. BP <140/90 mm Hg reduces long-term chronic diseases, such as HF, stroke, and chronic kidney disease. A 2017 ACC/AHA task force for management of high BP in adults recommends that "patients planning elective major surgery with systolic BP ≥180 mm Hg or diastolic BP ≥110 mm Hg, deferring surgery may be considered."[17] No recommendations exist for low-risk surgery. A preinduction systolic blood pressure (SBP) greater than 200 mm Hg is associated with postoperative myocardial injury and death after major surgery.[18] *Baseline* versus *preinduction* BP is considered when deciding to defer surgery. Anxiety typically elevates BP. Optimal conditions for BP measurement, including a relaxed environment, patient seated with arm outstretched for 1 minute, repeat measurements, ambulatory BP monitoring, and manual determination if the heart rate is irregular,

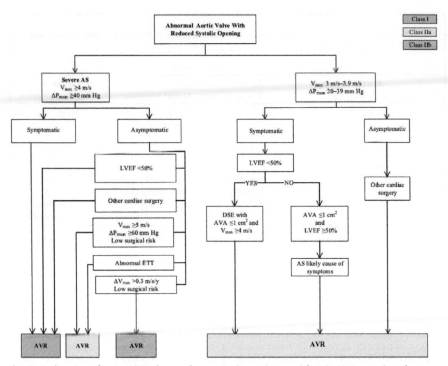

Fig. 3. Indications for aortic valve replacement in patients with AS. AVA, aortic valve area; AVR, aortic valve replacement by either surgical or transcatheter approach; DP_mean, mean pressure gradient; DSE, dobutamine stress echocardiography; ETT, exercise treadmill test; LVEF, left ventricular ejection fraction; V_max, maximum velocity. (*Adapted from* Nishimura RA, Otto CM, Bonow RO, et al. 2014 AHA/ACC guideline for the management of patients with valvular heart disease: a report of the American College of Cardiology/American Heart Association task force on practice guidelines. J Am Coll Cardiol 2014;63(22):e77; with permission.)

are seldom met on the DOS. If BP as measured by ambulatory monitoring or in a primary care provider's office is controlled, a single elevated reading preoperatively does not warrant delaying surgery.

A joint guideline published by the Association of Anaesthetists of Great Britain and Ireland and the British Hypertension Society provides pragmatic recommendations.[19] To improve resource utilization and prevent unnecessary cancellations on the DOS due to hypertension, they recommend screening in the primary care setting, and only patients with documented SBP less than 160 mm Hg and diastolic BP less than 100 mm Hg within the last year are referred for elective surgery. The guidelines advocate for adequate BP control before referring patients for surgery. For patients lacking documented primary care BP readings, noncompliant with treatment, or poorly controlled despite appropriate management, surgery may be reasonable if BP is less than 180/110 mm Hg in the preoperative clinic.[19] The argument for proceeding stems from understanding that cardiovascular morbidity reduction occurs over a period that is much longer than the time to achieve BP control.

If surgery is delayed for BP optimization, preoperative clinic providers should initiate medications when a diagnosis of hypertension is evident and coordinate care with primary care providers to continue therapy for 6 to 8 weeks to allow regression of vascular changes. Perioperative hypotension is more harmful than hypertension. Antihypertensive therapy is managed to avoid perioperative hypotension.[20,21] Angiotensin-converting enzyme inhibitors (ACEIs) and angiotensin II receptor antagonists (ARBs) cause intraoperative hypotension that can be refractory to treatment. Clinicians may be reluctant to hold these medications over concern for preinduction hypertension. A randomized trial demonstrated that discontinuing ACEIs and ARBs on the day of ambulatory surgery does not substantially increase preoperative BP or result in cancellations.[22] Patients should continue all other antihypertensive medications on the DOS. Initiating β-blockers immediately preoperatively is discouraged to avoid hypotension.[23]

Diabetes Mellitus

DM can cause systemic effects, such as gastroparesis, renal insufficiency, CAD, and neuropathy. Chronic hyperglycemia leads to altered metabolism, oxidative stress, and impaired leukocyte function, which contribute to poor wound healing, surgical site infections, and mortality.[24,25] Preoperative evaluation determines glycemic control, hemoglobin A1c (HbA_{1c}) levels, medications, and episodes of hypoglycemia and hyperglycemia. HbA_{1c} levels acceptable for surgery are controversial. An HbA_{1c} >8% is associated with significantly decreased wound healing.[26] A consensus guideline from the Joint British Diabetes Society suggests targeting an HbA_{1c} <8.5% before surgery.[27] The Society for Ambulatory Anesthesia recommends delaying surgery only if there is evidence of severe dehydration, ketoacidosis, or hyperosmolar nonketotic state, but not for a specific blood glucose level.[28]

The preoperative approach avoids hypoglycemia, maintains fluid and electrolyte balance, and prevents significant hyperglycemia or ketoacidosis.[29] **Table 3** details preoperative management of oral hypoglycemic agents and insulin. Oral agents are typically held on DOS, but surgery should not be delayed if patients take hypoglycemics. A 2018 French expert consensus suggests continuing oral hypoglycemics, including metformin, on DOS. Lactic acidosis from metformin is extremely rare without liver or kidney failure.[30] Metformin should not be restarted after contrast dye administration unless renal function is at baseline.

Table 3
Recommendations for the preoperative management of oral hypoglycemic agents and insulin

	Day Before Surgery	DOS
Insulin pump	No change	No change
Long-acting insulins	No change	75%–100% of morning dose
Intermediate-acting insulin	No change with daytime dose; 75% of dose if taken in the evening	50%–75% of morning dose
Fixed combination insulin	No change	50%–75% of morning dose
Short-acting insulin	No change	Hold the dose
Noninsulin injectables	No change	Hold the dose
Oral antiglycemic agents	No change	Hold the dose

Adapted from Joshi GP, Chung F, Vann MA, et al. Society for Ambulatory Anesthesia consensus statement on perioperative blood glucose management in diabetic patients undergoing ambulatory surgery. Anesth Analg 2010;111(6):1382; with permission.

Cataract surgery

Cataract surgery is the most common surgery in the United States. It is associated with very low morbidity, minimal physiologic stress, no blood loss or fluid shifts, and no need to interrupt routine medications. Most patients having cataract surgery are elderly with multiple comorbidities, but routine or screening preoperative testing does not improve safety.[31,32] Tests are indicated ONLY if the patient presents with a severe medical problem that warrants evaluation even without planned surgery.[31] If the patient is able to lie flat, stay still, communicate, follow simple commands, and local or regional anesthesia is planned, there are very few conditions that preclude surgery.[33] Before delaying cataract surgery, one must consider vision loss, increased rates of falls and hip fractures, and reduced quality of life with continued cataracts.[34]

Elderly patients

In 2017, the population of adults greater than 65 years was 15.2% of the US population,[35] and many will undergo surgery. Elderly patients have increased postoperative complications, including pulmonary, cardiovascular, and infectious events.[36] Patients greater than 70 years have increased hospital admissions following ambulatory surgery, with an odds ratio of 1.54 (1.29–1.84).[37] Elderly patients with renal failure, chronic obstructive pulmonary disease, current cancer treatment, DM, history of amputation, or revascularization are particularly at risk for unplanned admissions.[37] Care coordination to assist with discharge to home, including wound care, home medications, monitoring for complications, and adapting to limitations in daily function, is advantageous.

The American College of Surgeons and the American Geriatrics Society published guidelines for the optimal surgical care of older adults.[38,39] Recommendations are applicable to the ambulatory setting and include confirming outcome goals, identifying a surrogate decision-maker, minimizing perioperative fluids, limited fasting, and appropriate medication instructions. The guidelines specifically address comorbidities unique to the elderly. Frailty, cognitive impairment, decreased functional status, falls, and impaired nutrition are associated with postoperative morbidity and mortality.

PREOPERATIVE TESTING (NONCARDIAC)

Routine or screening preoperative blood tests, chest radiography, and electrocardiography (ECG) before ambulatory surgery have low clinical utility, have increased costs, and may unnecessarily delay surgery. Eliminating routine testing for ASA-PS I and II patients before ambulatory surgery does not increase adverse events.[40] Testing based on diseases or risk factors is indicated when it impacts decisions to proceed with surgery, the proper surgical venue, or anesthetic or surgical management. **Table 4** reviews testing indications for the ambulatory setting.

CARE COORDINATION FOR COMPLEX PATIENTS

Preoperative evaluation allows for coordination of care, choosing the appropriate venue (freestanding vs hospital-based facility), and ensures availability of resources. Patients benefitting from perioperative planning include those with CIEDs, dialysis dependency, or anticipated complex pain management.

Cardiac Implantable Electronic Devices

Ambulatory surgery is safe for patients with CIEDs with an appropriate plan for management of the device. Patients with CIEDs have significant cardiac pathologic

Table 4
Preoperative (noncardiac) testing in ambulatory surgery patients

Test	Indications
ECG	• Arrhythmias • Acute ischemia • Syncope
Complete blood count	• Anemia • Cirrhosis
Pregnancy test	May be offered to women of childbearing age for whom the result will alter management[55]
Coagulation studies (prothrombin time [PT], international normalized ratio [INR], partial thromboplastin time, platelet count)	• Personal/family history of bleeding diathesis • Warfarin use (PT, INR) • Cirrhosis • Significant malnutrition
Polysomnography	At risk for sleep apnea (per screen, such as STOP-Bang), and result may affect candidacy for outpatient surgery or alter management
Chest radiograph	Investigation of new or active pulmonary symptoms
Type and screen	For pregnancy termination (Rh) Anticipated blood loss >500 cc
Electrolytes	Diuretic use
Creatinine	Use of contrast dye
Glucose	When hypoglycemia, diabetic ketoacidosis, or hyperglycemic, hyperosmolar nonketosis is suspected[28]

Patients having cataract surgery do not require preoperative testing.

condition and may be dependent on uninterrupted device functioning. The Heart Rhythm Society and the ASA published consensus guidelines for safe perioperative management of these patients.[41] Electromagnetic interference (EMI) from monopolar cautery, radiofrequency ablation, therapeutic radiation, electroconvulsive therapy, MRI, transcutaneous electrical nerve stimulation, spinal cord stimulators, or intraoperative monitors[41] can lead to inappropriate therapy. EMI may cause a pacemaker to inappropriately withhold pacing, which may result in symptomatic bradycardia and hemodynamic instability. EMI may trigger inappropriate cardioversion, causing undesired patient movement, or a ventricular arrhythmia. The CIED may need reprogrammed to asynchronous pacing or disabled to "ignore" EMI. Monopolar cautery is the most common source of EMI in the operating room. Several factors reduce EMI effects on a CIED. If the return electrode is on the lower body, surgery below the umbilicus will not affect a CIED. Cautery bursts of 4 to 5 seconds minimize EMI impact. The return electrode is placed to prevent the current crossing the generator or leads. Only select patients require device reprogramming, and many are safely managed with no device modification, or the use of a magnet to temporarily alter functions. Information from an implantable cardioverter-defibrillator (ICD) interrogation within 6 months or pacemaker within 12 months is required and informs management. Essential information includes the type of device, indication for placement (eg, sick sinus syndrome, atrioventricular block, syncope, prevention of cardiac arrest), underlying heart rate and rhythm, battery longevity greater than 3 months, programmed rate-responsiveness, pacing mode or ICD therapy, and response to magnet placement (eg, pacing rate). The term "pacemaker dependent" may be in the report and signifies patients with very low or absent heart rates without pacing. Even those not pacemaker dependent may poorly tolerate inhibition of devices.

Fig. 4 details CIED management for the DOS. A magnet applied to a pacemaker temporarily causes asynchronous pacing at a rate that differs by manufacturer. A magnet applied to an ICD suspends antitachycardia therapy, but *will not* affect pacing. If EMI is not anticipated (eg, monopolar cautery below the umbilicus or bipolar cautery only), reprogramming or magnet application is unnecessary. If EMI is anticipated, patients with an ICD who are also pacer dependent require device reprogramming. Reprogramming is necessary when EMI is a concern and the device cannot be readily accessed, such as in a prone patient. CIEDs are only reprogrammed after arrival to a facility where a patient can be monitored. Immediate access to external defibrillators is required if EMI is a possibility or the device is altered. A CIED specialist is required to reprogram. It is not appropriate to discharge a patient before restoring original settings.[41] Patients with an ICD generally have cardiomyopathies, ischemic heart disease, or significant, lethal arrhythmias, which may preclude safe care in some office-based or ambulatory settings.

Dialysis-Dependent Patients

Dialysis-dependent patients are at risk of infectious, pulmonary, and vascular complications[42] and increased rates of unplanned admission following elective outpatient orthopedic surgery.[43] Significant comorbidities (eg, anemia, DM, hypertension, HF, CAD, electrolyte abnormalities, fluid overload, dialysis access site complications) are common.[43,44] Dialysis the day before surgery helps ensure acceptable volume status, normal electrolytes, and acid/base status. A policy for elective surgery to be scheduled within 24 hours of dialysis aids operating room workflow and avoidance of hyperkalemia.[45]

Dialysis access is the most common reason for surgery in dialysis-dependent patients, and hyperkalemia is common, particularly when surgery is for inadequate

A

No programing changes required for procedures *below umbilicus except for a subcutaneous ICD*

If a procedure is above the umbilicus OR IF THE PATIENT HAS AN LVAD:

- Determine if device is an implantable cardioverter-defibrillator (ICD) or pacemaker (PM).
- Who is the manufacturer of the device: Medtronic, St. Jude, Boston Scientific, Biotronik, or Boston Scientific/Cameron(S-ICD) [subcutaneous]
- Request MOST RECENT INTERROGATION from the patient's PM/ICD clinic.

MAGNET APPLICATION
- PM will pace at manufacturer-specific rate asynchronously with magnet
  - Biotronik & Boston Scientific, 100 bpm
  - Medtronic, 85 bpm
  - St. Jude, 98 bpm
- ICD shock therapy is suspended; PM function of ICD is unchanged.
- If patient is PM dependent and has ICD, the PM must be reprogrammed.
- Subcutaneous ICD has NO PM function, is located under the LUE; the wires are not in the heart. Magnet suspends shock therapy.
- Place the magnet over the pulse generator (can).
  - PM – cause asynchronous pacing or
  - ICD -- suspend shocks (does NOT affect pacing)

- During procedure, monitor vital signs for abnormalities.
- In a patient with an ICD, if ventricular tachycardia (VT) or ventricular fibrillation (VF) occurs, remove magnet immediately to reactivate ICD shocks. The ICD will shock the patient if needed. If the patient does not stabilize, call a CODE for additional support.
- Once cautery is done remove magnet to allow device reactivation.

Fig. 4. (*A–C*) Device management during procedures. EP, electrophysiology; LUE, left upper extremity. (*Adapted from* Boston Scientific. Using a Magnet to Temporarily Inhibit S-ICD Therapy. Available at: www.bostonscientific.com/content/dam/bostonscientific/quality/education-resources/english/US_ACL_SICD_Magnet_Use_20150413.pdf. Accessed January 7, 2019. Image provided courtesy of Boston Scientific. © 2019 Boston Scientific Corporation or its affiliates. All rights reserved.)

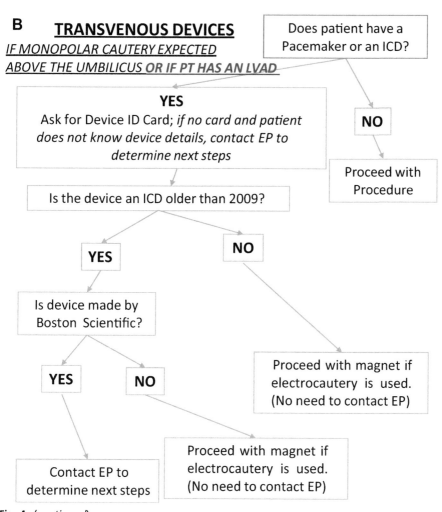

Fig. 4. (*continued*).

access. Moderate (5.7–6.3 mEq/L) to severe (>6.3 mEq/L) hyperkalemia is present in 14% of patients having outpatient hemodialysis access procedures. Recommendations are to proceed with procedures with mild (<5.7 mEq/L) potassium elevations, and delay surgery to treat patients with moderate to severe elevations.[46] In a study of 1350 vascular access procedures, 3.3% of patients had a potassium level greater than 6.0 mEq/L. Seventeen were treated with sodium polystyrene (Kayexelate) or dialyzed preprocedure; 7 had normal potassium levels on recheck, and 8 proceeded to surgery with potassium ranges of 6.1 to 8.0 mEq/L.[47] It is reasonable to proceed with ambulatory surgery with mild hyperkalemia without acidosis in a patient receiving regular dialysis.

Patients with Chronic Pain

Patients with chronic pain are at risk for delayed discharge from the postanesthesia care unit from inadequate pain control, excessive sedation, or respiratory depression from chronic opioid treatment. Patients with opioid dependence or abuse have

C SUBCUTANEOUS ICDs (S-ICD)

1. USE MAGNETS EVERY TIME ELECTROCAUTERY IS ANTICIPATED

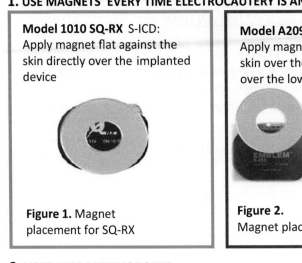

Model 1010 SQ-RX S-ICD:
Apply magnet flat against the skin directly over the implanted device

Figure 1. Magnet placement for SQ-RX

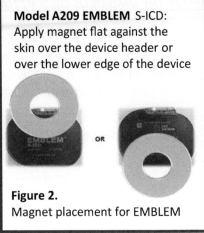

Model A209 EMBLEM S-ICD:
Apply magnet flat against the skin over the device header or over the lower edge of the device

OR

Figure 2.
Magnet placement for EMBLEM

2. LISTEN FOR BEEPING TONES

If magnet is correctly placed, beeping tones lasting 60 seconds are audible. Use a stethoscope or use 2 magnets stacked to hear beeping.
IF NO BEEPING HEARD, CONTACT EP TO REPROGRAM S-ICD.

3. KEEP MAGNET IN PLACE

Keep magnet in place to maintain suspended therapies (temporarily off).

4. REMOVE MAGNET

When magnet is removed, arrhythmia detection resumes and therapy delivery is now active (no longer suspended).

Fig. 4. (*continued*).

increased hospital admissions related to opioid overdose or acute pain.[48] Central sleep apnea is present in 25% of patients on chronic opioids, particularly those taking greater than 200 mg of morphine equivalents daily.[49] Taking opioids increases risk for postoperative respiratory depression. Methadone is used for treatment of chronic pain and opioid dependence, has a long half-life (8–59 hours), and is continued perioperatively to prevent withdrawal.[50] Methadone prolongs the QTc, and when combined with other QT prolonging agents (eg, antidepressants, quinolone and macrolide antibiotics, ondansetron, cocaine), can cause cardiac arrhythmias (eg, torsades de pointe).

Patients with anticipated difficult-to-control postoperative pain benefit from preoperative planning, including regional/neuraxial anesthesia, multimodal analgesia, and opioid alternatives. Preoperative nonsteroidal anti-inflammatory drugs, celecoxib, acetaminophen, gabapentin, or pregabalin, are beneficial.[51] Peripheral nerve catheters for postdischarge pain relief are useful.

Patients taking opioid agonist-antagonists require special management. Buprenorphine is a semisynthetic opioid that is a partial opioid mu-receptor agonist that provides analgesia, and a kappa-receptor antagonist that limits dysphoria. Buprenorphine has higher affinity for opioid receptors than fentanyl or morphine with slow dissociation, but low overall agonist activity.[52] Patients taking buprenorphine require large doses of opioids for analgesia. This effect persists for several days after discontinuation. The risk of substance abuse relapse with buprenorphine discontinuation is weighed against the challenge of managing postoperative pain. In consultation with the patient's pain or addiction specialist, buprenorphine may be held for at least 3 days preoperatively and resumed after postsurgical pain has diminished. Converting to methadone treatment is an alternative strategy in patients at risk for abuse relapse. If only mild to moderate postoperative pain is anticipated and adjunctive pain medication and regional analgesia are alternatives, buprenorphine may be continued. Supplemental sublingual buprenorphine may be used, although with limited efficacy because of a ceiling effect of the drug.

Buprenorphine is available in sublingual (Subutex), transdermal (Butrans), and parenteral (Buprenex) preparations, and combined with naloxone (Suboxone). Naloxone has limited oral bioavailability because of first-pass metabolism, so has limited systemic opioid antagonism but prevents constipation. Targiniq ER combines oxycodone with naloxone, whereas Embeda contains morphine sulfate and an opioid-antagonist naltrexone, which is chemically "sequestered" to prevent oral absorption.[53] Unlike Suboxone, Targiniq and Embeda contain full opioid agonists (oxycodone, morphine) and can be continued with minimal to no opioid antagonist activity. Patients exhibit tolerance to opioids proportional to the daily dose of oxycodone or morphine consumed.

Patients with opioid dependence or alcohol abuse may be prescribed Vivitrol, an extended release injectable suspension of naltrexone. This formulation blocks opioid receptors for 30 days, rendering opioids ineffective for analgesia except at extremely high doses. If possible, surgery is timed for the fourth week of treatment, when receptor blockade can be overcome with opioids if alternative analgesic strategies are ineffective.[54] The Food and Drug Administration advises a 7- to 10-day opioid-free period before administration to avoid withdrawal symptoms, so resumption postoperatively is coordinated with the patient's surgeon and addiction specialist.

SUMMARY

Many millions of ambulatory surgeries are successfully performed every year. Most patients safely undergo assessment immediately before surgery, because minimal advanced care planning or investigation is needed. Anesthesia providers must identify and manage clinical conditions that impact safety either on the DOS or in advance. Appropriate patient selection and coordination of care are essential for patients to reap the benefits of the added convenience and access offered by these centers.

REFERENCES

1. Majholm B, Engbaek J, Bartholdy J, et al. Is day surgery safe? A Danish multi-center study of morbidity after 57,709 day surgery procedures. Acta Anaesthesiol Scand 2012;56:323–31.

2. American Society of Anesthesiology Task Force on Preanesthesia Evaluation. Practice advisory for preanesthesia evaluation. A report by the ASA Task force on preanesthesia evaluation. Anesthesiology 2012;116:522–38.

3. Blitz JD, Kendale SM, Jain SK, et al. Preoperative evaluation clinic visit is associated with decreased risk of in-hospital postoperative mortality. Anesthesiology 2016;125:280–94.

4. Sessler DI, Sigl JC, Manberg PJ, et al. Broadly applicable risk stratification system for predicting duration of hospitalization and mortality. Anesthesiology 2010; 113:1026–37.
5. Ferschl MB, Tung A, Sweitzer B, et al. Preoperative clinic visits reduce operating room cancellations and delays. Anesthesiology 2005;103:855–9.
6. Fleisher LA, Fleischmann KE, Auerbach AD, et al. 2014 ACC/AHA guideline on perioperative cardiovascular evaluation and management of patients undergoing noncardiac surgery: a report of the American College of Cardiology/American Heart Association Task Force on practice guidelines. J Am Coll Cardiol 2014; 64:e77–137.
7. Gupta PK, Gupta H, Sundaram A, et al. Development and validation of a risk calculator for prediction of cardiac risk after surgery. Circulation 2011;124:381–7.
8. Bilimoria KY, Liu Y, Paruch JL, et al. Development and evaluation of the universal ACS NSQIP surgical risk calculator: a decision aid and informed consent tool for patients and surgeons. J Am Coll Surg 2013;217:833–42.
9. Lee TH, Marcantonio ER, Mangione CM, et al. Derivation and prospective validation of a simple index for prediction of cardiac risk of major noncardiac surgery. Circulation 1999;100:1043–9.
10. Glance LG, Faden E, Dutton RP, et al. Impact of the choice of risk model for identifying low-risk patients using the 2014 American College of Cardiology/American Heart Association perioperative guidelines. Anesthesiology 2018. https://doi.org/10.1097/ALN.0000000000002341.
11. Schiefermueller J, Myerson S, Handa A. Preoperative assessment and perioperative management of cardiovascular risk. Angiology 2013;64:146–50.
12. Levine GN, Bates ER, Bittl JA, et al. 2016 ACC/AHA guideline focused update on duration of dual antiplatelet therapy in patients with coronary artery disease: a Report of the American College of Cardiology/American Heart Association Task Force on Clinical practice guidelines. J Am Coll Cardiol 2016;68:1082–115.
13. Hernandez AF, Whellan DJ, Stroud S, et al. Outcomes in heart failure patients after major noncardiac surgery. J Am Coll Cardiol 2004;44:1446–53.
14. Yancy CW, Jessup M, Bozkurt B, et al. 2017 ACC/AHA/HFSA focused update of the 2013 accf/aha guideline for the management of heart failure: a report of the American College of Cardiology/American Heart Association Task Force on Clinical practice guidelines and the Heart Failure Society of America. J Am Coll Cardiol 2017;70:776–803.
15. Hennis PJ, Meale PM, Grocott MP. Cardiopulmonary exercise testing for the evaluation of perioperative risk in non-cardiopulmonary surgery. Postgrad Med J 2011;87:550–7.
16. Nishimura RA, Otto CM, Bonow RO, et al. 2014 AHA/ACC guideline for the management of patients with valvular heart disease. J Am Coll Cardiol 2014;63: e57–185.
17. Whelton PK, Carey RM, Aronow WS, et al. 2017 ACC/AHA/AAPA/ABC/ACPM/AGS/APhA/ASH/ASPC/NMA/PCNA guideline for the prevention, detection, evaluation, and management of high blood pressure in adults: a report of the American College of Cardiology/American Heart Association Task Force on clinical practice guidelines. J Am Coll Cardiol 2018;71:e127–248.
18. Wax DB, Porter SB, Lin HM, et al. Association of preanesthesia hypertension with adverse outcomes. J Cardiothorac Vasc Anesth 2010;24:927–30.
19. Hartle A, McCormack T, Carlisle J, et al. The measurement of adult blood pressure and management of hypertension before elective surgery Joint Guidelines

from the Association of Anaesthetists of Great Britain and Ireland and the British Hypertension Society. Anaesthesia 2016;71:326–37.

20. Bijker JB, van Klei WA, Vergouwe Y, et al. Intraoperative hypotension and 1-year mortality after noncardiac surgery. Anesthesiology 2009;111:1217–26.

21. Bijker JB, Persoon S, Peelen LM, et al. Intraoperative hypotension and perioperative ischemic stroke after general surgery: a nested case-control study. Anesthesiology 2012;116:658–64.

22. Twersky RS, Goel V, Narayan P, et al. The risk of hypertension after preoperative discontinuation of angiotensin-converting enzyme inhibitors or angiotensin receptor antagonists in ambulatory and same-day admission patients. Anesth Analg 2014;118:938–44.

23. POISE Study Group, Devereaux PJ, Yang H, Yusuf S, et al. Effects of extended-release metoprolol succinate in patients undergoing non-cardiac surgery (POISE trial): a randomized controlled trial. Lancet 2008;371:1839–47.

24. Akhtar S, Barash PG, Inzucchi SE. Scientific principles and clinical implications of perioperative glucose regulation and control. Anesth Analg 2010; 110:478–97.

25. Richards JE, Kauffmann RM, Zuckerman SL, et al. Relationship of hyperglycemia and surgical-site infection in orthopaedic surgery. J Bone Joint Surg Am 2012;94: 1181–6.

26. Christman AL, Selvin E, Margolis DJ, et al. Hemoglobin A1c predicts healing rate in diabetic wounds. J Invest Dermatol 2011;131:2121–7.

27. Dhatariya K, Levy N, Kilvert A. NHS Diabetes guideline for the perioperative management of the adult patient with diabetes. Diabet Med 2012;29:420–33.

28. Joshi GP, Chung F, Vann MA, et al. Society for Ambulatory Anesthesia consensus statement on perioperative blood glucose management in diabetic patients undergoing ambulatory surgery. Anesth Analg 2010;111:1378–87.

29. Cosson E, Catargi B, Cheisson G, et al. Practical management of diabetes patients before, during and after surgery: a joint French diabetology and anaesthesiology position statement. Diabetes Metab 2018;44:200–16.

30. Salpeter SR, Greyber E, Pasternak GA, et al. Risk of fatal and nonfatal lactic acidosis with metformin use in type 2 diabetes mellitus. Cochrane Database Syst Rev 2010;(4):CD002967.

31. Schein OD, Katz J, Bass EB, et al. The value of routine preoperative medical testing before cataract surgery. Study of Medical Testing for cataract surgery. N Engl J Med 2000;342:168–75.

32. Keay L, Lindsley K, Tielsch J, et al. Routine preoperative medical testing for cataract surgery. Cochrane Database Syst Rev 2012;(3):CD007293.

33. MacPherson R. Structured assessment tool to evaluate patient suitability for cataract surgery under local anaesthesia. Br J Anaesth 2004;93:521–4.

34. Hodge W, Horsley T, Albiani D. The consequences of waiting for cataract surgery: a systematic review. CMAJ 2007;176:1285–90.

35. United States Census Bureau. The nation's older population is still growing, Census Bureau Reports. Available at: www.census.gov/newsroom/press-releases/2017/cb17-100.html. Accessed May 31, 2018.

36. Oresanya LB, Lyons WL, Finlayson E. Preoperative assessment of the older patient: a narrative review. JAMA 2014;311:2110–20.

37. De Oliveira GS, Holl JL, Lindquist LA, et al. Older adults and unanticipated hospital admission within 30 days of ambulatory surgery: an analysis of 53,667 ambulatory surgical procedures. J Am Geriatr Soc 2015;63:1679–85.

38. Chow WB, Rosenthal RA, Merkow RP, et al. Optimal preoperative assessment of the geriatric surgical patient: a best practices guideline from the American College of Surgeons National Surgical Quality Improvement Program and the American Geriatrics Society. J Am Coll Surg 2012;215:453–66.

39. Mohanty S, Rosenthal RA, Russell MM, et al. Optimal perioperative management of the geriatric patient: a best practices guideline from the American College of Surgeons National Surgical Quality Improvement Program and the American Geriatrics Society. J Am Coll Surg 2016;222:930–47.

40. Chung F, Yuan H, Yin L, et al. Elimination of preoperative testing in ambulatory surgery. Anesth Analg 2009;108:467–75.

41. Crossley GH, Poole JE, Rozner MA, et al. The Heart Rhythm Society (HRS)/American Society of Anesthesiologists (ASA) expert consensus statement on the perioperative management of patients with implantable defibrillators, pacemakers and arrhythmia monitors: facilities and patient management. Heart Rhythm 2011;8:1114–54.

42. Tam SF, Au JT, Chung PJ, et al. Is it time to rethink our management of dialysis patients undergoing elective ventral hernia repair? Analysis of the ACS NSQIP database. Hernia 2015;19:827–33.

43. Noureldin M, Habermann EB, Ubl DS, et al. Unplanned readmissions following outpatient hand and elbow surgery. J Bone Joint Surg Am 2017;99:541–9.

44. Siracuse JJ, Shah NK, Peacock MR, et al. Thirty-day and 90-day hospital readmission after outpatient upper extremity hemodialysis access creation. J Vasc Surg 2017;65:1376–82.

45. Renew JR, Pai SL. A simple protocol to improve safety and reduce cost in hemodialysis patients undergoing elective surgery. Middle East J Anaesthesiol 2014;22:487–92.

46. Ross J, DeatherageHand D. Evaluation of potassium levels before hemodialysis access procedures. Semin Dial 2015;28:90–3.

47. Olson RP, Schow AJ, McCann R, et al. Absence of adverse outcomes in hyperkalemic patients undergoing vascular access surgery. Can J Anaesth 2003;50:553–7.

48. Gupta A, Nizamuddin J, Elmofty D, et al. Opioid abuse or dependence increases 30-day readmission rates after major operating room procedures: a National Readmissions Database Study. Anesthesiology 2018;128:880–90.

49. Correa D, Farney RJ, Chung F, et al. Chronic opioid use and central sleep apnea: a review of the prevalence, mechanisms, and perioperative considerations. Anesth Analg 2015;120:1273–85.

50. Vadivelu N, Mitra S, Kaye AD, et al. Perioperative analgesia and challenges in the drug-addicted and drug-dependent patient. Best Pract Res Clin Anaesthesiol 2014;28:91–101.

51. Chou R, Gordon DB, de Leon-Casasola OA, et al. Management of postoperative pain: a clinical practice guideline from the American Pain Society, the American Society of Regional Anesthesia and Pain Medicine, and the American Society of Anesthesiologists' Committee on Regional Anesthesia, Executive Committee, and Administrative Council. J Pain 2016;17:131–57.

52. Bryson EO, Lipson S, Gevirtz C. Anesthesia for patients on buprenorphine. Anesthesiol Clin 2010;28:611–7.

53. Vadivelu N, Chang D, Lumermann L, et al. Management of patients on abuse-deterrent opioids in the ambulatory surgery setting. Curr Pain Headache Rep 2017;21:1–7.

54. Curatolo C, Trinh M. Challenges in the perioperative management of the patient receiving extended-release naltrexone. A A Case Rep 2014;3:142–4.
55. American Society of Anesthesiologists. Pregnancy testing prior to anesthesia and surgery. Available at: http://www.asahq.org/quality-and-practice-management/ standards-guidelines-and-related-resources/pregnancy-testing-prior-to-anesthesia-and-surgery. Accessed July 25, 2018.

Obesity and Obstructive Sleep Apnea in the Ambulatory Patient

Gaganpreet Grewal, MD[a],*, Girish P. Joshi, MBBS, MD, FFARCSI[b]

KEYWORDS

- Obesity • Obstructive sleep apnea • Ambulatory surgery • Patient selection
- Perioperative outcomes • Patient safety

KEY POINTS

- Appropriate preoperative evaluation in selecting obese and obstructive sleep apnea (OSA) patients scheduled for ambulatory surgery includes the identification and optimization of comorbidities.
- Preoperative screening for OSA is essential in minimizing perioperative risk in undiagnosed patients.
- Obese and OSA patients may be at increased risk for difficult airway management.
- Anesthetic management strategies to reduce perioperative risk in obese and OSA patients presenting for ambulatory surgery include an emphasis on regional anesthesia, use of short-acting agents, and minimizing use of muscle relaxants and opioids.
- Two key discharge criteria for obese and OSA patients are the ability to maintain baseline oxygen saturations on room air and the management of pain with minimal opioids.

INTRODUCTION

Obesity is often associated with increased perioperative risks, particularly at extremes (ie, body mass index [BMI] >40 kg/m^2). However, BMI alone is a poor predictor of perioperative risk because obesity is a heterogeneous condition.[1,2] Morbid obesity has a strong association with obstructive sleep apnea (OSA), a common form of sleep-disordered breathing, which frequently remains undiagnosed.[2] OSA has been linked not only to adverse long-term health outcomes but also to increased perioperative

Disclosure Statement: Dr G. Grewal has no commercial or financial conflicts of interest or any funding sources. Dr G.P. Joshi has received honoraria from Baxter Pharmaceuticals, Pacira Pharmaceuticals, Mallinckrodt Pharmaceuticals, and Merck Pharmaceuticals.

a University of Texas Southwestern Medical Center, 5323 Harry Hines Boulevard, Dallas, TX 75390-9068, USA; b University of Texas Southwestern Medical Center, 5323 Harry Hines Boulevard, Dallas, TX 75390-7208, USA
* Corresponding author.
E-mail address: gaganpreet.grewal@utsouthwestern.edu

Anesthesiology Clin 37 (2019) 215–224
https://doi.org/10.1016/j.anclin.2019.01.001
1932-2275/19/© 2019 Elsevier Inc. All rights reserved.
anesthesiology.theclinics.com

risk, particularly respiratory complications.[3] Over recent years, there has been an increase in the rate of ambulatory surgery,[4] which coupled with the increasing prevalence of obesity and OSA, means that this patient population is increasingly presenting for ambulatory surgery. This article discusses the current controversies surrounding perioperative care of morbidly obese patients with or without OSA scheduled for ambulatory surgery, particularly in a free-standing ambulatory center.

PREOPERATIVE CONSIDERATIONS

Obese patients should be screened for comorbidities, including cardiovascular disease, respiratory disease (particularly OSA), and endocrine disorders (particularly diabetes mellitus).[5] Although ambulatory surgeries typically carry a low risk of perioperative cardiac complications (cardiac risk <1%), morbid obesity (BMI >40 kg/m^2) itself can lead to cardiomyopathy in the absence of coronary artery disease.[6] The American Heart Association and the American College of Cardiology have developed guidelines regarding the preoperative evaluation of severely obese patients.[6,7] The initial step should be a thorough history and physical examination, including an evaluation of functional status. However, in the severely obese, functional capacity may be difficult to assess and may be impaired due to reasons other than cardiac compromise. Therefore, an electrocardiogram should be obtained in patients with limited functional capacity and at least one risk factor for perioperative cardiovascular morbidity (ie, history of heart disease, history of congestive heart failure, history of cerebrovascular disease, preoperative insulin treatment, and preoperative serum creatinine >2 mg/dL).[5,6] The presence of left bundle branch block is unusual in uncomplicated obesity and may indicate underlying heart disease. The presence of right heart hypertrophy suggests pulmonary hypertension. A chest radiograph can reveal cardiac chamber enlargement suggestive of heart failure or abnormal pulmonary vascularity suggestive of pulmonary hypertension, and it is reasonable to have this information as a baseline in the event of postoperative respiratory compromise.[6] Further cardiovascular testing, such as stress test or echocardiography, may be indicated in patients with 3 or more risk factors for perioperative cardiovascular morbidity, but routine testing is not indicated.[5]

Approximately 70% of patients with a BMI greater than 40 kg/m^2 may have OSA.[2] Because a significant portion of OSA patients presenting for surgery do not have a formal diagnosis of OSA, identifying patients at risk for OSA has been recommended.[8,9] The Society for Ambulatory Anesthesia and the Society of Anesthesia and Sleep Medicine (SASM) recommend the use of the STOP-BANG questionnaire to screen patients for OSA, because it is the most validated tool.[8,9] A cutoff of ≥5 is suggested because scores of 5 to 8 identify patients with a high probability of moderate to severe OSA.[10,11]

Selection of Obese and Obstructive Sleep Apnea Patients for Ambulatory Surgery

It is well accepted that obesity alone is not a contradiction for ambulatory surgery.[12] Because of weight limitations on equipment, such as stretchers and operating tables, there are limits as to the total body weight (TBW) of a patient that can be taken care of at any given ambulatory center. Studies investigating perioperative outcomes in obese patients are of limited quantity, but seem to indicate that obese patients with BMI ≤40 kg/m^2 can undergo ambulatory surgery if comorbidities are optimized before surgery.[12] Patients with BMI greater than 50 kg/m^2 appear to be at increased risk for postdischarge readmission, and caution should be used when selecting these patients for ambulatory surgery, particularly those requiring general anesthesia.[12] For patients with BMI of 41 to 50 kg/m^2, the presence of OSA should be taken into consideration.[8] A recent study in patients undergoing elective ambulatory hernia repairs found that the readmission rates increased with increasing BMI.[13] Adjusting for age and comorbidities, the BMI threshold associated with increased readmission risk was 45.7 kg/m^2. However, the modest discriminating ability of the model indicates that in addition to BMI, patient comorbidity and surgical factors should also be taken into account.[13]

Patients with known OSA scheduled for ambulatory surgery should have other comorbidities optimized and be able to use continuous positive airway pressure (CPAP) after discharge.[8] If a patient is deemed to be at high risk for moderate to severe OSA based on a screening tool, the surgery or procedure should proceed with the assumption that the patient has OSA. Of note, there is no clear evidence to suggest that delaying a procedure to obtain a sleep study and initiate positive airway pressure therapy (eg, CPAP) would improve perioperative outcome.[8,9] Therefore, delaying surgery to obtain a sleep study is not recommended.

INTRAOPERATIVE CONSIDERATIONS
Sedation and Analgesia

Many ambulatory procedures can be performed with sedation/analgesia, avoiding some of the risks of general anesthesia. Benzodiazepines, most commonly midazolam, are frequently used for sedation; however, these agents may cause respiratory depression and decrease the arousal response to airway occlusion. Therefore, benzodiazepines should be used with caution.[14]

Propofol, a commonly used agent for sedation during gastrointestinal (GI) endoscopy procedures and drug-induced sleep endoscopy (DISE), is also associated with increased respiratory events and desaturation in OSA patients.[14] Studies examining propofol sedation during DISE procedures have found OSA and increasing BMI to be risk factors for airway obstruction and collapse.[14] Several studies have found that OSA, increased BMI, male gender, American Society of Anesthesiologists (ASA) physical status >3, and increased age to be independent risk factors for hypoxic events during procedural sedation with propofol.[14] In addition, in obese patients, there is uncertainty regarding the appropriate dosing,[14] with some studies supporting lean body weight (LBW)[15] and others supporting a scalar between LBW and TBW.[16] Therefore, careful titration is recommended when using propofol for sedation in patients with obesity or OSA.

Another common agent for procedural sedation is ketamine. Ketamine does not decrease upper airway muscle activity,[17] which may be a beneficial property for OSA patients. Studies in the general adult population have shown that when ketamine supplements propofol in procedural sedation, there are fewer adverse respiratory events.[18] Thus, it is reasonable to assume that obese and OSA patients could also benefit from ketamine, although there is no strong evidence in these populations.

Dexmedetomidine has a favorable respiratory profile, making it desirable in obese or OSA patients. However, there is limited evidence linking dexmedetomidine to improved outcomes in these patient populations. A systematic review of dexmedetomidine compared with propofol in patients undergoing DISE found that dexmedetomidine resulted in less airway obstruction and a more stable cardiopulmonary profile. However, propofol resulted in a quicker onset and shorter duration.[19] A prospective case series of patients at high risk for OSA undergoing sedation for upper endoscopy found that compared with propofol alone, a dexmedetomidine-propofol combination resulted in prolonged induction and recovery times.[20] The combination of dexmedetomidine and ketamine may provide adequate sedation/analgesia while maintaining airway patency. However, it has not been adequately studied in the obese and OSA populations.

Regardless of the anesthetic agents chosen for procedural sedation, it is important to use capnography to monitor respiratory status, because it allows early detection of apnea and decreases hypoxemic events.[21] The use of CPAP or an oral appliance during sedation in patients with OSA can be considered,[22] but there is limited evidence to support improved outcomes.

Regional Anesthesia

There are several reasons that regional anesthesia may be advantageous over general anesthesia in obese and OSA patients. With regional anesthesia, airway manipulation and airway difficulties are avoided. In addition, the effects of intraoperative anesthetic agents, neuromuscular blockade, and opioids are avoided. Regional anesthesia also offers pain relief, thereby reducing postoperative opioid requirements.[8,14,22] Therefore, regional anesthesia has been recommended as a safer alternative to general anesthesia in obese and OSA patients.[14,22] A systematic review of literature revealed 6 observational trials suggesting that regional anesthesia resulted in improved postoperative outcomes.[14] However, several studies included in this review were performed in hospitalized patients. A review of studies involving peripheral nerve blocks in obese and nonobese patients found a higher block failure rate in obese patients, although the overall rate of success was still high.[23] Overall, the superiority of regional anesthesia over general anesthesia in the ambulatory surgical population remains controversial, particularly with the use of "fast-track" general anesthesia techniques that include using shorter-acting anesthetics at the lowest possible doses.

Airway Management

Although several retrospective and prospective studies have supported that OSA is an independent risk factor for difficult airway management,[14] obesity itself has not consistently been shown to be an independent risk factor. Studies examining incidence of difficulty with tracheal intubation have found mixed results, with some studies associating obesity with difficult intubation and other studies finding no correlation with BMI, but finding correlation with high Mallampati score and neck circumference (characteristics associated with OSA).[24] These studies reiterate the importance of screening for OSA, especially in obese patients.

Because of the increased potential for difficult airway management, optimal preoxygenation is essential. There is a negative correlation between BMI and time to desaturation when apneic. Maneuvers to improve preoxygenation include head-up position and application of CPAP. In addition, appropriate positioning (ramping or stacking) reduces difficulty in tracheal intubation.[25] There is some debate as to the appropriateness of video laryngoscopy as a first-line intubation method in the obese. A meta-analysis found that video laryngoscopy in obese patients was superior to direct laryngoscopy in glottic visualization, success rate, and intubation time, but intubation time was only improved if the video laryngoscope had a tracheal tube guide channel.[26] Nevertheless, the investigators of this meta-analysis did not yet recommend routine use of video laryngoscopy in obese patients because of the limitations in studies analyzed. Because of decreased time to desaturation and possible difficult mask ventilation, there is argument for using succinylcholine for its rapid onset and short duration of action. However, it may be disadvantageous if difficulty intubating occurs, because fasciculations can decrease safe apnea time.[27] With the introduction of sugammadex, the use of large doses of rocuronium in patients with suspected difficult mask ventilation has been considered because spontaneous respirations may occur more quickly with rocuronium-sugammadex than with succinylcholine.[28] Unfortunately, pharmacologic simulation shows that in a significant portion of morbidly obese and obese patients, rocuronium-sugammadex will not result in return of spontaneous ventilation before significant desaturation occurs.[29]

Choice of General Anesthetic Technique

There is lack of scientific literature regarding the choice of anesthetic technique in the OSA population. The SASM analyzed studies in the obese population, because there is a strong association between obesity and OSA.[14] Studies in the obese population indicate that desflurane and sevoflurane have a superior recovery profile compared with isoflurane and propofol.[14] Studies comparing desflurane and sevoflurane have shown conflicting results, with some finding that desflurane results in quicker emergence, whereas other studies show no difference between the 2 inhalational agents.[14] A systematic review of randomized controlled trials in obese patients undergoing abdominal surgery found that desflurane is superior to sevoflurane, isoflurane, and propofol in providing a quicker recovery, but that there were no differences in postoperative nausea and vomiting (PONV) or postoperative pain scores.[15] Two randomized trials in bariatric surgery patients did show that total intravenous anesthesia (propofol and dexmedetomidine) resulted in less PONV.[30,31] Intraoperative monitoring of hypnosis (eg, bispectral index monitoring) may be particularly helpful in patients with obesity and/ or OSA, especially in titrating anesthetic agents. However, good evidence is lacking.

Neuromuscular Blockade

Residual neuromuscular blockade is a common problem, with studies showing that approximately 20% of patients in the postanesthesia care unit (PACU) have a train-of-4 ratio less than 0.9.[32] Residual neuromuscular blockade is associated with impaired pharyngeal function, airway obstruction, attenuation of hypoxic ventilatory response, and increased risk of postoperative pulmonary complications.[32] It is, therefore, important to take measures to reduce residual neuromuscular blockade. If possible, the use of neuromuscular blockade should be avoided or minimized, neuromuscular function monitored, and neuromuscular blockade reversed appropriately.[14] A Cochrane Review found that in the general adult surgical population receiving neuromuscular blocking drugs, sugammadex resulted in quicker recovery of twitches and decreased bradycardia and PONV when compared with neostigmine.[33] The studies included in this review did not report on OSA status, but 6 of the studies did include morbidly obese patients, which found that sugammadex resulted in faster recovery and decreased incidence of residual postoperative neuromuscular blockade.[33] Because of the paucity of evidence in the OSA population, the SASM has not recommended routine use of sugammadex over neostigmine at this time.[14] The recommended manufacturer dosing for sugammadex is based on TBW, but being a water-soluble drug, sugammadex may better dosed based on ideal body weight (IBW) or LBW. So far, studies show that in morbidly obese patients, ideal dose may be IBW + 40%.[34–36]

Perioperative Pain Management

It is recommended that perioperative opioid use must be limited because of adverse effects, particularly respiratory depressant effects.[37] Unfortunately, the intermittent hypoxia and sleep fragmentation seen in OSA can lead to hyperalgesia and increased analgesic requirements.[38] Studies examining if OSA patients are more likely to have adverse respiratory events in the setting of opioids have shown mixed results.[14] In fact, there is no high-quality evidence to support a direct link between OSA and opioid-induced ventilatory impairment.[14] Despite this, it is important to note that some studies, which found no increased respiratory impairment in OSA patients receiving opioids, did find increased GI impairment.[14] High-quality evidence regarding opioid risks in the obese population is also lacking. Opioid-free anesthesia has been increasingly used in recent years.[39] Several studies have used lidocaine, dexmedetomidine, ketamine, and magnesium, either alone or in combination.[40] However, the available evidence is limited. Furthermore, the adverse effects of these drugs and their combinations have not been adequately assessed. Thus, the risks and benefits of each agent need to be considered before administration.

Available studies do support superior outcomes with a multimodal, opioid-sparing approach.[40] Adequate postoperative pain management is necessary for enhanced recovery after surgery. Procedure- and patient-specific pain management strategies should be developed so that they can be incorporated in enhanced recovery protocols.[41] The aim of an analgesic technique should be to optimize pain relief and facilitate early ambulation and physical therapy. The choice of analgesic combinations should depend not only on analgesic efficacy but also on the overall side-effect profiles of these combinations. Regional/local analgesic techniques should form the basis of any optimal multimodal analgesic approach and should be supplemented with a combination of acetaminophen, traditional nonsteroidal anti-inflammatory drugs or cyclo-oxygenase-2–specific inhibitors, and dexamethasone, assuming there are no contraindications. Opioids should used as "rescue" analgesics on an "as-needed" basis rather than on a scheduled basis.[11]

POSTOPERATIVE CONSIDERATIONS
Postanesthesia Care Unit Care

Postoperatively, patients with OSA and/or obesity should be carefully monitored, particularly for respiratory compromise. In the PACU, the patient should be positioned in a semiupright position to decrease airway obstruction; continuous pulse oximetry should be used, and the patient should be observed for apneic events.[22]

If needed, supplemental oxygen should be used until the patient can maintain baseline saturations on room air. There has been some concern that supplemental oxygen can result in delayed detection of hypercapnia from respiratory depression. Although supplemental oxygen improves oxygen saturations, it can also increase the length of apneic episodes, because hypoxia is a trigger for arousal.[42] This potential for increased length of apneic episodes with supplemental oxygen has led to concerns that supplemental oxygen can actually increase respiratory depression[43] and impair detection of hypoventilation.[44] A recent study randomized untreated OSA patients to supplemental oxygen postoperatively and showed no difference in apnea-hypopnea event duration or incidence of hypercarbia.[45]

In addition to supplemental oxygen, CPAP therapy may be used in the PACU. It is prudent to have a CPAP device available should the need arise. Several studies have shown benefit in initiating CPAP therapy postoperatively in untreated patients,[46] but these studies are often in patients undergoing major surgery, not the type of surgery performed in the ambulatory setting. As an alternative to CPAP, high-flow nasal oxygen therapy is starting to show promise, because it can decrease apnea-hypopnea events and arousals from sleep in patients with OSA.[47]

Discharge

Patients should not be discharged until there is no longer a risk of postoperative respiratory depression. To meet this requirement, patients should be able to maintain adequate oxygen saturations while in an unstimulated environment, preferably asleep, and while breathing room air.[22] Pain should also be well controlled without opioids. Patients with CPAP therapy should be advised to use CPAP any time they sleep, whether day or night.[8] The use of at-home oxygen saturation monitoring has been considered in OSA patients, but in one study, severe postoperative desaturation at home occurred in one-quarter of patients, but did not result in any complications or required interventions.[48]

SUMMARY

Patients with morbid obesity and OSA can be at increased perioperative risk, and there is a large overlap between the 2 pathologic conditions. However, these patients can and do safely undergo ambulatory surgery provided appropriate precautions are taken. First, appropriate preoperative workup can ensure appropriate patient selection, excluding patients with nonoptimized comorbidities. Intraoperatively, precautions include appropriate management of a potentially difficult airway and careful selection of anesthetic techniques with an emphasis on using shorter-acting anesthetics, muscle relaxants, and opioids at lowest possible doses. Postoperatively, careful monitoring is essential in determining an appropriate discharge. With these concepts in mind, obese and OSA patients can do well in the ambulatory setting.

REFERENCES

1. Tsai A, Schumann R. Morbid obesity and perioperative complications. Curr Opin Anaesthesiol 2016;29:103–8.
2. Moon TS, Joshi GP. Are morbidly obese patients suitable for ambulatory surgery? Curr Opin Anaesthesiol 2016;29:141–5.
3. Opperer M, Cozowicz C, Bugada D, et al. Does obstructive sleep apnea influence perioperative outcome? A qualitative systematic review for the society of anesthesia and sleep medicine task force on preoperative preparation of patients with sleep-disordered breathing. Anesth Analg 2016;122:1321–34.
4. Hollenbeck BK, Dunn RL, Suskind AM, et al. Ambulatory surgery centers and outpatient procedure use among Medicare beneficiaries. Med Care 2014;52: 926–31.
5. Bohmer AB, Wappler F. Preoperative evaluation and preparation of the morbidly obese patient. Curr Opin Anaesthesiol 2017;30:126–32.
6. Poirier P, Alpert MA, Fleisher LA, et al. Cardiovascular evaluation and management of severely obese patients undergoing surgery. A Science Advisory from the American Heart Association. Circulation 2009;120:86–95.
7. Fleisher LA, Fleischmann KE, Auerbach AD, et al. 2014 ACC/AHA guideline & on perioperative cardiovascular evaluation and management of patients undergoing noncardiac surgery: a report of the American College of Cardiology/American Heart Association Task Force on practice guidelines. J Am Coll Cardiol 2014; 64:e77–137.
8. Joshi GP, Ankichetty SP, Gan TJ, et al. Society for Ambulatory Anesthesia consensus statement on preoperative selection of adult patients with obstructive sleep apnea scheduled for ambulatory surgery. Anesth Analg 2012;115:1060–8.
9. Chung F, Memtsoudis SG, Stavros G, et al. Society of anesthesia and sleep medicine guidelines on preoperative screening and assessment of adult patients with obstructive sleep apnea. Anesth Analg 2016;123:452–73.
10. Chung F, Subramanyam R, Liao P, et al. High STOP-Bang score indicates a high probability of obstructive sleep apnoea. Br J Anaesth 2012;108:768–75.

11. Farney RJ, Walker BS, Farney RM, et al. The STOP-Bang equivalent model and prediction of severity of obstructive sleep apnea: relation to polysomnographic measurements of the apnea/hypopnea index. J Clin Sleep Med 2011;7:459–65.

12. Joshi GP, Ahmad S, Riad W, et al. Selection of obese patients undergoing ambulatory surgery: a systematic review of the literature. Anesth Analg 2013;117: 1082–91.

13. Rosero EB, Joshi GP. Finding the body mass index threshold for selection of patients for ambulatory open hernia repair. Proceedings of the IARS 2018 Annual Meeting and International Science Symposium. Chicago (IL), April 28–May 1, 2018.

14. Memtsoudis SG, Cozowicz C, Nagappa M, et al. Society of anesthesia and sleep medicine guidelines on intraoperative management of adult patients with obstructive sleep apnea. Anesth Analg 2018;127(4):967–87.

15. Ingrande J, Lemmens HJ. Dose adjustment of anaesthetics in the morbidly obese. Br J Anaesth 2010;105(Suppl 1):i16–23.

16. Subramani Y, Riad W, Chung F, et al. Optimal propofol induction dose in morbidly obese patients: a randomized controlled trial comparing the bispectral index and lean body weight scalar. Can J Anaesth 2017;64:471–9.

17. Drummond G. Comparison of sedation with midazolam and ketamine: effects on airway muscle activity. Br J Anaesth 1996;76:663–7.

18. De Oliveira GS Jr, Fitzgerald PC, Hansen N, et al. The effect of ketamine on hypoventilation during deep sedation with midazolam and propofol: a randomised, double-blind, placebo-controlled trial. Eur J Anaesthesiol 2014;31:654–62.

19. Chang ET, Certal V, Song SA, et al. Dexmedetomidine versus propofol during drug-induced sleep endoscopy and sedation: a systematic review. Sleep Breath 2017;21:727–35.

20. Hannallah M, Rasmussen M, Carroll J, et al. Evaluation of dexmedetomidine/propofol anesthesia during upper gastrointestinal endoscopy in patients with high probability of having obstructive sleep apnea. Anaesth Pain Intensive Care 2013;17:257–60.

21. Friedrich-Rust M, Welte M, Welte C, et al. Capnographic monitoring of propofol-based sedation during colonoscopy. Endoscopy 2014;46:236–44.

22. Gross JB, Apfelbaum JL, Caplan RA, et al. Practice guidelines for the perioperative management of patients with obstructive sleep apnea an updated report by the American society of anesthesiologists task force on perioperative management of patients with obstructive sleep apnea. Anesthesiology 2014;120:268–86.

23. Ingrande J, Brodsky JB, Lemmens HJ. Regional anesthesia and obesity. Curr Opin Anaesthesiol 2009;22:683–6.

24. Hashim MM, Ismail MA, Esmat AM, et al. Difficult tracheal intubation in bariatric surgery patients, a myth or reality? Br J Anaesth 2016;116:557–8.

25. Cattano D, Melnikov V, Khalil Y, et al. An evaluation of the rapid airway management positioner in obese patients undergoing gastric bypass or laparoscopic gastric banding surgery. Obes Surg 2010;20:1436–41.

26. Hoshijima H, Denawa Y, Tominaga A, et al. Videolaryngoscopy versus Macintosh direct laryngoscopy in obese patients — a meta-analysis. J Clin Anesth 2018;44: 69–75.

27. Taha SK, El-Khatib MF, Baraka AS, et al. Effect of suxamethonium vs rocuronium on onset of oxygen desaturation during apnoea following rapid sequence induction. Anaesthesia 2010;65:358–61.

28. Sorensen ML, Bretlau C, Gatke MR, et al. Rapid sequence induction and intubation with rocuronium-sugammadex compared with succinylcholine: a randomized trial. Br J Anaesth 2012;108:682–9.

29. Naguib M, Brewer L, LaPierre C, et al. The myth of rescue reversal in "can't intubate, can't ventilate" scenarios. Anesth Analg 2016;123:82–92.

30. Ziemann-Gimmel P, Goldfarb A, Koppman J, et al. Opioid-free total intravenous anaesthesia reduces postoperative nausea and vomiting in bariatric surgery beyond triple prophylaxis. Br J Anaesth 2014;112:906–11.

31. Elbakry AE, Sultan WE, Ibrahim E. A comparison between inhalational (Desflurane) and total intravenous anaesthesia (Propofol and dexmedetomidine) in improving postoperative recovery for morbidly obese patients undergoing laparoscopic sleeve gastrectomy: a double-blinded randomised controlled trial. J Clin Anesth 2018;45:6–11.

32. Brull SJ, Kopman AF. Current status of neuromuscular reversal and monitoring: challenges and opportunities. Anesthesiology 2016;126:173–90.

33. Hristovska AM, Duch P, Allingstrup M, et al. Efficacy and safety of sugammadex versus neostigmine in reversing neuromuscular blockade in adults. Cochrane Database Syst Rev 2017;(8):CD012763.

34. Van Lancker P, Dillemans B, Bogaert T, et al. Ideal versus corrected body weight for dosage of sugammadex in morbidly obese patients. Anaesthesia 2011;66: 721–5.

35. Abd El-Rahman AM, Othman AH, El Sherif FA, et al. Comparison of three different doses sugammadex based on ideal body weight for reversal of moderate rocuronium-induced neuromuscular blockade in laparoscopic bariatric surgery. Minerva Anestesiol 2017;83:138–44.

36. Duarte NMDC, Caetano AMM, Neto SDSC, et al. Sugammadex by ideal body weight versus 20% and 40% corrected weight in bariatric surgery - double-blind randomized clinical trial. Rev Bras Anestesiol 2018;68:219–24.

37. Chung F, Liao P, Elsaid H, et al. Factors associated with postoperative exacerbation of sleep-disordered breathing. Anesthesiology 2014;120:299–311.

38. Lam KK, Kunder S, Wong J, et al. Obstructive sleep apnea, pain, and opioids: is the riddle solved? Curr Opin Anaesthesiol 2016;29:134–40.

39. Samuels DJ, Abou-samra A, Dalvi P, et al. Opioid-free anesthesia results in reduced post-operative opioid consumption. J Clin Anesth Pain Med 2017;1(2):5.

40. Budiansky AS, Margarson MP, Eipe N. Acute pain management in morbid obesity - an evidence based clinical update. Surg Obes Relat Dis 2017;13:523–32.

41. Joshi GP, Schug S, Kehlet H. Procedure specific pain management and outcome strategies. Best Pract Res Clin Anaesthesiol 2014;28:191–201.

42. Mehta V, Vasu TS, Phillips B, et al. Obstructive sleep apnea and oxygen therapy: a systematic review of the literature and meta-analysis. J Clin Sleep Med 2013;9: 271–9.

43. Nioctore M, Mahajan RP, Aarts L, et al. High-inspired oxygen concentration further impairs opioid-induced respiratory depression. Br J Anaesth 2013;110: 837–41.

44. Fu ES, Downs JB, Schweiger JW, et al. Supplemental oxygen impairs detection of hypoventilation by pulse oximetry. Chest 2004;126:1552–8.

45. Liao P, Wong J, Singh M, et al. Postoperative oxygen therapy in patients with OSA: a randomized controlled trial. Chest 2017;151:597–611.

46. Chung F, Nagappa M, Singh M, et al. CPAP in the perioperative setting: evidence of support. Chest 2016;149:586–97.

47. McGinley BM, Patil SP, Kirkness JP, et al. A nasal cannula can be used to treat obstructive sleep apnea. Am J Respir Crit Care Med 2007;176:194–200.
48. Eckert SR, Joshi GP, Vyas A. At-home overnight oxygen desaturation in obstructive sleep apnea patients after ambulatory surgery. Proceedings of the ASA 2010 Annual Meeting. San Diego (CA), October 16-20, 2010.

Enhanced Recovery Programs in Outpatient Surgery

Anoushka M. Afonso, MD[a],*, Hanae K. Tokita, MD[b],
Patrick J. McCormick, MD, MEng[c], Rebecca S. Twersky, MD, MPH[d]

KEYWORDS

- Enhanced recovery programs • Enhanced recovery after surgery
- Ambulatory surgery • Postdischarge nausea and vomiting • Quality of recovery
- Multimodal analgesia • Opioid-sparing pain management • Peripheral nerve blocks

KEY POINTS

- Multidisciplinary participation and team coordination are needed for optimal development of enhanced recovery programs in an ambulatory setting.
- Effective patient-centric education programs can improve patients' perioperative experience, reducing anxiety and improving patient satisfaction.
- Ambulatory pathways must be tailored to the patient, procedure, and institution.
- Multimodal analgesia and regional anesthesia are key for opioid-sparing pain management in an enhanced recovery protocol.
- Prophylactic treatment of postoperative nausea and vomiting is a prominent feature in the implementation of a successful surgical enhanced recovery pathway.

PRINCIPLES OF ENHANCED RECOVERY PROGRAMS AND THEIR APPLICATION TO OUTPATIENT SURGERY AND ADVANCED AMBULATORY PROCEDURES

Enhanced recovery after surgery or enhanced recovery program (ERP) is a surgical program designed to increase quality of patient care and satisfaction by integrating

Financial Disclosures: A.M. Afonso—Pacira Pharmaceutical (United States) Research grant, consulting. H.K. Tokita has no commercial or financial disclosures to make at this time. P.J. McCormick has no commercial or financial disclosures to make at this time. R.S. Twersky has no commercial or financial disclosures to make at this time.
Funding: Research reported in this publication was supported by the National Cancer Institute (United States) of the National Institutes of Health under Award Number P30CA008748. The content is solely the responsibility of the authors and does not necessarily represent the official views of the National Institutes of Health.
[a] Enhanced Recovery Programs (ERP), Department of Anesthesiology & Critical Care Medicine, Josie Robertson Surgery Center, Memorial Sloan Kettering Cancer Center, 1275 York Avenue, M-301, New York, NY 10065, USA; [b] Department of Anesthesiology & Critical Care, Josie Robertson Surgery Center, Memorial Sloan Kettering Cancer Center, 1275 York Avenue, New York, NY 10065, USA; [c] Department of Anesthesiology & Critical Care Medicine, Memorial Sloan Kettering Cancer Center, 1275 York Avenue, New York, NY 10065, USA; [d] Department of Anesthesiology & Critical Care Medicine, Josie Robertson Surgery Center, Memorial Sloan Kettering Cancer Center, 1133 York Avenue, Suite 312, New York, NY 10065, USA
* Corresponding author.
E-mail address: afonsoa@mskcc.org

evidence-based protocols to help standardize care and decrease health care expenditures, hospital length of stay (LOS), and morbidity associated with surgical stress.[1] The physiologic chain reaction brought on by direct surgical injury results in systemic release of cytokines and hormones as well as the local release of inflammatory mediators that contribute to the stress response to surgery.[2] If left untreated, patients may become catabolic, immobile, and weak and may develop gut dysfunction, which compounds the injury. These problems delay healing and can lead to complications.[3] The overall goal of ERP is to accelerate recovery by decreasing the body's physical, physiologic, and psychological responses to surgical stress.

Perioperative goals should strive to

1. Minimize the primary surgical injury and reduce blood loss by using minimally invasive techniques.
2. Individualize fluid therapy to maintain physiologic homeostasis: proper fluid therapy helps maintain cellular perfusion, reduce extracellular fluid flux, and avoid salt and water overload, which lead to gut ileus.
3. Optimize pain control by using multimodal analgesia techniques; manage early gut function and enteral feedings to help reduce insulin resistance and restore homeostasis.
4. Encourage early mobilization postoperatively to reduce complications, such as atelectasis, chest infection, and deep vein thrombosis, and stimulate muscle function to maintain strength.

These objectives rely on successful incorporation of key components of ERP (**Fig. 1**) at each stage of the perioperative period.

Each ERP requires a multidisciplinary team to plan and develop the most optimal protocol.

Key players that should be part of the multidisciplinary team include:

1. Patients
2. Anesthesiologists
3. Surgeons
4. Nursing staff
5. Administrations
6. Physiotherapists
7. Dieticians
8. Pharmacists
9. Research personnel

Preoperative	Intraoperative	Postoperative
• Preadmission counseling and education	• Short-acting anesthetic agents	• Appropriate regional anesthesia/analgesia
• Fluid and carbohydrate loading	• Multimodal analgesia and minimize opioid use	• Nonopioid oral analgesia/NSAIDs
• Unprolonged fasting	• Appropriate regional anesthesia/analgesia	• No nasogastric tubes
• No or selective bowel prep	• Maintenance of normothermia (body warmer or warm IV fluids)	• Minimize PONV
• Antibiotic prophylaxis and thromboprophylaxis		• Early oral nutrition
		• Early mobilization

Fig. 1. Key components of ERP. (*Modified from* Varadhan KK, Lobo DN, Ljungqvist O. Enhanced recovery after surgery: the future of improving surgical care. Crit Care Clin 2010;26(3):529; with permission.)

The challenges to successful implementation of an ERP include:

- Assembly of a multidisciplinary team
- Lack of consistency in staffing
- Achieving and maintaining high rates of protocol compliance
- Initial and recurrent staff education
- Variability in program elements due to different surgical procedures
- Audit to monitor staff compliance and measure outcomes
- Financial support for all of these challenges

How is Enhanced Recovery Program Relevant to the Ambulatory Setting?

Specific ERP pathways for ambulatory surgery are limited in the literature. Many of the principles for inpatient ERP, however, are relevant to patients undergoing ambulatory and short-stay surgery. As ambulatory surgery facilities expand their scope to involve more complex procedures, ERP pathways are key to ensure the success of expansion. Although shorter LOS is characteristic of successful inpatient ERP, this outcome is less relevant in the ambulatory context. The focus of ambulatory surgery ERP should be on reduced variance in other patient outcomes.[4]

Important patient outcomes for ambulatory surgery enhanced recovery program:

- Pain
- Opioid minimization
- Reduced postoperative nausea and vomiting (PONV) and postdischarge nausea and vomiting (PDNV)
- Early ambulation
- Improved quality of recovery

Implementation of Enhanced Recovery Program in Ambulatory Surgery Centers

The authors have successfully implemented ERP for nontraditional ambulatory surgery cancer procedures performed at the Josie Robertson Surgery Center, a freestanding ambulatory surgery facility of the Memorial Sloan Kettering Cancer Center, New York, New York. This was accomplished with a combination of extensive literature review, multidisciplinary collaborative efforts, and creation of surgery-specific pathways. Creating a standardized clinical care pathway enables the anesthesia team to systematically approach the patients care while minimizing variability and maximizing predictable outcomes. Specifically, 4 surgical procedures were identified as short-stay nontraditional ambulatory procedures for cancer surgery: mastectomy with and without reconstruction, robotic prostatectomy, minimally invasive robotic and laparoscopic hysterectomy, and thyroidectomy. Data from the authors' facility are forthcoming in future publications.

The following important elements in the authors' enhanced recovery after surgery ambulatory programs were identified:

1. Administration of standardized antiemetic protocol, which includes administration of dexamethasone and a serotonin receptor antagonist, such as ondansetron, for all patients. Aprepitant is given to high-risk patients
2. Minimization of opioid administration and supplementation with preoperative gabapentin, intravenous (IV) acetaminophen, and ketorolac, if appropriate
3. Use of regional anesthesia where appropriate
4. Minimal use of nasogastric tubes

5. Appropriate fluid administration
6. Standardized interventions related to the specific surgical procedure

Ambulatory surgical ERP should measure outcomes, including:

- LOS, measured in hours
- Need for pain management, in particular postoperative narcotic demand
- Need for immediate postoperative transfer to acute care hospital
- Visit to urgent care or the emergency room within 30 days
- Readmission within 30 days

In addition to early and intermediate outcomes, later outcomes, such as patient-reported outcomes and health-related quality-of-life assessment postdischarge, may be incorporated, although more research is needed in this respect. Auditing compliance of individual ERP elements can improve outcomes, such as postoperative LOS.[5]

Implementation of ambulatory surgery ERP provides improved outcomes with shortened postoperative LOS. Improved outcomes are only sustainable, however, through close cooperative interdisciplinary efforts, continuous education, and routine auditing of pathway compliance. More benchmark and outcome data are needed.

PATIENT EDUCATION AND POSTOPERATIVE EXPECTATIONS

Little has been written on the effectiveness of patient education regarding patient perioperative outcomes in ambulatory surgery. There are many benefits in educating patients (**Fig. 2**) about what to expect in their surgical and recovery pathway. A well-run preoperative education program is central to the success of a surgical ambulatory program with ERPs in place.

Emotional stress and preoperative anxiety are common in patients preoperatively. One study reported incidences of preoperative anxiety in 45.3% of inpatients and 38.3% of ambulatory patients.[6]

Appropriate preoperative education also can increase patient satisfaction. Younis and colleagues[7] showed in a retrospective study that improved quality

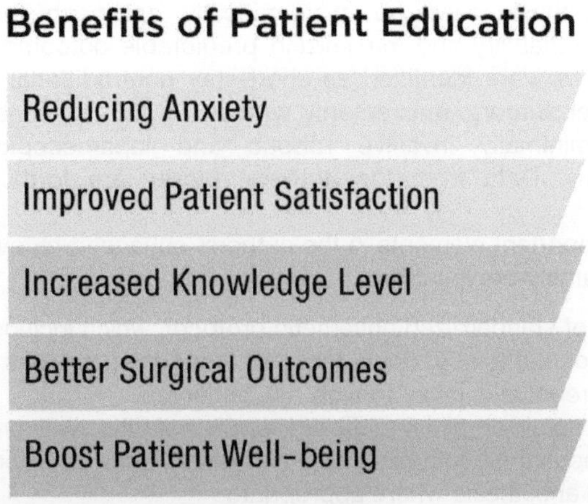

Benefits of Patient Education

Reducing Anxiety

Improved Patient Satisfaction

Increased Knowledge Level

Better Surgical Outcomes

Boost Patient Well-being

Fig. 2. Various benefits of patient education for ERPs.

of patient information for ambulatory hemorrhoidectomy resulted in increased patient satisfaction and fewer patients seeking medical attention postdischarge. An informed patient is more likely to be a satisfied patient in this process. Improving the manner in which key information is relayed to patients requires thorough and conscious effort with repeated reassessments, as in the example of patient adherence to preoperative fasting guidelines.[8] This simple improvement in education could lead to decreased cancellations, improved work flow, and decreased operating room delays, especially important in ambulatory ERPs.

Each patient encounter needs to be individualized, with the preoperative education being a forum for[9]:

1. Building patient-physician rapport and trust
2. Identifying potential problems to be addressed prior to surgery
3. Confirming and establishing diagnoses, options, and alternatives to surgical approach and overall treatment
4. Educating the patients and answering questions
5. Ensuring better outcomes for both surgeon and patient

In an ambulatory setting, pain management and early mobilization are imperative for patients to succeed on their enhanced recovery track. Patients should be educated on pain rating scales used in the postoperative setting and alternatives to opioid medications, and a plan should be made in chronic pain patients well in advance. Preoperative teaching needs to address expectations of performing activities and mobilizing postoperatively and strategies to make these tasks measurable for the patient.[10] Especially in an ambulatory ERP, patients need to anticipate their departure as soon as they meet their milestones for discharge.

The Educational Process and Types of Educational Tools for Enhanced Recovery Programs

Because there is a limited time to get salient information to patients, the multidisciplinary team needs to make sure information is repeated by all members of the team and reinforced along the process in the limited time available to the patient. Inclusion of patients (focus groups/patient interviews) when making educational content is helpful to understand what issues are of most concern to the patient.

Patient education must be complete, yet easy to understand for patients to follow through the pathway successfully. Adapting preoperative education material to patients' preferences (**Fig. 3**) affects patients' perception of the perioperative experience.

Comparisons of all these educational modalities need further research and clarification. Multimedia support should be considered worthwhile, according to a randomized controlled trial involving 203 patients scheduled for radical prostatectomy. Although anxiety and measures of decision making were comparable, knowledge and patient satisfaction were superior to those in the group without preoperative multimedia support.[11] Kearney and colleagues[12] compared outcome of 150 patients who did and did not attend a hospital-based preoperative education class. Although there was no significant difference between groups in LOS, ambulation distance, pain level, or complication rate, the patients scheduled for joint replacement surgery felt better prepared and were better able to control their pain after surgery. Comparisons of an in-person versus online source of education are needed to shed light on what is best for patients. In the breast reconstruction patients, the effectiveness of educational

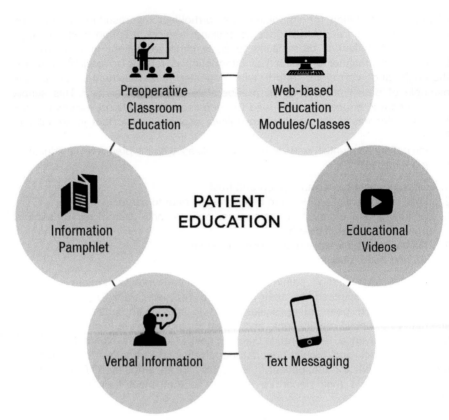

Fig. 3. Important components of patient education for ERPs.

programs is largely positive. Those women who used an interactive educational tool for breast reconstruction had significantly increased knowledge levels as well as increased satisfaction with experience, decision process, and the outcomes of the breast reconstruction.[13]

According to Ronco and colleagues,[14] these are some trends in preoperative education from a systematic review of 19 studies involving 3944 patients:

- Increased frequency of message exposure through several reinforcements and/or interventions
- Educational content frequently addressing postoperative management
- Measurement of patient outcomes (cognitive, experiential, and biophysiological aspects)

Postoperative Expectations

Understanding the type of information patients need from their perspective is key. Often, surgeons and anesthesia providers focus on those items most important to the perioperative team, failing to address issues significant to the patient.[15] As part of the ambulatory ERP, effective education tools in the preoperative setting can help patients have a clear understanding of expectations and realistic milestones in the postoperative setting. It is through careful planning and feedback from the multidisciplinary team and patients that improvements can be made in preoperative education programs. In addition, these programs serve as valuable tools for training staff members improving their own clinical practice. There is a need for better research in patient education, especially in the development of appropriate educational aids that are patient-specific for an improved ambulatory patient experience.

MULTIMODAL ANALGESIA IN AMBULATORY SURGERY: NONOPIOID ANALGESICS

A central tenet of ERPs is the minimization and/or elimination of opioids. To achieve this goal, ambulatory programs strive to achieve optimal analgesia though multimodal agents. Multimodal analgesia, combination of medications with different mechanisms of action, and fewer side-effect profiles can provide a more superior pain relief compared with a single agent. Use of this approach can improve the analgesic outcomes in ambulatory surgery, allowing for patients' rapid recovery after surgery. A few of the nonopioid options are examined, reserving discussion of opioids for breakthrough pain control.

Acetaminophen

Acetaminophen is one of the most common medications used in ambulatory ERPs with minimal side effects. Acetaminophen has a complex mechanism of action, which effects both peripheral (cyclooxygenase [COX] inhibition) and central antinociception processes.[16] Acetaminophen administered to patients in laparoscopic surgeries reduced total opioid dose perioperatively.[17] Combination of acetaminophen with a nonsteroidal anti-inflammatory drug is better than acetaminophen alone for postoperative pain.[18] Jibril and colleagues[19] reviewed IV acetaminophen and oral acetaminophen in a systematic review and found no clear indication for the IV form to be administered over oral if the patient has a functioning gastrointestinal tract and is able to take oral dosage forms. Of the 3 studies reporting efficacy outcomes, Pettersson and colleagues[20] showed lower opioid usage with IV form, but this did not translate to a difference in pain scores or rates of nausea and vomiting in coronary artery bypass grafting. In contrast to what Brett and colleagues[21] found in patients undergoing knee arthroscopy, pain scores were in favor of IV administration, but this did not translate into significant differences in opioid consumption or LOS. Although some centers give the oral form in the preoperative holding area, the authors administer IV acetaminophen preemptively before surgical incision in the operating room for a faster onset and more predictable absorption. These patients then postoperatively transition to standing oral medication as soon as patients can tolerate oral intake. Patients can then take around-the-clock oral medications at home to control acute postoperative pain with less reliance on opioids.

Nonsteroidal Anti-inflammatory Drugs and Cyclooxygenase 2 Inhibitors

The nonsteroidal anti-inflammatory drug and COX-2 agents are commonly used in ERP preoperatively and work by reducing inflammation, effectively treating postoperative pain. Ibuprofen and ketorolac are nonselective agents that work by COX-1 and COX-2 inhibition. Ketorolac is commonly used in ambulatory surgical centers, but renal dosage adjustments must be done in select patients. Both ibuprofen (1200 mg/d) and celecoxib (400 mg/d) significantly decreased the need for rescue analgesia in the early postoperative period in patients undergoing ambulatory surgery. Improvements in quality of recovery and patient satisfaction with their pain management were noted in this double-blinded placebo-controlled study.[22] Timing of use of COX-2 inhibitors is important, as most clinicians recommend *preemptive* administration rather than postoperative. Celecoxib (400 mg orally) administered on the day of surgery and continued 3 days postoperatively improves pain management as well as the speed and recovery after plastic surgery rather than just in the postoperative period.[23] In outpatient ambulatory orthopedic surgery, comparable analgesia with single doses of celecoxib and combination of hydrocodone/acetaminophen were noted in more than 400 patients.[24]

Gabapentinoids

Both gabapentin and pregabalin are γ-aminobutyric acid analogs that have been used in historically as antiepileptics but have anticonvulsant, analgesic, and anxiolytic effects. Pregabalin has better bioavailability and onset time but is more expensive than gabapentin. The addition of preemptive pregabalin at either dose (150 mg or 300 mg) decreased pain scores and postoperative fentanyl consumption in patients after laparoscopic surgery in a dose-dependent manner without any differences in side effects.[25] Although they are an effective tool for postoperative pain treatment, care must be taken in the outpatient domain. Although generally well tolerated, the side effects of sedation and dizziness can prove troublesome for certain ambulatory patients, such as the elderly. Schmidt and colleagues[26] summarize the use of gabapentinoids—choice of agent, dose, and timing, with effects on chronic postsurgical pain. In the authors' ambulatory surgery facility, patients who are less than 65 years old who undergo more complex outpatient procedures, such as robotic-assisted hysterectomy, robotic-assisted prostatectomy, mastectomy, and thyroidectomy, are given gabapentin, 300 mg orally, prior to surgery.

Lidocaine Intravenous Infusion

IV lidocaine has shown promise for inpatient enhanced recovery protocols due to its anti-inflammatory and analgesic properties. Although not common in the ambulatory space, it is easy to use and has minimal toxicity at typical doses (1.5–3 mg/kg/h). Kaba and colleagues[27] report that lidocaine infusions led to decreased postoperative opioid consumption and fewer opioid-related side effects, such as time to first bowel movement and time to first flatus, in laparoscopic colectomy patients. This study also reported decreased hospital LOS and decreased PONV. McKay and colleagues[28] reported that systemic lidocaine decreased the perioperative opioid analgesic requirements but failed to reduce discharge time after ambulatory surgery. Wu and Liu[29] discuss in an editorial that the usual outcome measurements (such as LOS) for hospitalized patients do not always apply to ambulatory anesthesia studies. To better understand the effects of lidocaine, more studies reporting patient-reported outcomes with a validated instrument appropriate for the ambulatory setting are needed.

REGIONAL ANESTHESIA AS PART OF A MULTIMODAL APPROACH IN ENHANCED RECOVERY PROGRAMS

A major focus of ERPs for ambulatory surgery should be opioid-sparing multimodal analgesia. Local anesthesia–based techniques, including wound infiltration, regional nerve blocks, and neuraxial anesthesia, have increasingly become a key component of an opioid-sparing pain management strategy for ambulatory surgery.[30] These techniques are recommended by the American Society of Anesthesiologists Task Force on Acute Pain Management.[31] Ultrasound guidance has transformed the clinical practice of regional anesthesia. More anesthesiologists are comfortable using this technology in their everyday practice.[32] The utility of regional anesthesia techniques for common nonorthopedic outpatient procedures is reviewed, with a focus on transversus abdominis plane (TAP) block for laparoscopic surgery and chest wall blocks for ambulatory breast surgery.

Transversus Abdominis Plane Blocks

The TAP block is a fascial plane block in which local anesthesia is infiltrated between the transversus abdominis and internal oblique muscles to provide analgesia to the anterior abdominal wall. TAP blocks have been described for postoperative pain management for a variety of procedures. As a component of an ERP, TAP blocks have been described in a small study of patients undergoing laparoscopic colorectal surgery. Patients who received TAP blocks had reduced mean hospital stay and overall opioid consumption compared with historic controls.[33] A study of TAP blocks in microvascular breast reconstruction found that ERP patients had shortened LOS and decreased postoperative opioid consumption compared with historic controls.[34] The benefit of TAP blocks has not been demonstrated in outpatient laparoscopic procedures. A meta-analysis of randomized controlled trials by De Oliveira and colleagues[35] in 2014 investigated pain outcomes after laparoscopic surgery with TAP blocks. This study found that patients who received preoperative TAP blocks had less pain at rest during both early and late stages of recovery but no improvement in pain with movement throughout recovery.[35] Furthermore, improved quality of recovery outcomes were found in patients who received preoperative TAP blocks for laparoscopic gynecologic surgery but no improvement in quality of recovery or pain outcomes was found in patients undergoing laparoscopic hysterectomy with postoperative TAP blocks.[35] A meta-analysis that sought to determine the efficacy of TAP blocks for a variety of abdominal surgeries found that TAP blocks provided only minimal analgesic efficacy.[36] This meta-analysis had significant heterogeneity in procedure types, which made it challenging to draw any meaningful conclusions. Importantly, no major cases of local anesthetic toxicity were noted in these meta-analyses. Although more evidence is needed to support routine use of TAP blocks for outpatient laparoscopic surgery, they have minimal risk to the patient and may prove to have a role in a multimodal analgesic plan. Despite these promising findings, there are several parameters that need to be further evaluated and addressed in future studies:

1. Appropriate choice in local anesthetic
2. Dosing
3. Use of adjuvant medications, such as dexamethasone and clonidine
4. Preoperative versus postoperative administration
5. Ultrasound-guided versus surgeon infiltration
6. Pain and quality outcomes after discharge

Chest Wall Blocks

Increasingly, complex breast surgery is being performed in the outpatient setting.[37] Pain—both acute and chronic—is a significant complication of breast surgery.[38] The paravertebral block (PVB) is considered the gold standard regional anesthetic technique for breast surgery. Use of PVB in conjunction with total intravenous anesthesia or general anesthesia is associated with decreased pain scores, postoperative analgesic consumption, PONV, LOS, incidence of chronic pain, and higher patient satisfaction and superior quality of recovery compared with general anesthesia alone.[39] Although the classic approach was a landmark-based technique, an ultrasound guidance approach has also been described.[40] Risk of pneumothorax with PVB using ultrasound guidance is rare. A retrospective analysis of 856 patients who received ultrasound guided thoracic PVB for mastectomy with immediate reconstruction found no incidence of suspected pneumothorax.[41] More recently, fascial plane blocks have emerged as alternative regional anesthetic options for breast surgery.[39] Abdallah and colleagues[42] found that both pectoralis and serratus blocks reduced opioid consumption and PONV after ambulatory breast surgery. In recent years, the erector spinae block (ESB) has generated interest as an alternative regional technique for breast surgery and has been described in a case report for breast surgery.[43] The ESB is a novel fascial plane block initially used for thoracic neuropathic pain. Recently, Chiu and colleagues[44] reported that an ERP that incorporated pectoralis nerve blocks or PVBs in patients undergoing mastectomy with reconstruction led to decreased opioid consumption and PONV compared with historic controls at a 23-hour short stay surgery center. Although more data are needed to determine the analgesic efficacy of the newer fascial plane blocks, PVBs improve outcomes in patients undergoing complex breast surgery and should be incorporated into multimodal analgesic pathways for these patients. More studies are needed to determine how pectoralis nerve blocks, serratus plane blocks, and ESBs compared with PVBs in quality and safety outcomes.

POSTOPERATIVE NAUSEA AND VOMITING

Prophylactic treatment of PONV has been a prominent feature of nearly every surgical ERP. The landmark International Multicenter Protocol to Assess Antiemetic Combinations Trial demonstrated that antiemetic interventions have similar effectiveness and that high-risk patients benefit from multiple interventions.[45] Data from this study and other related investigations have been used by the Society for Ambulatory Anesthesia to generate a consensus guideline for PONV management.[46] Current evidence does not support giving PONV prophylaxis to everyone. The low cost and favorable side-effect profile, however, of these medications has led many ERPs to include antiemetic medications for all patients.

One of the reasons for adding PONV therapies to an ERP is to improve compliance. Historically, compliance with PONV treatment has been poor. A study examining a computerized decision support tool for PONV prophylaxis found that the intervention raised appropriate prescriptions in eligible patients from 38% to 73%.[47] The rate fell to 37% after the intervention was discontinued. Another issue is that complex PONV guidelines can lead to poor results. A recent before-and-after study tested a radically simplified PONV protocol using only patient gender. The incidence of PONV within 24 hours after surgery went from 33% to 22% ($P = .02$).[48]

In ambulatory surgery patients, PDNV is a serious concern. These patients do not usually have easy access to antiemetic therapies at home. In a multicenter trial of PDNV in patients discharged on the day of surgery, patient-reported nausea and/or vomiting went from 20.7% to 37.1% after discharge.[49] Antiemetics with a short half-life are not effective for PDNV. Patients need to be given longer acting agents, such as dexamethasone, aprepitant, palonosetron, and transdermal scopolamine. Rolapitant is an neurokinin-1 antagonist with a very long half-life of 180 hours. A trial of rolapitant compared with ondansetron found that there was a higher rate of no emesis compared to placebo in the rolapitant 200-mg and 70-mg groups at all time points up to 120 hours after surgery.[50] In a study of 1041 pediatric ambulatory surgery patients, intraoperative and postdischarge opioids increased the nausea and vomiting risk.[51] Long-acting opioids carried an odds ratio of 3.093 (95% CI, 1.634–5.874) and postdischarge opioids had an odds ratio of 2.037 (95% CI, 1.142–3.632.) A recent study in Switzerland of 222 brief ambulatory surgeries treated with a propofol-based anesthetic and a standard antiemetic prophylaxis ladder found a PDNV rate of 11.3% on postoperative day 1 and 0.7% on postoperative day 2.[52] This extremely low rate is partially due to the low rate of postoperative opioid prescriptions in Switzerland and due to the exclusion of gynecologic surgeries, which are known are have a higher PONV rate.

Breast surgery patients are a subgroup of ambulatory surgery patients at an elevated risk of PONV. In 1 study, 59% of breast surgery patients experienced PONV when no prophylaxis was given.[53] A comprehensive ERP for mastectomy that included high-dose dexamethasone (8 mg IV) and regional anesthesia reduced PONV from 50% to 28% (P<.001).[44] It seems, however, that there may be a limit to how low the PONV rate can go. A recent prospective study of PONV in breast surgery patients found a 29.9% PONV rate and a 35% PDNV rate despite aggressive guideline-driven prophylaxis.[54]

In tandem with genetic techniques to diagnose and treat cancer in the near future, the authors hope to identify patients with a genetic predisposition to PONV who would not be otherwise given extra treatment. Polymorphisms in the serotonin receptor 3B, the dopamine D2 receptor, and the cytochrome P450 2D6 enzyme all have been associated with a higher incidence of PONV.[55] If PONV risk evaluation systems are extended to include these polymorphisms, further reducing the rates of PONV and PDNV may be possible.

SUMMARY

Enhanced recovery pathways have been shown to improve surgical outcomes. Although most research in ERPs has focused on inpatients, many of the principles are relevant to surgical procedures with same-day discharge or 23-hour stay. Success of an ERP depends on monitoring pathway compliance and patient outcomes, such as pain, opioid requirements, nausea and vomiting, and early ambulation. To reduce opioid need, ERPs rely on multimodal analgesia, including regional anesthesia. Robust preoperative education programs are integral to the success of ambulatory ERPs. Rather than measurements of LOS, as in traditional inpatient programs, the focus of ERP in ambulatory surgery should be on improved quality of recovery, pain management, and early ambulation.

ACKNOWLEDGMENTS

The authors wish to acknowledge Lucia Salamanca-Cardona, PhD for her technical writing and editing contribution.

REFERENCES

1. Varadhan K, Lobo D, Ljungqvist O. Enhanced recovery after surgery: the future of improving surgical care. Clin Care Clin 2010;26:527–47.
2. Kehlet H. Multimodal approach to control postoperative pathophysiology and rehabilitation. Br J Anaesth 1997;78(5):606–17.
3. Carli F. Physiologic considerations of Enhanced Recovery After Surgery (ERAS) programs: implications of the stress response. Can J Anaesth 2015;62(2):110–9.
4. Gan TJ, Scott M, Thaokor J, et al. American Society for Enhanced Recovery: advancing enhanced recovery and perioperative medicine. Anesth Analg 2018; 126(6):1870–3.
5. Bakker N, Cakir H, Doodeman HJ, et al. Eight years of experience with Enhanced Recovery After Surgery in patients with colon cancer: impact of measures to improve adherence. Surgery 2015;157(6):1130–6.
6. Wetsch WA, Pircher I, Lederer W, et al. Preoperative stress and anxiety in day-care patients and inpatients undergoing fast-track surgery. Br J Anaesth 2009; 103(2):199–205.

7. Younis J, Salerno G, Chaudhary A, et al. Reduction in hospital reattendance due to improved preoperative patient education following hemorrhoidectomy. J Healthc Qual 2013;35(6):24–9.

8. Kyrtatos PG, Constandinou N, Loizides S, et al. Improved patient education facilitates adherence to preoperative fasting guidelines. J Perioper Pract 2014;24(10): 228–31.

9. McGillis ST, Stanton-Hicks U. The preoperative patient evaluation: preparing for surgery. Dermatol Clin 1998;16(1):1–15.

10. Tollefson J. Essential clinical skills. 2nd edition. Cengage Learning Australia; 2012.

11. Huber J, Ihrig A, Yass M, et al. Multimedia support for improving preoperative patient education: a randomized controlled trial using the example of radical prostatectomy. Ann Surg Oncol 2013;20(1):15–23.

12. Kearney M, Jennrich MK, Lyons S, et al. Effects of preoperative education on patient outcomes after joint replacement surgery. Orthop Nurs 2011;30(6):391–6.

13. Heller L, Parker PA, Youssef A, et al. Interactive digital education aid in breast reconstruction. Plast Reconstr Surg 2008;122(3):717–24.

14. Ronco M, Iona L, Fabbro C, et al. Patient education outcomes in surgery: a systematic review from 2004 to 2010. Int J Evid Based Healthc 2012;10(4):309–23.

15. Preminger BA, Lemaine V, Sulimanoff I, et al. Preoperative patient education for breast reconstruction: a systematic review of the literature. J Cancer Educ 2011;26(2):270–6.

16. Jozwiak-Bebenista M, Nowak JZ. Paracetamol: mechanism of action, applications and safety concern. Acta Pol Pharm 2014;71(1):11–23.

17. Elvir-Lazo OL, White PF. The role of multimodal analgesia in pain management after ambulatory surgery. Curr Opin Anaesthesiol 2010;23(6):697–703.

18. Ong CK, Seymour RA, Lirk P, et al. Combining paracetamol (acetaminophen) with nonsteroidal antiinflammatory drugs: a qualitative systematic review of analgesic efficacy for acute postoperative pain. Anesth Analg 2010;110(4):1170–9.

19. Jibril F, Sharaby S, Mohamed A, et al. Intravenous versus oral acetaminophen for pain: systematic review of current evidence to support clinical decision-making. Can J Hosp Pharm 2015;68(3):238–47.

20. Pettersson PH, Jakobsson J, Owall A. Intravenous acetaminophen reduced the use of opioids compared with oral administration after coronary artery bypass grafting. J Cardiothorac Vasc Anesth 2005;19(3):306–9.

21. Brett CN, Barnett SG, Pearson J. Postoperative plasma paracetamol levels following oral or intravenous paracetamol administration: a double-blind randomised controlled trial. Anaesth Intensive Care 2012;40(1):166–71.

22. White PF, Tang J, Wender RH, et al. The effects of oral ibuprofen and celecoxib in preventing pain, improving recovery outcomes and patient satisfaction after ambulatory surgery. Anesth Analg 2011;112(2):323–9.

23. Sun T, Sacan O, White PF, et al. Perioperative versus postoperative celecoxib on patient outcomes after major plastic surgery procedures. Anesth Analg 2008; 106(3):950–8.

24. Gimbel JS, Brugger A, Zhao W, et al. Efficacy and tolerability of celecoxib versus hydrocodone/acetaminophen in the treatment of pain after ambulatory orthopedic surgery in adults. Clin Ther 2001;23(2):228–41.

25. Balaban F, Yagar S, Ozgok A, et al. A randomized, placebo-controlled study of pregabalin for postoperative pain intensity after laparoscopic cholecystectomy. J Clin Anesth 2012;24(3):175–8.

26. Schmidt PC, Ruchelli G, Mackey SC, et al. Perioperative gabapentinoids: choice of agent, dose, timing, and effects on chronic postsurgical pain. Anesthesiology 2013;119(5):1215–21.
27. Kaba A, Laurent SR, Detroz BJ, et al. Intravenous lidocaine infusion facilitates acute rehabilitation after laparoscopic colectomy. Anesthesiology 2007;106(1): 11–8 [discussion 15–6].
28. McKay A, Gottschalk A, Ploppa A, et al. Systemic lidocaine decreased the perioperative opioid analgesic requirements but failed to reduce discharge time after ambulatory surgery. Anesth Analg 2009;109(6):1805–8.
29. Wu CL, Liu SS. Intravenous lidocaine for ambulatory anesthesia: good to go or not so fast? Anesth Analg 2009;109(6):1718–9.
30. Carli F, Kehlet H, Baldini G, et al. Evidence basis for regional anesthesia in multidisciplinary fast-track surgical care pathways. Reg Anesth Pain Med 2011;36(1):63–72.
31. American Society of Anesthesiologists Task Force on Acute Pain Management. Practice guidelines for acute pain management in the perioperative setting: an updated report by the American Society of Anesthesiologists Task Force on Acute Pain Management. Anesthesiology 2012;116(2):248–73.
32. Marhofer P, Willschke H, Kettner S. Current concepts and future trends in ultrasound-guided regional anesthesia. Curr Opin Anaesthesiol 2010;23(5):632–6.
33. Favuzza J, Brady K, Delaney CP. Transversus abdominis plane blocks and enhanced recovery pathways: making the 23-h hospital stay a realistic goal after laparoscopic colorectal surgery. Surg Endosc 2013;27(7):2481–6.
34. Afonso A, Oskar S, Tan KS, et al. Is enhanced recovery the new standard of care in microsurgical breast reconstruction? Plast Reconstr Surg 2017;139(5):1053 61.
35. De Oliveira GS Jr, Castro-Alves LJ, Nader A, et al. Transversus abdominis plane block to ameliorate postoperative pain outcomes after laparoscopic surgery: a meta-analysis of randomized controlled trials. Anesth Analg 2014;118(2):454–63.
36. Baeriswyl M, Kirkham KR, Kern C, et al. The analgesic efficacy of ultrasound-guided transversus abdominis plane block in adult patients: a meta-analysis. Anesth Analg 2015;121(6):1640–54.
37. Miller AM, Steiner CA, Barrett ML, et al. Breast reconstruction surgery for mastectomy in hospital inpatient and ambulatory settings, 2009-2014: statistical brief #228. In: Healthcare Cost and Utilization Project (HCUP) statistical briefs. Rockville (MD): Agency for Healthcare Research and Quality; 2017. p. 1–20.
38. Jung BF, Ahrendt GM, Oaklander AL, et al. Neuropathic pain following breast cancer surgery: proposed classification and research update. Pain 2003; 104(1–2):1–13.
39. Woodworth GE, Ivie RMJ, Nelson SM, et al. Perioperative breast analgesia: a qualitative review of anatomy and regional techniques. Reg Anesth Pain Med 2017;42(5):609–31.
40. Tighe S, Greene MD, Rajadurai N. Paravertebral block. BJA Educ 2010;10(5):133–7.
41. Pace MM, Sharma B, Anderson-Dam J, et al. Ultrasound-guided thoracic paravertebral blockade: a retrocpective study of the incidence of complications. Anesth Analg 2016;122(4):1186–91.
42. Abdallah FW, MacLean D, Madjdpour C, et al. Pectoralis and serratus fascial plane blocks each provide early analgesic benefits following ambulatory breast cancer surgery: a retrospective propensity-matched cohort study. Anesth Analg 2017;125(1):294–302.
43. Kumar A, Hulsey A, Martinez-Wilson H, et al. The use of liposomal bupivacaine in erector spinae plane block to minimize opioid consumption for breast surgery: a case report. A A Pract 2018;10(9):239–41.

44. Chiu C, Aleshi P, Esserman LJ, et al. Improved analgesia and reduced post-operative nausea and vomiting after implementation of an enhanced recovery after surgery (ERAS) pathway for total mastectomy. BMC Anesthesiol 2018; 18(1):41.

45. Apfel CC, Korttila K, Abdalla M, et al. A factorial trial of six interventions for the prevention of postoperative nausea and vomiting. N Engl J Med 2004;350(24): 2441–51.

46. Gan TJ, Diemunsch P, Habib AS, et al. Consensus guidelines for the management of postoperative nausea and vomiting. Anesth Analg 2014;118(1):85–113.

47. Kooij FO, Klok T, Hollmann MW, et al. Decision support increases guideline adherence for prescribing postoperative nausea and vomiting prophylaxis. Anesth Analg 2008;106(3):893–8 [table of contents].

48. Dewinter G, Staelens W, Veef E, et al. Simplified algorithm for the prevention of postoperative nausea and vomiting: a before-and-after study. Br J Anaesth 2018;120(1):156–63.

49. Apfel CC, Philip BK, Cakmakkaya OS, et al. Who is at risk for postdischarge nausea and vomiting after ambulatory surgery? Anesthesiology 2012;117(3): 475–86.

50. Gan TJ, Gu J, Singla N, et al. Rolapitant for the prevention of postoperative nausea and vomiting: a prospective, double-blinded, placebo-controlled randomized trial. Anesth Analg 2011;112(4):804–12.

51. Efune PN, Minhajuddin A, Szmuk P. Incidence and factors contributing to postdischarge nausea and vomiting in pediatric ambulatory surgical cases. Paediatr Anaesth 2018;28(3):257–63.

52. Bruderer U, Fisler A, Steurer MP, et al. Post-discharge nausea and vomiting after total intravenous anaesthesia and standardised PONV prophylaxis for ambulatory surgery. Acta Anaesthesiol Scand 2017;61(7):758–66.

53. Layeeque R, Siegel E, Kass R, et al. Prevention of nausea and vomiting following breast surgery. Am J Surg 2006;191(6):767–72.

54. Wesmiller SW, Sereika SM, Bender CM, et al. Exploring the multifactorial nature of postoperative nausea and vomiting in women following surgery for breast cancer. Auton Neurosci 2017;202:102–7.

55. Lopez-Morales P, Flores-Funes D, Sanchez-Migallon EG, et al. Genetic factors associated with postoperative nausea and vomiting: a systematic review. J Gastrointest Surg 2018;22(9):1645–51.

Emergency Response in the Ambulatory Surgery Center

Vikram K. Bansal, MD[a],*, Katherine H. Dobie, MD[b], Evelyn Jane Brock, DO[c]

KEYWORDS

- Ambulatory surgery center • Emergencies • Local anesthetic systemic toxicity
- Myocardial infarction • Malignant hyperthermia • Anaphylaxis • Delayed emergence
- Airway fire

KEY POINTS

- Perioperative emergencies in ambulatory surgery centers can be uniquely challenging due to rarity of occurrence, fast-paced environment, and limited resources.
- Preparedness through education and simulation-based training is essential for effective emergency response.
- In addition to accreditation requirements, many surgery centers implement their own education, training, and simulation schedules for emergency response.
- Rapid recognition, stabilization, and transfer to the nearest hospital for invasive monitoring, testing, and treatment is the goal.

INTRODUCTION

In 2017, the US Department of Health and Human Services released a report estimating that 22.5 million ambulatory procedures and surgeries were performed at ambulatory surgery centers. Only 2% of those patients were admitted to the hospital.[1] The significant surgical volume shift to ambulatory centers can be attributed to advances in surgical and anesthetic care. The development of safer and shorter-acting drugs, regional anesthesia, multimodal analgesia, and minimally invasive surgery has significantly improved pain control, allowing patients to go home shortly after their surgery or procedure.[1,2] As advances in anesthetic care are allowing more complex cases and patients with comorbidities, such as extremes of age, obesity, and

Disclosure Statement: No disclosures for all authors.
a Department of Anesthesiology, Division of Ambulatory Anesthesiology, Vanderbilt University Medical Center, 1211 Medical Center Drive, Nashville, TN 37232, USA; b Department of Anesthesiology, Vanderbilt University Medical Center, 1211 Medical Center Drive, Nashville, TN 37232, USA; c Department of Anesthesiology, Division of Ambulatory Anesthesiology, Vanderbilt University Medical Center, 1301 Medical Center Drive, 4648 TVC, Nashville, TN 37232, USA
* Corresponding author.
E-mail address: vikram.bansal@vumc.org

Anesthesiology Clin 37 (2019) 239–250
https://doi.org/10.1016/j.anclin.2019.01.012
1932-2275/19/© 2019 Elsevier Inc. All rights reserved.

obstructive sleep apnea, into the surgery center, patient-related emergencies will likely increase. Response to emergencies in these environments relies on a relatively limited staff and resources, making ambulatory surgery centers more vulnerable to inadequate response. Preparedness for such emergencies in the ambulatory surgery setting is currently addressed by accreditation agencies, such as the Accreditation Association for Ambulatory Health Care and Joint Commission on Accreditation of Hospital Organizations. Each requires evidence of one cardiopulmonary resuscitation drill per year, yet ambulatory surgery centers are not required to, and typically do not have, "code teams." Simulation-based training increases emergency response preparedness through practice using "real-life" scenarios.[3] Preparing for a rare event can be difficult, but individuals who trained with simulation performed better with technical and nontechnical skills and were able to transfer those skills better to the operating room (OR) compared with traditional interactive seminars.[3] It is important to have individualized and structured debriefing to address any issues to improve personal performance.[3]

With pressures to maximize throughput, increasing surgical complexity, and patients with increasing comorbidities, all in the setting of limited resources and staff, preparedness for unexpected emergencies in the ambulatory setting is essential.

ANAPHYLAXIS

Anaphylaxis is a severe, life-threatening generalized or systemic hypersensitivity reaction with an incidence of 1:3500 to 20,000 and holds a mortality of 3% to 9%.[4]

The most common anaphylactic reactions seen in the OR include the following[5-7]:

Latex, 20%
Antibiotics, 15%
Neuromuscular blocking drugs, 10%

Rarely are there anaphylactic reactions to opioids, local anesthetics, propofol (even in egg or soy allergic individuals), or halogenated volatile anesthetics. Reactions also may be seen with protamine, heparin, contrast dye, oxytocin, nonsteroidal drugs (PGE2 pathway), and some preservatives, such as methyl-paraben.[6,8]

Anaphylaxis is divided into allergic and nonallergic. The clinical features of allergic and nonallergic anaphylaxis may be identical. Allergic anaphylaxis is mediated by an immunologic mechanism, often immunoglobulin (Ig)E, IgG, or complement activation by immune complexes. Nonallergic anaphylaxis is non-IgE mediated but produces a similar clinical picture.[5,8]

Anaphylaxis is not a homogeneous process: the pathways, mediators, time course, and response to treatment depend on the triggering agent, its route and rate of administration, the nature of the patient's hypersensitivity, and the health of the patient.[5]

Anaphylaxis may present with respiratory, circulatory, and/or cutaneous changes. The clinical diagnosis may include the following[5]:

- Hypotension
- Tachycardia
- Bradycardia
- Cutaneous flushing
- Rash
- Bronchospasm
- Hypoxia
- Angioedema
- Cardiac arrest

Intravascular volume redistribution and a decrease in cardiac output may occur, as well as a drop in coronary artery perfusion pressure and decreased venous return. Asphyxia may occur due to angioedema, bronchospasm, and mucus plugging. Anaphylaxis usually resolves in 2 to 8 hours, but secondary pathology arising from the reaction or its treatment may prolong the reaction and symptoms.

Management of Anaphylaxis in the Operating Room

Epinephrine is the cornerstone of treatment and should be given as soon as possible. It is a beta-agonist, inotrope, and bronchodilator. Epinephrine also reduces further mediator release by preventing mast cell degranulation. All potential causal agents should be removed. The airway should be maintained (intubate if necessary on 100% oxygen). Place the patient in Trendelenburg to improve venous return and start cardiopulmonary resuscitation (CPR) if indicated. Administer intravenous (IV) fluids, continue to repeat epinephrine according to Advanced Cardiac Life Support (ACLS) protocol or start an infusion. Obtain large-bore IV access and/or central access if needed. Diphenhydramine, steroids, and albuterol may be considered. Arrange for transfer to a hospital with a critical care facility due to the potential for recurrence even if the initial episode has been treated satisfactorily.[9,10]

MYOCARDIAL INFARCTION (ACUTE CORONARY SYNDROME)

Currently, the incidence of a perioperative cardiac events in low-risk patients is approximately 1% to 3%.[11] Most perioperative myocardial infractions are "silent" and occur in the immediate postoperative period, meaning the same or next day. As the complexity of cases performed in an ambulatory surgery setting increase, along with the comorbidities of patients accepted, there is expectation that the incidence of acute coronary events may increase.

Some of the common factors that increase the risk of having a perioperative myocardial infarction include the following[11]:

- Prior cardiac history
  - Coronary artery disease
  - Cardiac stents
  - History of congestive heart failure
- Poor exercise tolerance
- Other comorbidities including the following:
  - Diabetes requiring insulin therapy
  - Previous stroke
  - Renal insufficiency
- Intraoperative or postoperative hypotension
- New-onset, prolonged duration (meaning more than 10 minutes) of intraoperative ST and/or T-wave changes

Mechanisms involved in a perioperative myocardial infarction include the following[11]:

- There is a catecholamine surge that causes increases in heart rate and blood pressure.
- This is combined with an increased thrombotic risk due to many factors including increased platelet activation and decreased fibrinolysis.
- There can also be anemia, inflammation, tissue hypoxia, and fluid mobilization. This combination can induce both plaque rupture and produce cardiac ischemia.

Immediate medical management of perioperative myocardial infarction in the ambulatory surgery center should include the following[11,12]:

- High-flow oxygen
- Verify diagnosis (12-lead electrocardiogram [ECG] + troponin blood levels if available)
- Treat hypotension or hypertension
- Beta blockers to slow heart rate
- Aggressive pain management
- Consideration of nitroglycerin
- Aspirin administration
- Early transfer to hospital facility with interventional cardiology services
- Communication (complete report to accepting physician/facility), fax ECG, and so forth

Typically, in the ambulatory surgery center, especially freestanding, there is limited availability of laboratory testing or other equipment, such as a transesophageal echocardiography.

DELAYED EMERGENCE

Delayed emergence from anesthesia presents one of the biggest challenges for anesthesiologists. By definition, delayed emergence from anesthesia is persistent somnolence or unresponsiveness after an anesthetic.[13]

Risk factors should be broken down into the following[13]:

- Patient factors (age, genetic and preexisting conditions)
- Drug factors
- Surgical and anesthetic factors, including metabolic factors

Patient factors include extremes of age, geriatric and pediatric. Older individuals have an increased sensitivity toward anesthetics and a slow return of consciousness because of a decline in central nervous system function. Pediatric patients have a greater body surface area and are at risk for hypothermia, which slows drug metabolism.[13]

Genetic factors include gender (men are 1.4 times more likely to have delayed recovery than women), obesity, and other patient comorbidities (preexisting cardiac, pulmonary, hepatic, thyroid, or kidney disease). In some cases, other genetic causes, such as pseudocholinesterase deficiency, can prolong emergence if a depolarizing muscle relaxant is used.[14] Preexisting neurologic conditions include cognitive dysfunction, seizures (postictal state), and stroke. Other neurologic causes may include preexisting increased intracranial pressure, and preexisting mental disorder.[14]

Drug effect considerations may include prior illicit drug use, preoperative sedatives (such as midazolam), excess opioids, scopolamine, residual paralysis, and drug interactions, such as monoamine oxidase inhibitors or selective serotonin reuptake inhibitors. There are a large number of pharmacologic interactions that can potentiate the effects of neuromuscular blocking agents, such as aminoglycosides, diuretics, calcium channel antagonists, lithium, and some chemotherapeutic drugs.[13,14]

Surgical and anesthetic factors may include the following:

Metabolic disorders, such as hypercarbia, hypoxemia, hypoglycemia/hyperglycemia, and hypothermia/hyperthermia, and electrolyte imbalance, such as acidosis, hypernatremia/hyponatremia, hypokalemia, hypomagnesemia/hypermagnesemia, and hypocalcemia.[14]

Other surgical/anesthetic complications should be considered, such as hypoperfusion, air/gas/thrombic emboli, including pulmonary embolism. A new neurologic event may have occurred, including a new ischemic event or cerebral hemorrhage.[14]

A rapid assessment should be performed to rule out and identify cause of delayed emergence[13]:

- Check the IV site and ensure that it has not infiltrated
- Confirm that all anesthetic agents are OFF
- Change the airway circuit and ventilate with 100% oxygen to make sure all inhalation agents are eliminated
- Re-check all medications given
- Re-check patient temperature
- Review patient history
- Check vital signs
- Check twitch monitor to access residual paralysis, neurologic examination (pupils, cranial nerves, reflexes, and response to pain)
- Glucose should be checked as well as arterial blood gas and electrolytes if available
- Reversal agents should be available, including naloxone, flumazenil, physostigmine (anticholinergic), neostigmine, or sugammadex for residual paralysis

Transfer to nearest hospital if mental status does not improve.

MALIGNANT HYPERTHERMIA

Malignant hyperthermia (MH) is one of the anesthetic emergencies that every anesthesiologist reads about but hopes to never experience. Immediate diagnosis and treatment are imperative to save the patient's life. MH is a potentially fatal condition. The true incidence of MH is unknown due to variable reporting, but it is anywhere from 1 to 5000 to 50,000 cases.[15] Mortality before dantrolene and aggressive treatment was more than 70% and now is less than 5%,[15] but may be higher in freestanding ambulatory surgery centers.

Causes

MH is caused by a defect in the ryanodine receptor in skeletal muscle. The regulation of calcium is altered due to the defect and causes a buildup of calcium, creating a chain reaction and a massive metabolic reaction. The most common gene that is altered is the *RYR 1* gene, but more than 100 mutations have been discovered with this gene.[15] Trigging agents for MH include volatile agents, such as desflurane, sevoflurane, isoflurane, halothane, and depolarizing neuromuscular blocking agents.[15]

Diagnosis and Presentation

The diagnosis of MH can be difficult. The initial signs of MH are tachycardia, hypercarbia, hypertension, muscle rigidity, and hyperthermia. It can be confused with sepsis, thyroid storm, or any hypermetabolic state.

Criteria to help with the diagnosis[15,16]:

- Respiratory acidosis, ETCO2 greater than 55
- Arrhythmia
- Metabolic acidosis, pH <7.25
- Muscle rigidity

- Creatine kinase greater than 20,000 or myoglobinuria
- Temperature greater than 38.8°C
- Family history
- Rapid improvement with dantrolene

Management

- Initiate treatment immediately and have another person work on immediate transfer to a hospital setting with potential for intensive care admission[16–18]
- Dantrolene or Ryanodex should be given as soon as possible and must be given before transfer
  - An improvement in patient outcomes is seen with early treatment
- Stop any volatile anesthetics and start IV sedation
- Place the patient on 100% oxygen and hyperventilate using a bag valve and/or a new anesthetic circuit (after flushing the machine for at least 90 seconds)
  - Hyperventilate to decrease hypercarbia
- Place charcoal filters on anesthetic circuit
- Call the MH hotline: 1-800-644-9737
- Cool patient with ice packs, decrease room temperature, administer cold IV fluids
- Draw a complete blood count, basic metabolic panel, urinalysis, and arterial blood gas
- Treat acidosis and hyperkalemia if present
- Transfer to the nearest facility

In the freestanding ambulatory center where there is limited availability for laboratory testing guidance, stabilize to the best of one's ability and transfer.

LOCAL ANESTHETIC SYSTEMIC TOXICITY

Local anesthetic systemic toxicity (LAST) is an anesthetic emergency that can lead to cardiovascular collapse.[19] Ambulatory surgery centers are at a relatively high risk of LAST due to the commonality of regional anesthesia and local injection by the surgical team to provide postoperative analgesia. It is important to know the signs of LAST and to warn our surgical colleagues that local anesthetic doses are cumulative. With the use of ultrasound, regional anesthesia has become very popular in ambulatory surgery centers, but the incidence of local anesthetic uptake is not zero. The use of ultrasound decreases the risk of LAST and may be contributing to a trend in delayed presentation, but it does not prevent toxicity.

Causes, Risk Factors, and Prevention

LAST is likely caused by the local anesthetic absorption and the reduction of sodium influx in neurons. Local anesthetics also can inhibit cardiac sodium channels and the necessary action potential leading to disturbances, arrhythmias, and decreased cardiac contractility.[19]

Risk factors of LAST include patients with extremes of age, hepatic dysfunction, pregnancy, any patient with decreased plasma proteins, and high and low cardiac output states.[19]

The most common causes of LAST are peripheral nerve blocks, local infiltration, and tumescence.

The best way to prevent toxicity is to use the lowest dose needed to achieve the desired effect. The use of ultrasound during regional anesthesia can monitor the spread of local anesthetic and help prevent intravascular injections.

However, ultrasound will not eliminate the risks due to artifacts and loss of needle visualization during injection.[20] Another way to minimize toxicity is with incremental injections and frequent aspirations.[19,20] This allows you to monitor the patient's vital signs and neurologic signs and monitor for any intravascular injections.[20]

Diagnosis and Presentation

Classically neurologic signs precede the cardiovascular signs, but not always.

Signs[19]:
- Neurologic signs:
  - Perioral numbness
  - Metallic taste
  - Tinnitus
  - Seizures
  - Agitation
  - Loss of consciousness
- Cardiac signs:
  - Bradycardia
  - Hypotension
  - Arrhythmias

Treatment

After diagnosis, treatment should begin immediately.[19,21–23]
- Call for help
- Alert nearest facility for transfer
- Airway management: 100% Fio_2, intubation if indicated
- Seizure suppression with midazolam
- ACLS
- 20% lipid emulsion: bolus of 1.5 mL/kg if <70 kg and 100 mL if >70 kg given over 2 to 3 minutes
- 20% lipid emulsion continuous infusion at 0.25 mL/kg
- Can repeat 20% lipid bolus as needed (upper limit approximately 12 mL/kg over 30 minutes)
- Consider central and arterial access and additional IV access for resuscitation
- Goal is to avoid acidosis and hypoxia
- Transfer to nearest facility, when stable
Patients should be monitored for at least 12 hours after LAST due to the potential for recurrence
Per the American Society of Regional Anesthesia 2017 updated guidelines: lipid emulsion therapy should be initiated soon after airway management in any LAST event that is judged to be potentially serious

(AIRWAY) FIRE

A fire can occur during any surgery, but an airway fire has important preventive measures and treatment plans. For a fire to occur, 3 components are necessary: an oxidizer, ignition, and fuel.[24,25] The oxidizer is usually oxygen or nitrous oxide in a closed system. The ignition is usually a surgical source, such as a laser, heat probes, or cautery. The fuel can be sponges, drapes, gowns, alcohol-based solutions, and endotracheal tubes.[24,25] The highest risk surgeries for airway fire include tonsillectomy, head and neck surgery, tracheostomy, and removal of laryngeal papillomas.[26]

Prevention

Prevention is always best and takes coordination with the OR team, anesthesiologist, and surgeon to minimize airway fire risks.

Goals[24,26–28]:
- Fraction of inspired oxygen (Fio_2) less than 30% for any open delivery system
- Avoid nitrous oxide
- Use a sealed gas delivery system-cuffed endotracheal tube (ETT) (especially if patient requires high Fio_2)
- Flammable skin prep must dry before draping
- Minimize drapes around the airway
- Gauze and sponges moistened
- Close communication between surgeon and anesthesiologist
- Monitor inspired and exhaled oxygen
- For laser procedures, use a laser-resistant tracheal tube and cuff filled with saline or indicator dye

Treatment

If an airway fire is suspected, immediate action should be followed[26]:
- Call for help and inform the surgeon and OR team
- The surgeon should remove the ETT and pour saline down the airway
- The anesthesiologist should disconnect the circuit from the machine to remove the oxygen source
- The surgeon should assess the airway for debris and for injury
- Reestablish ventilation with room air and reintubate the patient
- The OR team should remove all drapes and any potential flammable materials away from the patient
- Extinguish burning materials with saline, water, or smothering
- Transfer the patient to the nearest facility for further care and to monitor for any airway edema

POWER FAILURE

There is no central reporting servicer for OR power failure so the occurrence is unknown. The most common causes of power failure involve the simultaneous failure of backup generators and is often related to construction work.[29] Extreme weather events and regional power failures are the usual causes of primary power failure. When backup power fails, it is important to know what equipment can be affected and what equipment has backup power if needed:

- Equipment that can be affected
  - Telephones, pagers, Wi-Fi, electronic medical record
- Equipment that has backup power (intrinsic backup power)
  - Anesthesia machine, vaporizers, medical gases, and portable monitors, portable suction, portable infusion pumps
- Equipment that has limited backup power (no backup power)
  - Lights, fluid warmers, transesophageal echocardiography, wall suction, video towers, gas analyzers, electrosurgical units

When a power failure occurs,[30]

- Confirm ventilator is working and on backup power with vaporizers and oxygen supply[30]
  - If not, change to total intravenous anesthesia with infusion pump and use a bag valve mask with oxygen E-cylinder
    - May need to change due to exhaustion of battery
  - Obtain additional light, via flashlights, cellphones, and laryngoscopes
    - Open doors and shades
  - If monitors fail, use portable monitors or defibrillator or check pulse and manual blood pressure regularly[30]
    - Call engineering for the building and determine if other ORs have lost power as well
      - If no other OR has lost power, check circuit breaker and unplug the piece of equipment last plugged in
        - Determine the need to evacuate building due to fire

SIMULATION-BASED TRAINING AND PREPAREDNESS

It is important for every ambulatory surgery center to develop an emergency and disaster plan that is tailored to their specific patient population and surgical facility. To assess the plan, it is necessary to implement simulation-based training with clinically relevant scenarios. Leaders of the surgery center should develop corrective plans and hold debriefing sessions to identify issues and to address them before an emergency occurs. Regular and repeated simulation sessions have been shown to improve readiness and ensure the best patient outcome.[3]

Effective preparedness includes creating a standard response algorithm, role delegations for staff, and requires consistent simulation-based drills.[31] The emergency manual by Stanford anesthesia cognitive aid group[32] is an excellent resource that provides information on crisis management. Being prepared for an emergency is the best way to limit complications and ease the transition of care from the ambulatory surgery center to the hospital. Preparedness at the individual level is also critical to optimize responses, and should be part of simulation-based training. Ambulatory center staff should know where all the emergency drugs, the difficult airway equipment, and emergency carts are located. These need to be checked daily to make sure they are present, secure, and functioning. It is recommended to participate in full-scale community exercise and not table-top drills.[3]

In addition, it is helpful to develop a facility-based checklist, as well as a calendar for emergency drills. This checklist helps ensure that nothing is missed medically but also makes sure that everyone has a defined role. The center must know who will alert the nearest hospital, who will go with the patient to the hospital if needed, and who will help to monitor other patients in the OR. All of these roles should be predetermined to prevent confusion during an emergency.

Finally, communication and documentation are very important and often challenging during crisis management, especially when rapid transfer to another facility is involved. It is essential that staff at the receiving facility obtain important information with regard to the patient's medical conditions and recent events and interventions. Any significant delay in transfer and failure to communicate relevant information can potentially contribute to poor patient outcomes.

SIMULATION DRILLS

- Identify roles for CPR[31]
  - ○ Facilitator
    - ■ Plans and evaluates the drill
    - ■ Develops corrective action
    - ■ Debriefs team
  - ○ Runner
    - ■ Obtains emergency equipment and other items
  - ○ Team Leader
    - ■ Activates plan and gives orders
  - ○ Responder
    - ■ Initiates CPR pathway
  - ○ Documenter
    - ■ Records times, drugs, sequence of events
  - ○ Communicator
    - ■ Gathers patient chart, information
    - ■ Communicates emergency to others
- Run the scenario
  - ○ Provide instructions to staff
  - ○ Identify everyone's role
  - ○ Provide the emergency situation
  - ○ Begin the scenario
    - ■ Each individual should carry out his or her role
- Facilitator develops a checklist of the events and develops a corrective plan
- Debriefing
  - ○ Completed immediately after the drill
  - ○ Obtain feedback on how to improve the drill
  - ○ Ask questions
    - ■ What went wrong?
    - ■ What was successful?
    - ■ How can we improve?
- Implement corrective plan
  - ○ Communicate the changes to all staff

SUMMARY

Ambulatory surgery centers, where emergencies are less common and resources are limited, can be more vulnerable to inadequate emergency response. It is essential that every ambulatory surgery center is prepared for these rare events and that staff are educated and participate in routine simulation-based drilling. The limited resources in an ambulatory surgery center must be used to the fullest with stabilization of the patient for transfer to a higher-acuity facility for further testing, medications, and interventions as the ultimate goal. Ambulatory surgery center emergency response standardization through frequently scheduled simulation drilling could potentially optimize response in the setting of leaner resources.

REFERENCES

1. Hall MJ, Schwartzman A, Zhang J, et al. Ambulatory surgery data from hospitals and ambulatory surgery centers: United States, 2010. Natl Health Stat Report 2017;(102):1–15.

2. Urman RD, Desai SP. History of anesthesia for ambulatory surgery. Curr Opin Anaesthesiol 2012;25(6):641–7.
3. Bruppacher HR, Alam SK, LeBlanc VR, et al. Simulation-based training improves physicians' performance in patient care in high-stakes clinical setting of cardiac surgery. Anesthesiology 2010;112(4):985–92.
4. Caimmi S, Caimmi D, Bernardini R, et al. Perioperative anaphylaxis: epidemiology. Int J Immunopathol Pharmacol 2011;24(3 Suppl):S21–6.
5. Kannan JA, Bernstein JA. Perioperative anaphylaxis: diagnosis, evaluation, and management. Immunol Allergy Clin North Am 2015;35(2):321–34.
6. Lagopoulos V, Gigi E. Anaphylactic and anaphylactoid reactions during the perioperative period. Hippokratia 2011;15(2):138–40.
7. Sarkar U, Lopez A, Maselli JH, et al. Adverse drug events in U.S. adult ambulatory medical care. Health Serv Res 2011;46(5):1517–33.
8. Sampson HA, Munoz-Furlong A, Campbell RL, et al. Second symposium on the definition and management of anaphylaxis: summary report–Second National Institute of Allergy and Infectious Disease/Food Allergy and Anaphylaxis Network symposium. J Allergy Clin Immunol 2006;117(2):391–7.
9. Mertes PM, Malinovsky JM, Jouffroy L, et al, Working Group of the SFAR and SFA. Reducing the risk of anaphylaxis during anesthesia: 2011 updated guidelines for clinical practice. J Investig Allergol Clin Immunol 2011;21(6):442–53.
10. Simons FE, Ardusso LR, Dimov V, et al. World Allergy Organization Anaphylaxis Guidelines: 2013 update of the evidence base. Int Arch Allergy Immunol 2013; 162(3):193–204.
11. O'Gara PT, Kushner FG, Ascheim DD, et al. 2013 ACCF/AHA guideline for the management of ST-elevation myocardial infarction: a report of the American College of Cardiology Foundation/American Heart Association Task Force on practice guidelines. Circulation 2013;127(4):e362–425.
12. Ryu DR, Choi JW, Lee BK, et al. Effects of critical pathway on the management of patients with ST-elevation acute myocardial infarction in an emergency department. Crit Pathw Cardiol 2015;14(1):31–5.
13. Tzabazis A, Miller C, Dobrow MF, et al. Delayed emergence after anesthesia. J Clin Anesth 2015;27(4):353–60.
14. Misal US, Joshi SA, Shaikh MM. Delayed recovery from anesthesia: a postgraduate educational review. Anesth Essays Res 2016;10(2):164–72.
15. Rosenberg H, Pollock N, Schiemann A, et al. Malignant hyperthermia: a review. Orphanet J Rare Dis 2015;10:93.
16. Glahn KP, Ellis FR, Halsall PJ, et al. Recognizing and managing a malignant hyperthermia crisis: guidelines from the European Malignant Hyperthermia Group. Br J Anaesth 2010;105(4):417–20.
17. Larach MG, Dirksen SJ, Belani KG, et al. Special article: Creation of a guide for the transfer of care of the malignant hyperthermia patient from ambulatory surgery centers to receiving hospital facilities. Anesth Analg 2012;114(1):94–100.
18. Litman RS, Joshi GP. Malignant hyperthermia in the ambulatory surgery center: how should we prepare? Anesthesiology 2014;120(6):1306–8.
19. Mercado P, Weinberg GL. Local anesthetic systemic toxicity: prevention and treatment. Anesthesiol Clin 2011;29(2):233–42.
20. Neal JM, Mulroy MF, Weinberg GL, et al. American Society of Regional Anesthesia and Pain Medicine checklist for managing local anesthetic systemic toxicity: 2012 version. Reg Anesth Pain Med 2012;37(1):16–8.
21. Burch MS, McAllister RK, Meyer TA. Treatment of local-anesthetic toxicity with lipid emulsion therapy. Am J Health Syst Pharm 2011;68(2):125–9.

22. Neal JM, Bernards CM, Butterworth JFT, et al. ASRA practice advisory on local anesthetic systemic toxicity. Reg Anesth Pain Med 2010;35(2):152–61.
23. Fencl JL. Local anesthetic systemic toxicity: perioperative implications. AORN J 2015;101(6):697–700.
24. Smith LP, Roy S. Operating room fires in otolaryngology: risk factors and prevention. Am J Otolaryngol 2011;32(2):109–14.
25. Rinder CS. Fire safety in the operating room. Curr Opin Anaesthesiol 2008;21(6): 790–5.
26. American Society of Anesthesiologists Task Force on Operating Room Fires, Caplan RA, Barker SJ, Connis RT, et al. Practice advisory for the prevention and management of operating room fires. Anesthesiology 2008;108(5): 786–801, quiz: 971–2.
27. Rogers ML, Nickalls RW, Brackenbury ET, et al. Airway fire during tracheostomy: prevention strategies for surgeons and anaesthetists. Ann R Coll Surg Engl 2001; 83(6):376–80.
28. Gorphe P, Sarfati B, Janot F, et al. Airway fire during tracheostomy. Eur Ann Oto-rhinolaryngol Head Neck Dis 2014;131(3):197–9.
29. Eichhorn JH, Hessel EA 2nd. Electrical power failure in the operating room: a neglected topic in anesthesia safety. Anesth Analg 2010;110(6):1519–21.
30. Carpenter T, Robinson ST. Case reports: response to a partial power failure in the operating room. Anesth Analg 2010;110(6):1644–6.
31. Kusler-Jensen JA. Cardiac emergency simulation: drilling for success in the ambulatory setting. AORN J 2014;99(3):385–94.
32. Stanford Anesthesia Cognitive Aid Group. Emergency Manual: Cognitive aids for perioperative critical events. Creative Commons BY-NC-ND. 2016.

Anesthesia for Same-Day Total Joint Replacement

Adam W. Amundson, MD, Jason K. Panchamia, DO, Adam K. Jacob, MD*

KEYWORDS

- Outpatient • Ambulatory • Arthroplasty • Total knee replacement
- Total hip replacement

KEY POINTS

- Appropriate patient screening and selection, medical optimization, and defining expectations about pain control, home care, and rehabilitation goals should be initiated in the preoperative setting.
- Multimodal, opiate-sparing analgesic regimens should be initiated the morning of surgery.
- Intraoperative anesthetic care should be tailored to facilitate rapid recovery, nausea control, and early ambulation.
- A system should be developed for early, postdischarge follow-up to monitor pain management, progress with physical therapy, and address questions or concerns.

INTRODUCTION

Total knee arthroplasty (TKA) and total hip arthroplasty (THA) are 2 of the most commonly performed surgical procedures in the United States. Historically, most providers and patients believed a multiple-day hospital stay was needed following total joint replacement (TJR) because of pain, limited mobility, and infection risk.[1] New payment models and demand for lower-cost health care has forced the TJR industry to evaluate and mitigate the highest variable costs in an episode of care for THA or TKA.[2] The largest variable costs include daily hospital and skilled nursing facility (SNF) charges during the hospitalization and postdischarge inpatient rehabilitation. Therefore, minimizing hospital stay and avoiding SNF dismissal can have significant reductions in total cost of care.[3] Importantly, shortening the hospital stay and SNF disposition does not compromise patient safety or satisfaction, and may result in fewer perioperative complications than previous multiple-day hospital stays.[4–6]

Disclosure Statement: The authors have no disclosures or conflicts of interest.
Department of Anesthesiology and Perioperative Medicine, Mayo Clinic, 200 First Street Southwest, Rochester, MN 55905, USA
* Corresponding author.
E-mail address: jacob.adam@mayo.edu

Anesthesiology Clin 37 (2019) 251–264
https://doi.org/10.1016/j.anclin.2019.01.006
1932-2275/19/© 2019 Elsevier Inc. All rights reserved.

anesthesiology.theclinics.com

The most common reasons patients are hesitant for early discharge include a fear of poorly controlled pain, a slower recovery, complications, and being dependent on someone else.[7] When these concerns are addressed, most patients would rather recover at home instead of the hospital.[8] Through the use of enhanced recovery clinical pathways, hospital length of stay has been progressively reduced to the point of performing ambulatory TJR. Successful outpatient TJR has been accomplished through advances in surgical technique, presurgical education, muscle-sparing regional anesthetic techniques, opioid-sparing multimodal pain medications, and a progressive rehabilitation program.[7,9–11]

PATIENT SELECTION AND SUCCESS RATES

Many orthopedic practices are striving to create outpatient or ambulatory TJR programs. However, undergoing TJR in an ambulatory setting may not be feasible or reasonable for all patients. An experienced multidisciplinary team managing care is essential to the success of the outpatient TJR program.[9] Prescreening eligible patients is among the most important components to ensure a safe and productive process.[12] Several studies evaluating outpatient TJR have identified various comorbid and surgical risk factors as barriers to same-day discharge, as shown in **Table 1**.

Specifically, patients with coronary artery disease,[4,13] diabetes,[6] preoperative opioid use,[10] pain catastrophizers, body mass index greater than 40,[13] peripheral vascular disease,[14] chronic obstructive pulmonary disease,[4,13] congestive heart failure,[4,15] cirrhosis,[4,15] chronic kidney disease,[16] age greater than 70 years of age,[6] or a higher Charlson Comorbidity Index score[17–19] have a higher risk for failure to discharge or higher readmission rates after surgery, and may be poor candidates for ambulatory joint replacement. Also, lower surgical volume hospitals and operative times greater than 120 minutes are less likely to be compatible with outpatient TJR.[4,14] To prepare patients who are eligible for ambulatory TJR, patients should be medically optimized and educated about expectations for pain management and physical therapy (PT) before surgery.[10] In the last 5 years, program success rates have substantially improved, likely due to stronger adherence to the eligibility criteria, developing procedure-specific clinical pathways, and gaining experience in addressing common barriers to discharge.[4,12]

Table 1	
Common inclusion and exclusion criteria for same-day discharge	
Inclusion	**Exclusion**
≤70 y of age	Coronary artery disease
American Society of Anesthesiologists physical status I or II	Chronic obstructive pulmonary disease
Primary unilateral total knee or hip	Heart failure
Hemoglobin >10 g/dL	Cirrhosis
Assistance at home	Chronic renal disease
Independent ambulation	Human immunodeficiency virus positive
Body mass index <40 kg/m^2	Preoperative opioid consumption
No fracture present	Chronic pain syndrome (eg, fibromyalgia)

Preoperative Evaluation

After passing the initial screening process, patients should undergo a formal medical evaluation for several reasons:

1. Identify relevant history and/or physical examination findings that may preclude same-day discharge
2. Surgical risk assessment
3. Medical optimization

A thorough medical examination may reveal areas affecting perioperative surgical outcomes specific to orthopedic surgery. For example, preoperative anemia or history of anticoagulant use can increase risk for perioperative blood transfusion. Presence of chronic kidney disease may require alterations to the multimodal pain management protocol, particularly judicious use of nonsteroidal antiinflammatory medications. Undocumented preoperative opioid dependence may result in higher postoperative pain scores and opioid consumption, potentially requiring unanticipated hospital admission. Although some of these conditions may initially preclude patients from undergoing same-day TJR, addressing these concerns in the preoperative medicine clinic via medical optimization and rehabilitation provides patients the opportunity to succeed in the ambulatory surgical program. Although anesthetic management should be individualized based on patient comorbidities, compliance with the enhanced recovery pathway is essential to a program's success.[12]

Multimodal Analgesia and Opiate-Sparing Anesthetic Techniques

The use of peripheral nerve blocks in a comprehensive multimodal pathway for lower extremity total joint reconstruction practice has demonstrated improved pain control, minimized opioid exposure and opioid-related adverse drug events, reduced hospital length of stay, and improved patient outcomes.[1] In accordance with the recent movement for quicker hospital discharge, procedure-specific clinical pathways incorporating a variety of muscle-sparing analgesic techniques have evolved to facilitate early PT and ambulation.[20,21] The concept behind these techniques is preferential blockade of sensory nerves while preserving motor strength to the surgical extremity. Techniques may be used alone or, more commonly, in combination to produce comprehensive analgesia.[22,23]

Periarticular injection (local infiltration analgesia)

Periarticular infiltration (PAI), also known as local infiltration analgesia or arthroplasty block, is a surgeon-administered local anesthetic injection in the tissues around and within the knee or hip joint, as shown in **Fig. 1**, often placed just before component placement during THA or TKA. Common anatomic structures targeted during PAI for TKA include the posterior capsule; synovium overlying the distal femur medially and laterally; suprapatellar pouch; arthrotomy, including the medial and lateral retinaculum; and the subcutaneous tissue.[20] The PAI technique for THA involves a series of injections into the femoral neck periosteum; anterior, inferior, and posterior hip capsule; trochanteric bursa; superficial tissue overlying the iliotibial fascia; and subcutaneous tissue. Though there is significant variability in injection technique, as well as the individual medication components of the injectate, the use of PAI has consistently been demonstrated to provide effective analgesia of the surgical joint when used alone or in combination with other regional anesthetic techniques.[20] Most PAI solutions include a weight-based long-acting local anesthetic dose (bupivacaine, ropivacaine, liposomal bupivacaine) mixed together with multiple adjuvants (epinephrine, ketorolac, methylprednisone, morphine) in a large total volume (80–120 mL). Though the

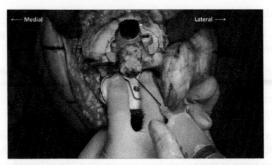

Fig. 1. PAI. An 18-gauge needle is used to inject local anesthetic solution around the knee joint for postoperative pain control. The needle tip is in the posterior capsule.

type of long-acting local anesthetics chosen may not affect overall pain control,[20,21] the adjuvant mixture within the PAI solution may enhance analgesia.[24] The duration of analgesia for a single-injection technique is estimated to be approximately 8 to 11 hours.[25]

Adductor canal block

Adductor canal block (ACB) provides pain relief similar to a traditional femoral nerve block without sacrificing quadriceps motor function,[26,27] which is essential for rehabilitation. Consequently, ACB has replaced femoral nerve blocks in most updated enhanced recovery pathways for primary TKA. The adductor canal is formed when the medial border of the sartorius muscle meets the medial border of the adductor longus muscle, and extends to the adductor hiatus where the saphenous nerve exits the canal along with the saphenous branch of descending genicular artery.[28] This point is slightly distal to the half-way point between the anterior superior iliac spine and patella. An aponeurotic vastoadductor membrane (VAM) overlies the roof of the canal, which can serve as a confirmatory sonographic finding to identify the adductor canal.[28] The ACB is performed by injecting local anesthetic deep to the VAM and adjacent to the superficial femoral artery (**Fig. 2**). The vastus medialis nerve lies just outside

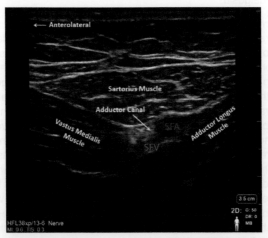

Fig. 2. Adductor canal sonoanatomy in the low thigh to midthigh. SFA, superficial femoral artery; SFV, superficial femoral vein.

of this canal and could also be blocked separately with an additional injection or proximal spread in the canal (see **Fig. 2**).

An alternative to the ACB is the subsartorial femoral nerve block (also known as low femoral triangle), which is located in the midthigh, approximately halfway between the anterior superior iliac spine and the base of the patella (proximal to the origin of the adductor canal).[29] The femoral triangle contains the saphenous nerve, nerve to vastus medialis, and medial femoral cutaneous nerve.[28] Blocking these nerves may provide improved analgesic coverage to the anteromedial aspect of the knee compared with the ACB; however, there is minimal information comparing these techniques in a clinical trial. The subsartorial femoral nerve block is performed by injecting local anesthetic deep to the posterior border of the sartorius muscle, adjacent to the superficial femoral artery.

Continuous catheter devices can be placed for extended pain control. There are several considerations to placing a continuous catheter:

1. Placing a continuous catheter within the adductor canal may interfere with the surgical prepping site; therefore, a more proximal location should be considered for catheter placement.
2. Although ACB catheters can extend analgesia beyond the 24-hour postoperative period, it may not provide any additional analgesic benefit compared with a single-injection technique. Because No analgesic differences have been found between these approaches.[30,31]
3. Home-going continuous catheter and pump devices involve patient and family participation, and a dedicated acute pain service team should be available for follow-up care.

Interspace between the popliteal artery and capsule of the posterior knee block
The interspace between popliteal artery and capsule of the posterior knee (IPACK) block is a relatively novel technique for TKA that targets the articular branches of the sciatic nerve innervating the posterior knee joint.[32] The IPACK block is performed by placing local anesthetic under live ultrasound guidance in the area between the popliteal artery and the proximal femoral condyles[25] (**Fig. 3**), which captures the sensory nerves that supply the posterior capsule of the knee. A recent study showed that this block in combination with an ACB and lateral femoral cutaneous nerve block

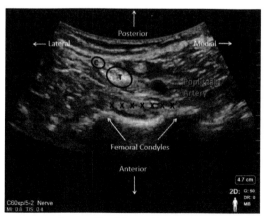

Fig. 3. IPACK sonoanatomy in the popliteal fossa. C, common peroneal nerve; T, tibial nerve; X, targeted area.

compared with a PAI provided a slightly longer analgesic profile in the immediate post-operative period.[25] IPACK is routinely combined with ACB and PAI for a complete analgesic coverage of the knee joint.

Selective tibial nerve block

Selective tibial nerve blockade is another relatively novel technique for TKA that involves preferentially blocking the tibial nerve as it separates from the common peroneal nerve in the popliteal fossa (**Fig. 4**).[33] Although tibial nerve blockade will result in motor blockade of inversion and plantar flexion of foot, preservation of dorsiflexion and eversion of the foot will still facilitate rehabilitation after TKA.[33] With the advent of the IPACK block and extensive research on PAI into the posterior capsule, this injection technique is less commonly used.

Multimodal Analgesia

Multimodal analgesic protocols are designed to target pain transmission signals from the peripheral nociceptors to the central nervous system by using a combination of oral analgesics, regional anesthesia, and/or surgical infiltrative techniques. The goal of these protocols is to maximize pain control while reducing or avoiding opioid consumption. Although the optimal combination of pain-relieving medications have yet to be established, common medications found within multimodal analgesia protocols include dexmedetomidine, dexamethasone, acetaminophen, nonsteroidal antiinflammatory drugs (NSAIDs), ketamine, and gabapentinoids.[34]

Dexmedetomidine

Dexmedetomidine is an alpha-2 receptor agonist that, when used as a perineural adjuvant (dose 50–100 mcg), has been shown to prolong duration of analgesia and improve postoperative pain scores following single-injection peripheral nerve blockade.[35] Though most studies have evaluated perineural dexmedetomidine for brachial plexus blocks, it has been recently been extended to lower extremity peripheral nerve blocks.[36,37] Furthermore, intravenous (IV) use of this medication has been used to the prolong spinal anesthesia, as well as decrease the incidence of

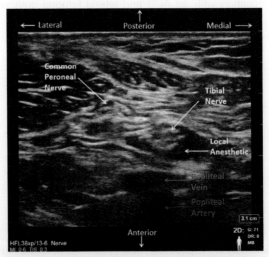

Fig. 4. Selective tibial nerve block sonoanatomy. Local anesthetic surrounds the tibial nerve.

postoperative delirium and opioid consumption after TJR.[38–40] Bradycardia and/or hypotension can occur via perineural and IV route.

Dexamethasone

Dexamethasone is a long-acting steroid with multiple potential uses in the perioperative period. First, dexamethasone (4–5 mg) is a well-known, potent, and long-acting antiemetic when given at induction of anesthesia. Second, low-dose dexamethasone (≤ 1 mg) has been used as a perineural adjuvant in an attempt to prolong duration of analgesia following single-injection peripheral nerve blockade.[41] Finally, intermediate-dose systemic dexamethasone (8–10 mg; 1 mg/kg) has been used as a component of multimodal analgesia in TJR surgery.[42] In a recent investigation comparing 8 mg IV dexamethasone with placebo (administered at incision and 24 hours after surgery) in patients undergoing TKA and THA, patients who received dexamethasone achieved discharge readiness criteria earlier and encountered a 27% reduction in morphine consumption.[43] Of note, all patients received multimodal analgesia (including PAI) and no differences were seen in complications between the groups. Furthermore, a recent meta-analysis investigating the use of dexamethasone in TKA or THA patients confirmed that patients receiving long-acting corticosteroid experienced less pain, less nausea, and consumed fewer opioids in the perioperative period.[44]

Acetaminophen

Regular acetaminophen dosing is a necessary component of any opioid-sparing, multimodal analgesic pathway. However, the optimal route of administration for acetaminophen (IV vs oral) in patients undergoing TJR is debatable.[45] Pharmacokinetically, IV administration results in a quicker increase in plasma and cerebral spinal fluid drug levels compared with an equivalent oral dose.[46] However, a randomized trial of 120 subjects undergoing TKA or THA tested the analgesic effect of IV acetaminophen (vs oral) in the setting of multimodal analgesic pathway. Specifically, subjects were randomized to receive either acetaminophen 1 g IV or oral preoperatively, then every 6 hours postoperatively for 24 hours. Subjects receiving IV acetaminophen had statistically better pain control during the first 4 hours after surgery; however, pain scores were not significantly different beyond 4 hours, suggesting that regular use of IV (vs oral) acetaminophen may be unnecessary if dosed appropriately.[47]

Nonsteroidal antiinflammatory medications

Historically, orthopedic surgeons were reluctant to use perioperative NSAIDs during TJR due to concerns about bone healing. Recent evidence has suggested that NSAID administration in the perioperative period may not significantly affect bone-healing and withholding this medication may contribute to other unwanted consequences. The synergistic analgesic benefit of NSAIDs and acetaminophen is well-known,[48] not to mention the potential for an opioid-sparing effect. Furthermore, low-dose ketorolac is a common adjuvant in many PAI solutions.[20,21]

Ketamine

Perioperative use of low-dose (0.15-1 mg/kg) ketamine has been shown to reduce opioid consumption in the perioperative period while also improving postoperative pain scores.[34,49] Although higher doses (>1 mg/kg) have been associated with the negative side effects such as sedation, hallucinations, and cognitive impairment, lower doses of ketamine have not shown to exhibit this negative profile. Furthermore, low-dose ketamine has shown no effect on nausea, vomiting, urinary retention, ileus, or constipation.[34]

Gabapentinoids

Gabapentinoid drugs (gabapentin and pregabalin) were originally developed and marketed as anticonvulsant medications; however, these have subsequently been found to be effective for neuropathic and acute pain management. Specifically, gabapentinoids reduce the hyperexcitability of dorsal horn neurons induced by tissue damage, stimulate descending inhibition, inhibit inflammatory mediators, and influence the affective component of pain. Compared with gabapentin, pregabalin has a better pharmacokinetic profile with rapid absorption, higher bioavailability, and less intersubject variability. Gabapentinoids are effective analgesics in most animal models of inflammation and postoperative pain; however, effects in human models are variable.[50] The risk of adverse effects, particularly sedation and dizziness, increases with higher doses and with concurrent opiate use. Meta-analyses indicate that a single dose of gabapentin or pregabalin administered preoperatively is associated with a decrease in postoperative pain and opioid consumption at 24 hours, although the optimal dosing regimen and duration of administration is unclear.[51,52]

Spinal Versus General Anesthesia

Several large studies have investigated outcomes related to anesthesia type for lower extremity TJR. The results, although not conclusive, marginally favor spinal anesthesia. One large study of nearly 400,000 subjects undergoing lower extremity TJR reported lower morbidity and mortality at 30 days, and lower risk of infections, pneumonia, and acute ronal failure.[53] A meta-analysis of 29 studies comparing general versus spinal anesthesia for TKA or THA also showed a reduction in length of stay.[54]

Though large-scale studies support the use of spinal anesthesia for TJR, its use must be balanced against the desire to initiate PT as soon as possible after surgery. Residual spinal-induced motor blockade and orthostasis can interfere with productive PT sessions. Therefore, the use of shorter-acting local anesthetics (eg, chloroprocaine, lidocaine, mepivacaine) or low-dose bupivacaine with or without adjuvants (eg, fentanyl) must be considered if performing spinal anesthesia. Chloroprocaine is generally recommended for procedures lasting 30 minutes or less, whereas lidocaine and mepivacaine can provide variable duration depending on the dose administered.[55,56] Historically, an overriding concern when performing lidocaine or mepivacaine spinal anesthesia is the potential for developing a transient neurologic symptom (TNS), which can develop 0 to 10 days after surgery. The characteristic symptoms representing a TNS entail buttock, leg, and thigh pain without neurologic dysfunction or deficit. A previous large observation study demonstrated a TNS incidence of 7.4% with spinal mepivacaine; however, recent literature has reported a lower incidence.[55]

Antifibrinolytic Therapy

Historically, intraoperative blood loss during TJR surgery has been associated with higher risk for postoperative transfusion. Stricter transfusion guidelines and greater tolerance of postoperative anemia have helped decrease transfusion rates. In addition, the use of intraoperative antifibrinolytic medications has further reduced perioperative blood loss. A recent investigation of ambulatory outpatient THA observed that 0.7% of 145 procedures required hospital transfer due to the requirement of a postoperative blood transfusion.[57] Although significant intraoperative blood loss may occur, adherence to strict inclusion criteria and active blood loss preservation techniques will allow the patient's hemodynamics to better accommodate these unexpected events.

The use of antifibrinolytic medications, such as tranexamic acid (TXA) given either orally, topically, or IV to patients undergoing lower extremity arthroplasty, have significantly reduced the frequency of intraoperative transfusions and their associated complications.[58] Routine perioperative TXA administration for eligible TKA and THA patients has been endorsed by the American Society of Regional Anesthesia and Pain Medicine, the American Association of Hip and Knee Surgeons, the American Academy of Orthopedic Surgeons, the Hip Society, and the Knee Society.[58] Different doses and routes have been extensively studied in TJR, and all seem to result in decreased perioperative blood loss and transfusion risk. However, specific evidence-based dose and route recommendations are currently not available.

Physical Therapy

PT and active rehabilitation is the cornerstone of early hospital discharge for lower extremity joint replacement surgery. Implementation of same-day PT may significantly improve short-term outcomes such as achieving rehabilitation goals and reduced hospital length of stay while also improving long-term functional outcomes after TJR.[59,60] Early mobilization allows medical staff to assess pain with active movement and better anticipate a patient's need for additional pain medicines. PT protocols may require patients to independently transfer into and out of bed and/or a chair, walk a specified distance, and ambulate on stairs.[11] Some protocols have transitioned to better accommodate outpatient procedures in which PT is initiated in recovery and continued at home where goals are achieved.

Discharge Criteria

Criteria for hospital or ambulatory center dismissal may vary across institutions; however, the same broad principles apply to each patient. As shown in **Table 2**, common criteria include:

1. Able to tolerate oral intake without significant nausea
2. Pain well-controlled on oral pain medicines
3. PT evaluation and treatment
4. Ability to climb steps if they are present at home
5. Hemodynamically stable
6. Able to urinate
7. Discharge to a safe environment[10,57]

Anesthesiologists have an important role in facilitating early hospital discharge through innovative pain techniques and measures to prevent common barriers to discharge and PT, as shown in **Table 3**.[61]

In a recent study of 106 subjects undergoing elective THA, the most common reason for failure to discharge on postoperative day 0 was subject preference (12),

Table 2	
Common outpatient discharge criteria	
Walk with minimal assistance 100 feet	Pain well-controlled on oral medicine
Stair walking (if present at home)	Voiding
Transfer from bed to standing, and toilet	Tolerating solid foods
Hemodynamically stable	Well-controlled nausea, lack of vomiting
Understanding of home therapy	Discharge to safe environment with active support

Modified from Fraser JF, Danoff JR, Manrique J, et al. Identifying reasons for failed same-day discharge following primary total hip arthroplasty. J Arthroplasty 2018;33(12):3625; with permission.

Table 3
Common barriers to same-day discharge

Pain	Urinary Retention
Nausea or vomiting	Medical complications
Orthostatic hypotension	Muscle weakness or poor mobility
Bleeding	Confusion
Sedation	Patient refusal

followed by dizziness or hypotension (8), failure to achieve PT goals (5), urinary retention (2), and poorly controlled pain (1).[10] In a 2009 study evaluating 150 subjects who underwent outpatient primary THA, 38 subjects were delayed in their recovery secondary to nausea (12), hypotension (10), combined nausea and hypotension (9), and oversedation (7).[11] Other studies have shown similar results, supporting the point that health care teams should anticipate and preemptively manage common postoperative obstacles. For example, nausea is a common symptom after anesthesia and can be further exacerbated by orthostatic hypotension. Similar to analgesia, a preemptive and multimodal approach should be used to mitigate the risk of postoperative and postdischarge nausea and vomiting. Careful attention to a patient's hemodynamic state in recovery and administering additional fluid boluses to prevent orthostatic hypotension may further improve uneventful discharge. Furthermore, opioid-sparing techniques and minimizing long-acting sedatives and opioids may have a profound effect on limiting postoperative sedation. These medicines include long-acting intrathecal opioid, oxycodone extended-release, and morphine extended-release.[62] Caution may be advised when administering high doses of gabapentinoids because they have also been associated with increased somnolence in the recovery period.[62] Furthermore, research has emerged to better counteract the sedating properties of anesthesia and pain medications, including the use caffeine to accelerate anesthetic emergence.[63] A common barrier to PT and early ambulation is numb extremities or muscle weakness, which is most often related to a residual spinal anesthetic. With the reemergence of short-acting local anesthetics such as lidocaine and mepivacaine, a more predictable recovery time period has emerged to allow for early postoperative recovery.[64] Urinary retention is also a common barrier to discharge after spinal anesthesia and the use of systemic opioids. Special attention should be implemented to reduce this side effect and mitigate potential factors that may be contributing.

SUMMARY

There is growing recognition of providing cost-effective, high-value care for patients undergoing TJR. One of the most costly variables in an episode of TJR care is postoperative hospitalization. The total cost of care may be reduced by 20% or more if inpatient care can be avoided. Fortunately, orthopedic outcomes and perioperative complications are not adversely affected, and may be improved by reducing or eliminating hospital stay. Therefore, there is a nationwide trend to create outpatient TJR programs.

Anesthesiologists play a critical role in the perioperative care of these patients. Appropriate screening and selection, medical optimization, and defining expectations about pain control, home care, and rehabilitation goals should be initiated in the preoperative setting. Multimodal, opiate-sparing analgesic regimens should be initiated the morning of surgery, and intraoperative anesthetic care should be tailored to facilitate rapid recovery, nausea control, and early ambulation with a goal of meeting dismissal criteria later that day. Finally, to minimize the possibility of readmission or emergency room visits, it is necessary to have a system in place for early post-discharge follow-up to monitor pain management, progress with PT, and address questions or concerns that patients and families may have.

REFERENCES

1. Hebl JR, Dilger JA, Byer DE, et al. A pre-emptive multimodal pathway featuring peripheral nerve block improves perioperative outcomes after major orthopedic surgery. Reg Anesth Pain Med 2008;33:510–7.
2. Bert JM, Hooper J, Moen S. Outpatient total joint arthroplasty. Curr Rev Musculoskelet Med 2017;10:567–74.
3. Lovald ST, Ong KL, Malkani AL, et al. Complications, mortality, and costs for outpatient and short-stay total knee arthroplasty patients in comparison to standard-stay patients. J Arthroplasty 2014;29:510–5.
4. Hoffmann JD, Kusnezov NA, Dunn JC, et al. The shift to same-day outpatient joint arthroplasty: a systematic review. J Arthroplasty 2018;33:1265–74.
5. Kort NP, Bemelmans YFL, Schotanus MGM. Outpatient surgery for unicompartmental knee arthroplasty is effective and safe. Knee Surg Sports Traumatol Arthrosc 2017;25:2659–67.
6. Courtney PM, Boniello AJ, Berger RA. Complications following outpatient total joint arthroplasty: an analysis of a national database. J Arthroplasty 2017;32:1426–30.
7. Berger RA, Sanders S, Gerlinger T, et al. Outpatient total knee arthroplasty with a minimally invasive technique. J Arthroplasty 2005;20:33–8.
8. Meneghini RM, Ziemba-Davis M. Patient perceptions regarding outpatient hip and knee arthroplasties. J Arthroplasty 2017;32:2701–2705 e1.
9. Cullom C, Weed JT. Anesthetic and analgesic management for outpatient knee arthroplasty. Curr Pain Headache Rep 2017;21:23.
10. Fraser JF, Danoff JR, Manrique J, et al. Identifying reasons for failed same-day discharge following primary total hip arthroplasty. J Arthroplasty 2018;33(12):3624–8.
11. Berger RA, Sanders SA, Thill ES, et al. Newer anesthesia and rehabilitation protocols enable outpatient hip replacement in selected patients. Clin Orthop Relat Res 2009;467:1424–30.
12. Berend ME, Lackey WG, Carter JL. Outpatient-focused joint arthroplasty is the future: the Midwest Center for Joint Replacement experience. J Arthroplasty 2018;33:1647–8.
13. Sher A, Keswani A, Yao DH, et al. Predictors of same-day discharge in primary total joint arthroplasty patients and risk factors for post-discharge complications. J Arthroplasty 2017;32:S150–156 e1
14. Fleisher LA, Pasternak LR, Lyles A. A novel index of elevated risk of inpatient hospital admission immediately following outpatient surgery. Arch Surg 2007;142:263–8.
15. Courtney PM, Rozell JC, Melnic CM, et al. Who should not undergo short stay hip and knee arthroplasty? Risk factors associated with major medical complications following primary total joint arthroplasty. J Arthroplasty 2015;30:1–4.
16. Warth LC, Pugely AJ, Martin CT, et al. Total joint arthroplasty in patients with chronic renal disease: is it worth the risk? J Arthroplasty 2015;30:51–4.

17. SooHoo NF, Farng E, Lieberman JR, et al. Factors that predict short-term complication rates after total hip arthroplasty. Clin Orthop Relat Res 2010;468:2363–71.

18. SooHoo NF, Lieberman JR, Ko CY, et al. Factors predicting complication rates following total knee replacement. J Bone Joint Surg Am 2006;88:480–5.

19. Lovald S, Ong K, Lau E, et al. Patient selection in outpatient and short-stay total knee arthroplasty. J Surg Orthop Adv 2014;23:2–8.

20. Amundson AW, Johnson RL, Abdel MP, et al. A Three-arm randomized clinical trial comparing continuous femoral plus single-injection sciatic peripheral nerve blocks versus periarticular injection with ropivacaine or liposomal bupivacaine for patients undergoing total knee arthroplasty. Anesthesiology 2017;126: 1139–50.

21. Johnson RL, Amundson AW, Abdel MP, et al. Continuous posterior lumbar plexus nerve block versus periarticular injection with ropivacaine or liposomal bupivacaine for total hip arthroplasty: a three-arm randomized clinical trial. J Bone Joint Surg Am 2017;99:1836–45.

22. Mariano ER, Perlas A. Adductor canal block for total knee arthroplasty: the perfect recipe or just one ingredient? Anesthesiology 2014;120:530–2.

23. Perlas A, Kirkham KR, Billing R, et al. The impact of analgesic modality on early ambulation following total knee arthroplasty. Reg Anesth Pain Med 2013;38: 334–9.

24. Kim TW, Park SJ, Lim SH, et al. Which analgesic mixture is appropriate for periarticular injection after total knee arthroplasty? Prospective, randomized, double-blind study. Knee Surg Sports Traumatol Arthrosc 2015;23:838–45.

25. Sogbein OA, Sondekoppam RV, Bryant D, et al. Ultrasound-guided motor-sparing knee blocks for postoperative analgesia following total knee arthroplasty: a randomized blinded study. J Bone Joint Surg Am 2017;99:1274–81.

26. Jaeger P, Nielsen ZJ, Henningsen MH, et al. Adductor canal block versus femoral nerve block and quadriceps strength: a randomized, double-blind, placebo-controlled, crossover study in healthy volunteers. Anesthesiology 2013;118: 409–15.

27. Jaeger P, Zaric D, Fomsgaard JS, et al. Adductor canal block versus femoral nerve block for analgesia after total knee arthroplasty: a randomized, double-blind study. Reg Anesth Pain Med 2013;38:526–32.

28. Wong WY, Bjorn S, Strid JM, et al. Defining the location of the adductor canal using ultrasound. Reg Anesth Pain Med 2017;42:241–5.

29. Panchamia JK, Niesen AD, Amundson AW. Adductor canal versus femoral triangle: let us all get on the same page. Anesth Analg 2018;127:e50.

30. Lee S, Rooban N, Vaghadia H, et al. A randomized non-inferiority trial of adductor canal block for analgesia after total knee arthroplasty: single injection versus catheter technique. J Arthroplasty 2018;33:1045–51.

31. Turner JD, Dobson SW, Henshaw DS, et al. Single-injection adductor canal block with multiple adjuvants provides equivalent analgesia when compared with continuous adductor canal blockade for primary total knee arthroplasty: a double-blinded, randomized, controlled, equivalency trial. J Arthroplasty 2018; 33(10):3160–6.e1.

32. Niesen AD, Harris DJ, Johnson CS, et al. Interspace between Popliteal Artery and posterior Capsule of the Knee (IPACK) injectate spread: a cadaver study. J Ultrasound Med 2019;38(3):741–5.

33. Sinha SK, Abrams JH, Arumugam S, et al. Femoral nerve block with selective tibial nerve block provides effective analgesia without foot drop after total knee

arthroplasty: a prospective, randomized, observer-blinded study. Anesth Analg 2012;115:202–6.

34. Kopp SL, Borglum J, Buvanendran A, et al. Anesthesia and analgesia practice pathway options for total knee arthroplasty: an evidence-based review by the american and european societies of regional anesthesia and pain medicine. Reg Anesth Pain Med 2017;42:683–97.

35. Fritsch G, Danninger T, Allerberger K, et al. Dexmedetomidine added to ropivacaine extends the duration of interscalene brachial plexus blocks for elective shoulder surgery when compared with ropivacaine alone: a single-center, prospective, triple-blind, randomized controlled trial. Reg Anesth Pain Med 2014; 39:37–47.

36. Andersen JH, Grevstad U, Siegel H, et al. Does dexmedetomidine have a perineural mechanism of action when used as an adjuvant to ropivacaine? A paired, blinded, randomized trial in healthy volunteers. Anesthesiology 2017;126:66–73.

37. Abdulatif M, Fawzy M, Nassar H, et al. The effects of perineural dexmedetomidine on the pharmacodynamic profile of femoral nerve block: a dose-finding randomised, controlled, double-blind study. Anaesthesia 2016;71:1177–85.

38. Shin HJ, Do SH, Lee JS, et al. Comparison of intraoperative sedation with dexmedetomidine versus propofol on acute postoperative pain in total knee arthroplasty under spinal anesthesia: a randomized trial. Anesth Analg 2018. [Epub ahead of print].

39. Sun S, Wang J, Bao N, et al. Comparison of dexmedetomidine and fentanyl as local anesthetic adjuvants in spinal anesthesia: a systematic review and meta-analysis of randomized controlled trials. Drug Des Devel Ther 2017;11:3413–24.

40. Mei B, Meng G, Xu G, et al. Intraoperative sedation with dexmedetomidine is superior to propofol for elderly patients undergoing hip arthroplasty: a prospective randomized controlled study. Clin J Pain 2018;34:811–7.

41. Williams BA, Schott NJ, Mangione MP, et al. Perineural dexamethasone and multimodal perineural analgesia: how much is too much? Anesth Analg 2014;118: 912–4.

42. De Oliveira GS Jr, Almeida MD, Benzon HT, et al. Perioperative single dose systemic dexamethasone for postoperative pain: a meta-analysis of randomized controlled trials. Anesthesiology 2011;115:575–88.

43. Dissanayake R, Du HN, Robertson IK, et al. Does dexamethasone reduce hospital readiness for discharge, pain, nausea, and early patient satisfaction in hip and knee arthroplasty? A randomized, controlled trial. J Arthroplasty 2018;33(11): 3429–36.

44. Li D, Wang C, Yang Z, et al. Effect of intravenous corticosteroids on pain management and early rehabilitation in patients undergoing total knee or hip arthroplasty: a meta-analysis of randomized controlled trials. Pain Pract 2018;18:487–99.

45. Politi J, Davis RL 2nd, Matrka A. Response to letter to the editor on "randomized prospective trial comparing the use of intravenous vs oral acetaminophen in total joint arthroplasty. J Arthroplasty 2017;32:3257.

46. Singla NK, Parulan C, Samson R, et al. Plasma and cerebrospinal fluid pharmacokinetic parameters after single-dose administration of intravenous, oral, or rectal acetaminophen. Pain Pract 2012;12:523–32.

47. Politi JR, Davis RL 2nd, Matrka AK. Randomized prospective trial comparing the use of intravenous versus oral acetaminophen in total joint arthroplasty. J Arthroplasty 2017;32:1125–7.

48. Moore RA, Wiffen PJ, Derry S, et al. Non-prescription (OTC) oral analgesics for acute pain - an overview of Cochrane reviews. Cochrane Database Syst Rev 2015;(11):CD010794.
49. Zeballos JL, Lirk P, Rathmell JP. Low-dose ketamine for acute pain management: a timely nudge toward multimodal analgesia. Reg Anesth Pain Med 2018;43: 453–5.
50. Chincholkar M. Analgesic mechanisms of gabapentinoids and effects in experimental pain models: a narrative review. Br J Anaesth 2018;120:1315–34.
51. Hurley RW, Cohen SP, Williams KA, et al. The analgesic effects of perioperative gabapentin on postoperative pain: a meta-analysis. Reg Anesth Pain Med 2006;31:237–47.
52. Mishriky BM, Waldron NH, Habib AS. Impact of pregabalin on acute and persistent postoperative pain: a systematic review and meta-analysis. Br J Anaesth 2015;114:10–31.
53. Memtsoudis SG, Sun X, Chiu YL, et al. Perioperative comparative effectiveness of anesthetic technique in orthopedic patients. Anesthesiology 2013;118:1046–58.
54. Johnson RL, Kopp SL, Burkle CM, et al. Neuraxial vs general anaesthesia for total hip and total knee arthroplasty: a systematic review of comparative-effectiveness research. Br J Anaesth 2016;116:163–76.
55. Frisch NB, Darrith B, Hansen DC, et al. Single-dose lidocaine spinal anesthesia in hip and knee arthroplasty. Arthroplast Today 2018;4:236–9.
56. Mahan MC, Jildeh TR, Tonbrunool TN, et al. Mepivacaine spinal anesthesia facilitates rapid recovery in total knee arthroplasty compared to bupivacaine. J Arthroplasty 2018;33:1699–704.
57. Toy PC, Fournier MN, Throckmorton TW, et al. Low rates of adverse events following ambulatory outpatient total hip arthroplasty at a free-standing surgery center. J Arthroplasty 2018;33:46–50.
58. Fillingham YA, Ramkumar DB, Jevsevar DS, et al. Tranexamic acid in total joint arthroplasty: the endorsed clinical practice guides of the American Association of Hip and Knee Surgeons, American Society of Regional Anesthesia and Pain Medicine, American Academy of Orthopaedic Surgeons, Hip Society, and Knee Society. J Arthroplasty 2018;44(1):7–11.
59. Guerra ML, Singh PJ, Taylor NF. Early mobilization of patients who have had a hip or knee joint replacement reduces length of stay in hospital: a systematic review. Clin Rehabil 2015;29:844–54.
60. Auyong DB, Allen CJ, Pahang JA, et al. Reduced length of hospitalization in primary total knee arthroplasty patients using an updated Enhanced Recovery after Orthopedic Surgery (ERAS) pathway. J Arthroplasty 2015;30:1705–9.
61. Raphael M, Jaeger M, van Vlymen J. Easily adoptable total joint arthroplasty program allows discharge home in two days. Can J Anaesth 2011;58:902–10.
62. Weingarten TN, Jacob AK, Njathi CW, et al. Multimodal analgesic protocol and postanesthesia respiratory depression during phase i recovery after total joint arthroplasty. Reg Anesth Pain Med 2015;40:330–6.
63. Fong R, Wang L, Zacny JP, et al. Caffeine accelerates emergence from isoflurane anesthesia in humans: a randomized, double-blind, crossover study. Anesthesiology 2018;129(5):912–20.
64. Ali Hassan HI. Comparison between two different selective spinal anesthesia techniques in ambulatory knee arthroscopy as fast-track anesthesia. Anesth Essays Res 2015;9:21–7.

Regional Anesthesia for Ambulatory Anesthesiologists

Alberto E. Ardon, MD, MPH[a],*, Arun Prasad, MBBS, FRCA, FRCPC[b],
Robert Lewis McClain, MD[c], M. Stephen Melton, MD[d],
Karen C. Nielsen, MD[d], Roy Greengrass, MD, FRCP[e]

KEYWORDS

- Regional anesthesia • Ambulatory analgesia • Peripheral nerve blocks
- Brachial plexus • PECS • TAP • PVB • Popliteal

KEY POINTS

- Regional anesthesia can enhance postoperative pain control and perioperative outcomes in an ambulatory surgical setting.
- Many surgeries commonly performed in ambulatory surgical centers are amenable to nerve blocks.
- Proper needling technique, discussed in this article, helps minimize risk of adverse events.

INTRODUCTION

Proper pain control is critical for ambulatory surgery. Uncontrolled postoperative pain can delay recovery, inhibit physical activity, and increase the risk of chronic postsurgical pain.[1] The use of regional anesthesia can be one of the most powerful tools in ambulatory anesthesiologists' armamentarium against severe postoperative pain. Regional anesthesia has been shown to enhance postoperative analgesia and improve patient satisfaction.[1] By decreasing the need for opioid agents, peripheral nerve blockade can decrease the risk of postoperative nausea/vomiting, altered

Disclosure: The authors have nothing to disclose.
[a] Department of Anesthesiology, University of Florida Jacksonville, 655 West 8th Street, Jacksonville, FL 32209, USA; [b] Department of Anesthesiology, University of Toronto, Women's College Hospital, Mc L 2-405, 399, Bathurst Street, Toronto, Ontario M5T 2S8, Canada; [c] Department of Anesthesiology and Perioperative Medicine, Mayo Clinic Jacksonville, 4500 San Pablo Road, Jacksonville, FL 32224, USA; [d] Department of Anesthesiology, Duke University Medical Center, Duke University Medical Center, DUMC Box #3094, Stop #4, Durham, NC 27710, USA; [e] Department of Anesthesiology and Perioperative Medicine, Mayo Clinic Jacksonville, 4500 San Pablo Road, Jacksonville, FL 32224, USA
* Corresponding author.
E-mail address: alberto.ardon@jax.ufl.edu

mental status, and pruritus, thus facilitating ambulatory surgical center discharge.[2,3] This article reviews those upper extremity, truncal, and lower extremity blocks that provide the best balance of clinical benefit to the patient and practicality in the ambulatory anesthesia clinical setting.

UPPER EXTREMITY BLOCKADE
Interscalene Brachial Plexus Block

The interscalene block (ISB), which is performed at the level of the roots, encompasses mainly C5 to C7 blockade and can involve C3 to C4. Benefits of ISB include potential avoidance of volatile anesthetics, reduced opioid consumption and opioid-related side effects, fewer awakenings from pain, and improved postoperative analgesia and rehabilitation.[2,4] In patients undergoing rotator cuff repair, continuous interscalene block has shown improved analgesia and reduced opioid requirements compared with single-injection ISB for up to 7 days.[5,6] Analgesia for outpatient shoulder arthroplasty can be accomplished with a continuous interscalene infusion at home.[7]

Surgical indications
An ISB provides surgical anesthesia and postoperative analgesia for shoulder and proximal arm surgery.

Ultrasonography-guided block technique
Scanning technique A 6-MHz to 15-MHz linear ultrasound probe is placed in the coronal oblique plane at the supraclavicular fossa. The hypoechoic brachial plexus trunks/divisions can be visualized in cross section, posterior-lateral to the hypoechoic subclavian artery seen in cross section above the hyperechoic first rib. Moving the ultrasound probe in a cephalad direction allows visualization of the brachial plexus trunks and nerve roots positioned between the anterior and middle scalene muscles. The traditional so-called stoplight presentation of the nerve roots between the anterior and middle scalene muscles can be C5, C6, and C7 but can also represent C5 and a bifid C6[8] (**Fig. 1**). Alternatively, C5 and C6 may course through, or anterior to, the anterior scalene muscle.

Needle technique and end point Introducing the block needle from the lateral end of the ultrasound probe, in plane with the beam, allows direct visualization of needle tip advancement, local anesthetic spread, and threading of the perineural catheter. The needle end point should be positioned in the space posterior-lateral to the C5 to C6

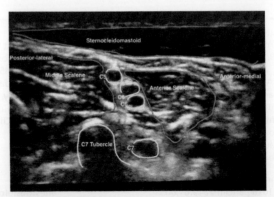

Fig. 1. Interscalene brachial plexus block. The nerve root of C5 can be seen overlying a bifid C6.

nerve roots, anterior-medial to the middle scalene muscle, avoiding intraneural injection. Alternatively, the needle may be introduced in the midline of the ultrasound probe, out of plane with the beam. The needle should be advanced in a cephalocaudad direction, with the needle end point at the C6 nerve root.

Typical local anesthetic dose
Typical dose is 15 to 20 mL of 0.5% ropivacaine.

Clinical pearls and possible complications
After ISB, transient phrenic nerve (C3–C5) blockade resulting in 100% incidence of ipsilateral hemidiaphragmatic paresis occurs when typical volumes are used.[9] As a result, ISB should be avoided in patients with preexisting pulmonary disease who are unable to tolerate a potential 25% reduction in pulmonary function.[10] Other side effects after ISB may include transient block of the cervical sympathetics resulting in Horner syndrome and transient recurrent laryngeal nerve block resulting in hoarseness.

Supraclavicular Brachial Plexus Block

The supraclavicular brachial plexus block is performed at the level of the trunks and divisions. This block provides reliable, complete anesthesia of the upper extremity below the midarm. Supraclavicular catheters can be used for postoperative analgesia in distal upper extremity surgery.[11]

Surgical indications
A supraclavicular brachial plexus block can be used for operations on the distal humerus, elbow, forearm, wrist, or hand.

Description of ultrasonography-guided block technique
Scanning technique A 6-MHz to 15-MHz linear ultrasound probe is placed in the coronal oblique plane at the supraclavicular fossa. The perivascular position of the brachial plexus can then be visualized in cross section anterior to the hyperechoic first rib. At this level, the trunks/divisions appear posterior-lateral and superior to the hypoechoic subclavian artery (**Fig. 2**).

Needle technique and end point Introducing the block needle from the lateral end of the ultrasound probe and advancing in line with the plane of the beam allows direct visualization of needle tip advancement and local anesthetic spread. The needle tip

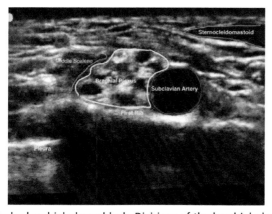

Fig. 2. Supraclavicular brachial plexus block. Divisions of the brachial plexus are observed.

is advanced into the space between the middle scalene muscle and the posterior-lateral lower third of the brachial plexus sheath.[12] This is typically accompanied by a palpable fascial click, and local anesthetic is then incrementally injected to open the perineural space and create a safe pathway for further needle advancement along the anterior-medial border of the middle scalene toward the corner pocket. The needle end point is subfascial at the corner pocket location.[13,14]

Typical local anesthetic dose
Typical local anesthetic dose is 20 to 25 mL of 0.5% ropivacaine or bupivacaine.

Clinical pearls and possible complications
Compared with the ISB, supraclavicular brachial plexus block is associated with a reduced incidence of phrenic nerve (C3–C5) blockade and resultant ipsilateral hemidiaphragmatic paresis. Nevertheless, care should be taken when considering this block in patients with preexisting pulmonary disease who may be unable to tolerate any reduction in pulmonary function.

Infraclavicular Brachial Plexus Block

The infraclavicular brachial plexus block targets the brachial plexus at the level of the cords, providing anesthesia to the upper extremity below the midarm. The lateral, posterior, and medial cords are named for their positions around the axillary artery. Perineural catheters at this level are very stable because of limited movement at the catheter insertion site below the clavicle.

Surgical indications
The infraclavicular block can be used for operations on the elbow, forearm, wrist, or hand.

Ultrasonography-guided block technique
Scanning technique A 6-MHz to 15-MHz linear ultrasound probe is placed in the parasagittal plane at the deltopectoral groove. At this level, the hyperechoic cords of the brachial plexus, the hypoechoic pulsatile axillary artery, and the hypoechoic compressible axillary vein can be identified in cross section, deep to the pectoralis major and minor muscles (**Fig. 3**).

Needle technique and end point Introducing the block needle from the superior end of the ultrasound probe and advancing in line with the plane of the beam allows direct visualization of needle tip advancement and local anesthetic spread. Needle tip placement posterior to the artery with local anesthetic spread circumferentially around the artery indicates a high likelihood of success.

Typical local anesthetic dose
Typical dose is 20 to 30 mL of 0.5% ropivacaine.

Clinical pearls and possible complications
Compared with the ISB and supraclavicular brachial plexus block, infraclavicular block is associated with a very low incidence of phrenic nerve (C3–C5) blockade and resultant ipsilateral hemidiaphragmatic paresis. Pneumothorax is a possible complication if the needle is advanced too far.

Axillary Brachial Plexus Block

The axillary block targets the terminal branches of the brachial plexus. An additional musculocutaneous nerve block is typically necessary to provide analgesia of the entire forearm.

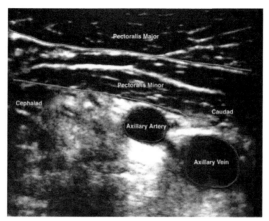

Fig. 3. Infraclavicular brachial plexus block. The hyperechoic (white) structures surrounding the axillary artery denote posterior, medial, and lateral cords of the brachial plexus.

Surgical indications
The axillary block can be used for operations of the elbow, forearm, wrist, and hand.

Ultrasonography-guided block technique
Scanning technique A 6-MHz to 15-MHz linear ultrasound probe is placed at the axillary fold in an anterior-posterior orientation. The nerves may appear as round to oval hypoechoic or hyperechoic structures in close proximity to the hypoechoic axillary artery (**Fig. 4**). The terminal branches are variable in their positions around the artery; however, the radial nerve is most commonly identified in a posterior position, the median nerve in an anterior position, and the ulnar nerve in a medial position. The musculocutaneous nerve may be identified within the coracobrachialis muscle or at a more perivascular position.

Needle technique and end point The block needle is introduced at the anterolateral end of the ultrasound probe and advanced in line with the plane of the beam, allowing visualization of needle tip advancement and local anesthetic spread. If individual

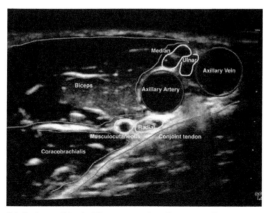

Fig. 4. Axillary brachial plexus block. The nerve structures can be seen surrounding the axillary artery. The musculocutaneous nerve lies anteriorly within the coracobrachialis muscle.

nerves cannot be identified, local anesthetic should be injected circumferentially around the artery. Before and on injection, pressure on the probe can be released to evaluate for perivascular (but not intravascular) spread of local anesthetic.

Typical local anesthetic dose
Typical dose is 20 to 30 mL of 0.5% ropivacaine.

Clinical pearls and possible complications
Phrenic nerve paralysis with axillary brachial plexus block has not been described, making this technique an excellent choice for patients with significant preexisting pulmonary disease. In addition, the axillary block is a reasonable option in anticoagulated patients, because any inadvertent hematoma can be rapidly and extensively compressed.

TRUNCAL BLOCKADE
Paravertebral Block

Paravertebral nerve blocks (PVBs) present an opportunity to block multiple mixed nerve roots soon after they emerge from the intervertebral foramina, thus delivering analgesia that follows a dermatomal distribution. The paravertebral space is a wedge-shaped anatomic compartment adjacent to the vertebral bodies. The space is defined anterolaterally by the parietal pleura; posteriorly by the superior costotransverse ligament (thoracic levels); medially by the vertebra, vertobral disk, and intervertebral foramina; as well as superiorly and inferiorly by the heads of the ribs (**Fig. 5**). Paravertebral techniques can incorporate continuous catheters, which offer advantages versus primary central neuraxial techniques.

Surgical indications

- Breast cancer surgery
- Inguinal herniorrhaphy
- Incisional, umbilical, ventral hernia repair
- Any thoracic or abdominal wall procedure
- Open renal surgery, cholecystectomy, appendectomy
- Mastectomy with major reconstructive surgery

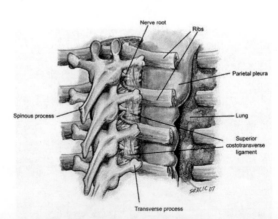

Fig. 5. The paravertebral space lies anterior to the superior costotransverse ligament. (*From* Greengrass RA, Duclas R. Paravertebral blocks. Int Anesthesiol Clin 2012;50(1):57; with permission.)

For repair of inguinal herniorrhaphy, PVB is associated with significantly reduced opioid requirements, significantly reduced pain, and enhanced recovery compared with general anesthesia.[15] PVB may also decrease time to first void, postoperative urinary retention, and recovery room and hospital stay compared with general anesthesia.[16]

Ultrasonography-guided block technique

PVB can be performed using either anatomic or ultrasonography-guided technique. Because many providers now use ultrasonography to perform this block, the authors refer readers to the review article by Greengrass and Duclas[17] for a detailed description of the landmark-based technique.

Landmarks The anesthesiologist should identify which dermatomes will be involved in the operative field. For example, for mastectomy with axillary dissection, T1 to T6 is routinely blocked. For inguinal herniorrhaphy, levels T11, T12, and L1 are blocked. The spinous process of each level is identified and a mark is placed at the most superior aspect. From the midpoint of these marks, a needle entry site is marked 2.5 cm laterally (**Fig. 6**).

Scanning technique A 6-MHz to 15-MHz linear ultrasound probe is adequate for most patients, but a curvilinear probe may be beneficial in obese patients. After determining the appropriate surgical dermatomes, the probe is initially placed transversely to confirm spine position. The probe is then placed parasagittally approximately 2.5 to 3 cm from the midline to image the lateral part of the transverse process (TP) and the TP rib junction. The TP is imaged just below the midpoint of the probe (**Fig. 7**).

Needle technique and end point A 22-gauge Tuohy needle is inserted at the midpoint of the probe parasagittally in a cephalad to caudad direction and directed to traverse the superior costotransverse ligament (**Fig. 8**) of the intended paravertebral space. Whether using anatomic or ultrasonography-guided techniques, it is essential that the needle be directed caudally to minimize contact with the neurovascular bundle. After negative aspiration, local anesthetic injection results in a downward displacement of the pleura on the ultrasonography screen.

Typical local anesthetic dose

Typical dose is 20 to 30 mL of 0.5% ropivacaine. Of note, large-volume single-injection PVB seems to produce less reliable anesthesia than multiple small-volume injections, each targeting specific dermatomes.

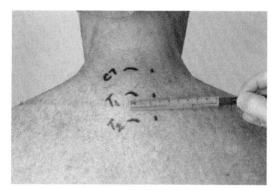

Fig. 6. Levels for axillary dissection. The needle entry site for a PVB is usually 2.5 cm lateral to the midline. (*From* Greengrass RA, Duclas R. Paravertebral blocks. Int Anesthesiol Clin 2012;50(1):62; with permission.)

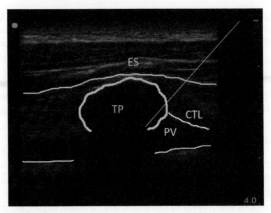

Fig. 7. Ultrasonography image for either a paravertebral block or erector spinae (ES) block. For a PVB, the needle is directed through the costotransverse ligament (CTL) to the paravertebral space (PV). For an ES block, local anesthetic is deposited between the ES muscle and the TP. The light blue line denotes pleura.

Clinical pearls and possible complications

Complications associated with PVB have traditionally been described as vascular puncture (3.8% incidence), pleural puncture (1.1%), and pneumothorax (0.5%).[18,19] However, these risks are less likely using proper landmark-based technique and use of ultrasonography guidance.

Erector Spinae Plane Block

The erector spinae plane block (ESP) is an interfascial plane block first described in 2016 in which local anesthetic is deposited below the fascia of the erector spinae (ES).[20] The ES is the deepest of the muscles near the midline superficial to the central neuraxis (see **Fig. 7**). The mechanism of action of ESP block is controversial. It was initially thought that injected local anesthetic spread into the paravertebral space to

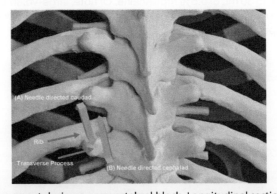

Fig. 8. Needle movement during a paravertebral block. Longitudinal section of the paravertebral space to show needle direction: (*A*) needle directed caudad, and (*B*) needle directed cephalad. Note: if initial bony contact was inadvertently rib, the needle would probably contact the TP (more superficial when directed caudad) versus the pleura (if the needle was directed cephalad). (*From* Greengrass RA, Duclas R. Paravertebral blocks. Int Anesthesiol Clin 2012;50(1):64; with permission.)

bathe the nerve roots,[20] but recent cadaveric dye injection studies contradict this concept. Injected local anesthetic seems to bathe the posterior roots only; sensory block is thought to occur via lateral spread of local anesthetic to bathe lateral cutaneous branches of intercostal nerves.[21]

Surgical indications

- Breast surgery
- Ventral hernia repair
- Postsurgical thoracic neuropathic pain

Ultrasonography-guided block technique

Landmarks As with PVB, the spinous processes relevant to the surgical dermatomes are determined and marked. Unlike PVB, in which three-fifths of the injectate is distributed caudad and two-fifths cephalad, most of the injectate after ESP block is distributed cranially and laterally, thus choosing a TP caudad in the surgical field seems most logical.

Scanning technique A 6-MHz to 15-MHz linear ultrasound probe (curvilinear for morbidly obese patients) is used initially transverse to confirm the spinous process. The probe is then moved parasagittally 2.5 cm lateral, to determine the lateral aspect of the TP; this is the same ultrasonography visualization technique as for PVB.

Needle technique and end point Using either an in-plane or parasagittal technique, the needle is directed to contact the TP. The needle is then moved a few millimeters back off the TP and local anesthetic incrementally injected. The local anesthetic spread should be visualized deep to the ES muscle, between it and the TP, expanding the interfascial plane.

Typical local anesthetic dose

Typical dose is 20 mL of 0.5% ropivacaine.

Clinical pearls and possible complications

No serious complications of ESP block have been reported as yet, but needle malposition and local anesthetic toxicity are among possible difficulties.

Pectoral Plane Blocks

The pectoral blocks (PECS I and PECS II and serratus plane block) were first described in 2011, 2012, and 2013 respectively.[22-24] The PECS II and serratus plane blocks are typically done in combination with PECS I.

PECS I Block

The PECS I block is a technique by which local anesthetic is injected between the pectoralis major and minor muscles. The block aims to block the medial and lateral pectoral nerves, which are branches of the brachial plexus that run between the pectoralis major and minor muscles.

Surgical indications

- Breast surgery (insertion of breast expanders, subpectoral prosthesis, implant insertion)
- Subpectoral pacemakers, port-a-cath, and intercostal chest drain insertions
- Traumatic chest injuries

Ultrasonography-guided block technique
Scanning technique A 6-MHz to 15-MHz linear ultrasound probe is placed below the clavicle along the sagittal plane and moved inferolateral to identify pectoralis major, pectoralis minor, and the thoracoacromial vessels in the plane between the muscles (**Fig. 9**A).

Needle technique and end point The block needle is introduced via an in-plane approach in a cephalad to caudad direction. The needle is advanced until the needle crosses the pectoralis major and lies just in between pectoralis major and minor. After negative aspiration, injection of local anesthetic should result in a visible separation of the two pectoral muscles, along the fascial plane in an ovoid manner.

Typical local anesthetic dose
Typical dose is 10 to 15 mL of 0.5% ropivacaine.

Clinical pearls and possible complications
Missing the fascial plane An intramuscular injection can be seen as a localized globular spread rather than an elliptical spread.

Vascular injury Verification that the pectoral branch of the thoracoacromial artery is not in the needle pathway should be performed.

PECS II/Modified Pectoral Block

In the PECS II block, local anesthetic is injected between the pectoralis minor and serratus anterior muscles. This technique blocks the lateral branches of the intercostal nerves and the long thoracic nerve, providing analgesia to the lateral aspect of the chest and the axilla.

Surgical indications
Mastectomy or wide local excision of breast with axillary dissection or sentinel node biopsy.

Ultrasonography-guided block technique
Scanning technique A 6-MHz to 15-MHz linear ultrasound probe is placed below the clavicle along the sagittal plane and moved inferolateral to identify pectoralis major, pectoralis minor, and serratus anterior muscles (usually around the level of the third or fourth rib) (**Fig. 9**B).

Needle technique and end point The block needle is introduced via an in-plane approach in a cephalad to caudad direction. The needle is advanced in a manner similar to that during a PECS I block. However, for a PECS II block the needle is advanced until it crosses the pectoralis minor and lies just in between pectoralis minor and serratus anterior. After negative aspiration, injection of local anesthetic should result in a visible separation of the two muscle layers.

Typical local anesthetic dose
Typical dose is 10 to 15 mL of 0.5% ropivacaine.

Clinical pearls and possible complications
Perform PECS II first It is normally advised to do PECS II rather than PECS I first so that the associated fascial plane is not pushed further posteriorly, which would increase the depth required for ultrasonography visualization.

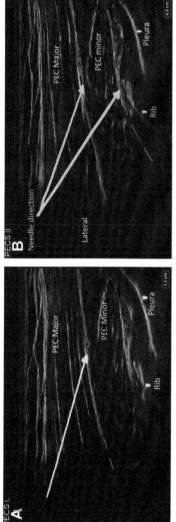

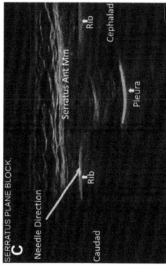

Fig. 9. (A) PECS I block. The orange line denotes the fascial layer between the pectoralis (PEC) major and minor muscles. (B) PECS II block. The most inferior orange line denotes the fascial layer between pectoralis minor and serratus anterior. (C) Serratus anterior plane block. The target of the injection is the fascial plane underneath the serratus anterior muscle (Serratus Ant Mm). Arrows denote needle direction.

Serratus Anterior Plane Block

The serratus anterior block is a technique in which local anesthetic is injected between the serratus anterior muscle and rib.[25,26] This block aims to anesthetize the intercostobrachial nerve, lateral cutaneous branches of the intercostal nerves (T3–T9), and thoracodorsal and long thoracic nerves.

Surgical indications
The serratus anterior plane block can be useful for surgeries involving an incision on the anterolateral chest wall, such as chest drain insertion, and for reconstructive or cosmetic breast surgery.

Ultrasonography-guided block technique
Scanning technique A 6-MHz to 15-MHz linear ultrasound probe is placed over the midaxillary region of the thoracic cage in a sagittal plane. The block is performed over the fourth rib (at the level of the nipple) where the rib and overlying serratus anterior muscle are identified (**Fig. 9C**).

Needle technique and end point The block needle is introduced via an in-plane approach in a cephalad to caudad direction. The needle is advanced until it crosses the serratus anterior muscle and lies in between the serratus anterior and rib. After negative aspiration, injection of local anesthetic should result in a visible expansion of the layer below the serratus anterior.

Typical local anesthetic dose
Typical dose is 20 to 25 mL of 0.5% ropivacaine.

Clinical pearls and possible complications
Using the rib as the end point Placing the needle tip over the rib offers some protection from injuring the pleura.

Transversus Abdominis Plane Block

The transversus abdominis plane (TAP) block was first described as an ultrasonography-guided technique in 2007.[27] The block aims to anesthetize the lower intercostal, the iliohypogastric, and the ilioinguinal nerves. The use of TAP blocks has also been described for areas above the umbilicus.[28]

Surgical indications
The TAP block can be useful for lower abdominal surgery (including appendectomy, hernia repair, umbilical surgery, and abdominal hysterectomy) and cesarean section.

Ultrasonography-guided block technique
Scanning technique A 6-MHz to 15-MHz linear ultrasound probe is placed in a transverse plane above the iliac crest and along the anterior axillary line. The transducer is moved laterally until 3 muscular layers of the abdominal wall are visible: the external oblique (most superficial), the internal oblique, and transversus abdominis. The peritoneal cavity lies deep to the transversus abdominis muscle layer and may be identified by the peristaltic movements of bowel loops (**Fig. 10**).

Needle technique and end point The block needle is introduced in an in-plane approach, in an anterior to posterolateral direction. The needle is advanced through the external and internal oblique muscles so that injectate can be seen in the fascial plane below the internal oblique and above the transversus abdominis.

Typical local anesthetic dose
Typical dose is 15 to 20 mL of 0.5% ropivacaine per side.

Clinical pearls and possible complications
Distinguishing muscle layers If difficulty is encountered in distinguishing the 3 muscle layers, it may be helpful to begin scanning near the midline over the rectus abdominis muscle and move the probe laterally to identify the correct 3 muscle layers. Accurate placement of the needle tip may be facilitated by injection of a small amount of saline to hydrodissect the appropriate plane.

Bowel injury Although rare, bowel injury is possible if care is not taken to avoid needle advancement into the peritoneal space.

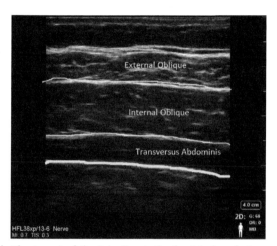

Fig. 10. TAP block. The target of the injection is the fascial plane between the internal oblique and transversus abdominis muscles. Hypoechoic bowel can be seen on the inferior portion of the image.

LOWER EXTREMITY BLOCKADE
Femoral Block

Blockade of the femoral nerve results in sensory deficit to the anterior medial thigh and medial leg to the foot. Motor blockade involves the muscles of the anterior thigh, including the vastus medialis, vastus lateralis, and vastus intermedius, along with the sartorius muscle and rectus femoris. A femoral nerve block can result in significant weakness of the quadriceps.

Surgical indications

- Total knee arthroplasty (TKA)
- Knee ligament repair
- Superficial surgery involving the distal anterior thigh and/or medial leg and ankle
- Surgery of the distal femur

Ultrasonography-guided block technique
Scanning technique An ultrasound probe is placed in the femoral crease in a transverse plane. The femoral artery should be visible on the screen; if not, more depth or medial movement of the probe may be required. The femoral nerve can be identified

as a hyperechoic structure lateral to the femoral artery and deep to the facia iliaca (**Fig. 11**).

Needle technique and end point The block needle is introduced via an in-plane or out-of-plane approach. As the needle is advanced toward the lateral aspect of the femoral nerve, tenting of the fascial lata or fascia iliaca may be visible. Concurrently, a pop may be felt as the needle is advanced through these fascial planes. The end point of needle advancement should be the moment the needle tip crosses the facia iliaca. After negative aspiration, injection of local anesthetic should result in visualization of anesthetic surrounding the nerve.

Typical local anesthetic dose
Typical dose is 20 to 25 mL of 0.5% ropivacaine.

Clinical pearls and possible complications
Weakness Significant sensory deficit and weakness of the lower extremity above the knee joint should be expected.

Injury to femoral artery Special attention should be paid to avoiding approximation of the needle to the artery because the structures often lie close to one another.

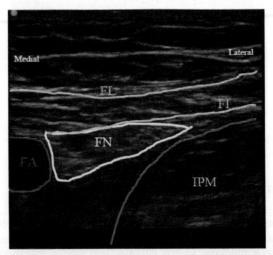

Fig. 11. Femoral nerve block. Deposition of local anesthetic just lateral to the femoral nerve (FN) and underneath fascia iliaca (FI) is desired. FA, femoral artery; FL, fascia lata; IPM, iliopsoas muscle.

Adductor Canal Block

The adductor canal is a triangular anatomic compartment bounded by the sartorius muscle medially, the vastus medialis muscle laterally, and the adductor magnus muscle posteriorly. In the area of the proximal thigh (circa the femoral triangle), both the saphenous nerve and the nerve to the vastus medialis lie within the same fascial plane. Moving to the mid/distal thigh, only the saphenous nerve remains in the adductor canal. Thus, a block at this level results in a sensory deficit along the distal anterior/medial thigh, anterior/medial knee, and a portion of the medial leg with little motor involvement.

Surgical indications

- TKA
- Knee ligament repair
- Superficial surgery involving the distal anterior thigh and/or medial leg and ankle
- Surgery of the distal femur

Ultrasonography-guided block technique

Scanning technique With the patient in the supine position, a line can be drawn from the anterior superior iliac spine to the medial condyle of the femur; the midpoint of this line approximates the initial position for the ultrasound probe. A 6-MHz to 15-MHz linear ultrasound probe (sheathed in a sterile cover) is placed at the midpoint of the thigh. The sartorius muscle and underlying superficial femoral artery and saphenous vein should be visible (**Fig. 12**). If these structures are not visible, cephalad or caudad movement of the probe may be necessary.

Needle technique and end point The block needle is introduced into the skin in an in-plane or out-of-plane fashion. The needle is advanced into the space below the sartorius muscle and adjacent to the superficial femoral artery. After negative aspiration, injection of local anesthetic should proceed in a slow fashion, such that the local anesthetic solution is injected to encompass the artery and fill the canal.

Typical local anesthetic dose

Typical dose is 10 to 15 mL of 0.5% ropivacaine.

Clinical pearls and possible complications

Both sensory and motor complications have been reported after high-volume adductor canal block.

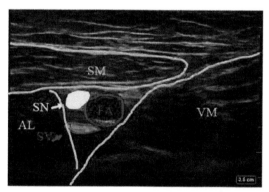

Fig. 12. Adductor canal block. The saphenous nerve (SN) lies in the adductor canal underneath the sartorius muscle (SM) and next to the FA. Care should be taken to identify the saphenous vein (SV). AL, adductor longus muscle; VM, vastus medialis muscle.

Popliteal Block

The popliteal block is a block of the sciatic nerve above the level of the popliteal fossa. Sensory deficit is expected in the distribution of the tibial and peroneal nerves; that is, in the entirety of the leg distal to the inferior aspect of the knee joint with the exception of the medial aspect of the leg and foot. Motor deficit is expected in all major musculature of the leg distal to the knee, preventing dorsiflexion and plantar flexion of the ankle.

Surgical indications

- Ankle arthroplasty
- Significant bony work of the ankle or proximal foot
- Achilles tendon repair
- Gastrocnemius recession
- Tibia or fibular repair
- Anterior cruciate ligament repair
- Total knee arthroplasty

Ultrasonography-guided block technique

Scanning technique Patients can be positioned either in the supine position with elevation of the leg or in a lateral decubitus position. A 6-MHz to 15-MHz linear ultrasound probe is placed directly on the popliteal fossa in a transverse plane. A hyperechoic nerve structure (tibial nerve) should be visible superficial to the popliteal artery (**Fig. 13**); if not, some tilting of the probe may be required. Once the nerve structure is in view, the probe is slid proximally until a second hyperechoic nerve structure (peroneal nerve) is observed to coalesce with the initially observed nerve. The desired point of nerve blockade is typically at the level of this bifurcation or immediately proximal to it (sciatic nerve; **Figs. 14 and 15**). A mental note of the depth of the nerve structures is made.

Needle technique and end point The block needle is introduced into the skin in an in-plane fashion and in a manner that is as equidistant as possible to the depth of the nerve structure on ultrasonography. An effort is made to maintain the needle as horizontal as possible to maximize visualization. The end point of needle advancement should be the moment the needle tip crosses the parasciatic sheath, which can be visualized on ultrasonography imaging as a tenting that progresses to a release of tissue, and can be felt as a pop as the needle is advanced into the parasciatic area. After negative aspiration, injection of local anesthetic should result in visualization of anesthetic surrounding the nerve and possibly expanding the potential space between the tibial nerve and peroneal nerve (if the needle injection is done at the level of the sciatic bifurcation).

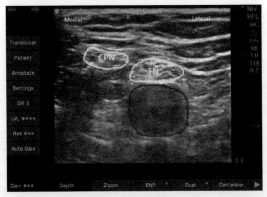

Fig. 13. Popliteal fossa image showing the common peroneal nerve (CPN) and tibial nerve (TN) as 2 separate components superficial to the popliteal artery (PA).

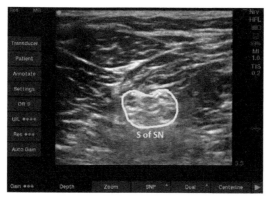

Fig. 14. As the ultrasound probe is moved in a cephalad direction, the split of the sciatic nerve (S of SN) becomes visible on the screen.

Typical local anesthetic dose
Typical dose is 20 to 25 mL of 0.5% ropivacaine.

Clinical pearls and possible complications
Fall risk Significant sensory deficit and weakness of the lower extremity distal to the knee joint should be expected.

Partial analgesia The sensory distribution of the foot and ankle may not follow expected sensory innervation patterns; a saphenous nerve block may also be required to achieve adequate postsurgical analgesia.

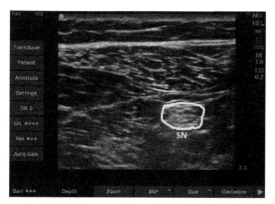

Fig. 15. Even more cephalad movement of the probe reveals a sciatic nerve (SN) that is singular and enveloped by a parasciatic sheath.

Interspace Between the Popliteal Artery and Capsule of the Knee Block

The iPACK (interspace between the popliteal artery and capsule of the knee) block is a block of the genicular nerves that give sensation to the posterior aspect of the knee joint. Sensory deficit is limited to the posterior knee. Because the involved nerves are purely sensory, no motor deficit is expected from this nerve block. Despite being a relatively new nerve block technique, the iPACK block has evidence supporting its use in total knee arthroplasty.[29,30]

Surgical indications

The iPACK block can be used for total knee arthroplasty, anterior cruciate ligament repair, and procedures involving the posterior aspect of the knee.

Ultrasonography-guided block technique

Scanning technique Patients can be positioned either in the supine position with elevation of the leg or in a lateral decubitus position. A 6-MHz to 15-MHz linear ultrasound probe (or 2-MHz to 5-MHz curvilinear probe) is placed directly on the popliteal fossa in a transverse plane, equivalent to initial visualization for a popliteal block. Once the popliteal artery is identified, an immediate increase in depth may be required to facilitate visualization of the medial and lateral femoral condyles. Likewise, movement of the probe in a medial or lateral fashion may be required to appreciate the concave osseous structures on either inferior corner of the screen (**Figs. 16** and **17**). Once the condyles have been identified, the probe is slid proximally until an almost-horizontal hyperechoic line is visualized on the inferior aspect of the screen (**Fig. 18**). This line represents the posterior aspect of the distal femur and is the site of local anesthetic infiltration.

Needle technique and end point The block needle is introduced into the skin in an in-plane fashion and in a manner that is as equidistant as possible to the depth of the target osseous structure on ultrasonography. The needle is advanced into the space in between the popliteal artery and the posterior aspect of the femur. The end point of needle advancement should be the inferior corner of the screen contralateral to the side of needle introduction. After negative aspiration, injection of local anesthetic should proceed in a slow fashion, such that, as the needle is withdrawn, the entirety of the anesthetic solution is injected along the entire transverse plane of the femur.

Typical local anesthetic dose

Typical dose is 15 to 20 mL of 0.5% ropivacaine.

Clinical pearls and possible complications

Feasibility Ultrasonography scanning may reveal a small distance between the popliteal artery and femoral line. Manipulation of the nerve block needle with adequate

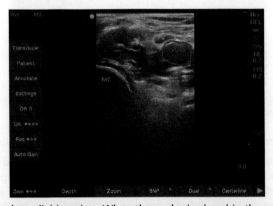

Fig. 16. iPACK block medial imaging. When the probe is placed in the popliteal fossa and moved in a medial direction, the medial condyle (MC) of the femur should be visualized. PV, popliteal vein.

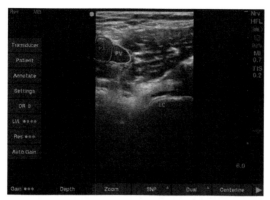

Fig. 17. iPACK block lateral imaging. When the probe is placed in the popliteal fossa and moved in a lateral direction, the lateral condyle (LC) of the femur should be visualized.

precautions to avoid arterial puncture may not be feasible in some patients. Likewise, performance of this block in morbidly obese patients may be significantly challenging.

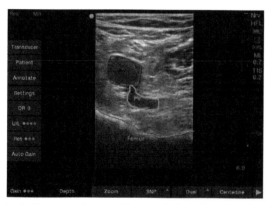

Fig. 18. iPACK block. As the probe is moved in a cephalad direction, the posterior border of the femur (*orange line*) is visible on the inferior portion of the screen. The needle end point is infiltration along this line.

Ankle Block

The ankle block provides anesthesia/analgesia to the entirety of the foot by blocking the sural, deep peroneal, superficial peroneal, posterior tibial, and saphenous nerves.

Surgical indications
An ankle block can be used for any surgery distal to the ankle, including bunionectomy, hammertoe correction, metatarsal surgery, and plantar foot surgery.

Ultrasonography-guided block technique
With the patient in the supine position, 2 or 3 blankets are placed underneath the surgical leg at the level of the distal calf to elevate the foot and allow for an ultrasound probe to be placed posterior to the malleoli. All nerves are blocked above the malleoli. Appropriate nerves are blocked using a 6-MHz to 15-MHz linear ultrasound probe.

Posterior tibial nerve block The probe is placed transversely, posterior to the medial malleolus, to image the posterior tibial artery. The nerve is imaged posterior to the artery. Using a 25-gauge needle, an in-plane or out-of-plane technique is used to deposit local anesthetic around the nerve (**Fig. 19**).

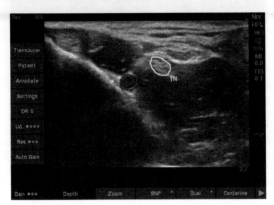

Fig. 19. Ankle block (medial aspect). The TN can be seen in close proximity to the tibial artery (TA).

Deep peroneal nerve block The probe is placed transversely across the dorsum of the foot to image the anterior tibial artery. The nerve is usually lateral to the artery but may divide above the vessel with branches on either side of it. A 25-gauge needle is inserted via an in-plane or out-of-plane technique to deposit local anesthetic on both sides of the vessel (**Fig. 20**).

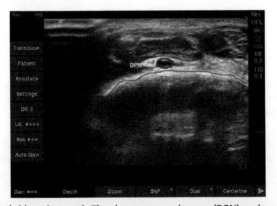

Fig. 20. Ankle block (dorsal aspect). The deep peroneal nerve (DPN) and superficial peroneal nerve (not elucidated) are in close proximity to the dorsalis pedis artery (DP). An infiltration of the area surrounding the artery is sufficient for adequate blockade.

Sural nerve block The probe is placed transversely posterior to the lateral malleolus to image the lesser saphenous vein. Using an in-plane or out-of-plane technique, local anesthetic is placed on both sides of the vein (**Fig. 21**).

The saphenous and superficial peroneal nerves are blocked using a subcutaneous injection from the posterior aspect of the medial malleolus across the foot to the posterior aspect of the lateral malleolus.

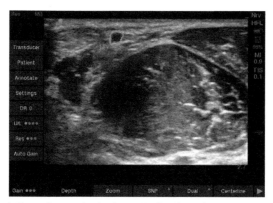

Fig. 21. Ankle block (lateral aspect). The lesser SV (LSV) can be appreciated when light pressure is applied to the ultrasound probe. Infiltration in this area results in anesthesia of the sural nerve.

Typical local anesthetic dose

Typical dose is 3 to 5 mL of 0.5% ropivacaine per nerve, plus 10 to 15 mL for subcutaneous injection.

SUMMARY

Regional anesthesia can provide extensive benefits for ambulatory surgical patients. Proper regional anesthetic techniques can maximize patient comfort, promote postoperative discharge, and form an integral part of an effective and efficient perioperative practice. Knowledgeable and skilled anesthesiologists performing regional anesthesia can be the driving force behind excellence in patient satisfaction at ambulatory surgical centers.

ACKNOWLEDGMENTS

The authors would like to thank Barys Ihnatsenka MD (Associate Professor of Anesthesiology, University of Florida) for his help in obtaining paravertebral images, and Shikha Bansal MBBS, MD (Fellow, Department of Anesthesiology, University of Toronto) for her contribution to the article.

REFERENCES

1. Chou R, Gordon DB, de Leon-Casasola OA, et al. Management of postoperative pain: a clinical practice guideline from the American Pain Society, the American Society of Regional Anesthesia and Pain Medicine, and the American Society of Anesthesiologists' Committee on Regional Anesthesia, Executive Committee, and Administrative Council. J Pain 2016;17(2):131–57.
2. Hadzic A, Williams BA, Karaca PE, et al. For outpatient rotator cuff surgery, nerve block anesthesia provides superior same-day recovery over general anesthesia. Anesthesiology 2005;102:1001–7.
3. Brummett CM, Williams BA. Additives to local anesthetics for peripheral nerve blockade. Int Anesthesiol Clin 2011;49(4):104–16.
4. Malhotra N, Madison SJ, Ward SR, et al. Continuous interscalene nerve block following adhesive capsulitis manipulation. Reg Anesth Pain Med 2013;38:171–2.

5. Ilfeld BM, Morey TE, Wright TW, et al. Continuous interscalene brachial plexus block for postoperative pain control at home: a randomized, double-blinded, placebo-controlled study. Anesth Analg 2003;96:1089–95.

6. Salviz EA, Xu D, Frulla A, et al. Continuous interscalene block in patients having outpatient rotator cuff repair surgery: a prospective randomized trial. Anesth Analg 2013;117:1485–92.

7. Ilfeld BM, Vandenborne K, Duncan PW, et al. Ambulatory continuous interscalene nerve blocks decrease the time to discharge readiness after total shoulder arthroplasty: a randomized, triple-masked, placebo-controlled study. Anesthesiology 2006;105:999–1007.

8. Franco CD. Ultrasound-guided interscalene block: reevaluation of the "stoplight" sign and clinical implications. Reg Anesth Pain Med 2016;41:452–9.

9. Urmey WF, Talts KH, Sharrock NE. One hundred percent incidence of hemidiaphragmatic paresis associated with interscalene brachial plexus anesthesia as diagnosed by ultrasonography. Anesth Analg 1991;72:498–503.

10. Urmey WF, McDonald M. Hemidiaphragmatic paresis during interscalene brachial plexus block: effects on pulmonary function and chest wall mechanics. Anesth Analg 1992;74:352–7.

11. Ahsan ZS, Carvalho B, Yao J. Incidence of failure of continuous peripheral nerve catheters for postoperative analgesia in upper extremity surgery. J Hand Surg 2014;39:324–9.

12. Brull R, Chan VWS. The corner pocket revisited. Reg Anesth Pain Med 2011;36:308.

13. Sivashanmugam T, Ray S, Ravishankar M, et al. Randomized comparison of extrafascial versus subfascial injection of local anesthetic during ultrasound-guided supraclavicular brachial plexus block. Reg Anesth Pain Med 2015;40:337–43.

14. Morfey D, Brull R. Ultrasound-guided supraclavicular block: what is intraneural? Anesthesiology 2010;112:250–1.

15. Hadzic A, Kerimoglu B, Loreio D, et al. Paravertebral blocks provide superior same day recovery over general anesthesia for patients undergoing inguinal hernia repair. Anesth Analg 2006;102(4):1076–81.

16. Bojaxhi E, Lee J, Bowers S, et al. Paravertebral blocks reduce the risk of postoperative urinary retention in inguinal hernia repair. Hernia 2018;22(5):871–9.

17. Greengrass RA, Duclas R. Paravertebral blocks. Int Anesthesiol Clin 2012;50(1):56–73.

18. Karmakar MK. Thoracic paravertebral block. Anesthesiology 2001;95:771–80.

19. Lonnqvist PA, MacKenzie J, Soni AK, et al. Paravertebral blockade: failure rate and complications. Anaesthesia 1995;50:813–5.

20. Forero M, Adhikary SD, Lopez H, et al. The erector spinae plane block: a novel analgesic technique in thoracic neuropathic pain. Reg Anesth Pain Med 2016;41:621–7.

21. Ivanusic J, Konishi Y, Barrington M. Cadaveric study investigating the mechanism of action of erector spinae blockade. Reg Anesth Acute Pain 2018;43:567–71.

22. Blanco R. The 'pecs block': a novel technique for providing analgesia after breast surgery. Anaesthesia 2011;66(9):847–8.

23. Blanco R, Fajardo M, Parras Maldonado T. Ultrasound description of Pecs II (modified Pecs I): a novel approach to breast surgery. Rev Esp Anestesiol Reanim 2012;59(9):470–5.

24. Blanco R, Parras T, McDonnell JG, et al. Serratus plane block: a novel ultrasound-guided thoracic wall nerve block. Anaesthesia 2013;68(11):1107–13.

25. Kunhabdulla NP, Agarwal A, Gaur A, et al. Serratus anterior plane block for multiple rib fractures. Pain Physician 2014;17(4):E553–5.
26. Madabushi R, Tewari S, Gautam SK, et al. Serratus anterior plane block: a new analgesic technique for post-thoracotomy pain. Pain Physician 2015;18(3): E421–4.
27. Hebbard P, Fujiwara Y, Shibata Y, et al. Ultrasound-guided transversus abdominis plane (TAP) block. Anaesth Intensive Care 2007;35(4):616–7.
28. Yoshida T, Furutani K, Watanabe Y, et al. Analgesic efficacy of bilateral continuous transversus abdominis plane blocks using an oblique subcostal approach in patients undergoing laparotomy for gynaecological cancer: a prospective, randomized, triple-blind, placebo-controlled study. Br J Anaesth 2016;117(6): 812–20.
29. Thobhani S, Scalercio L, Elliott CE, et al. Novel regional techniques for total knee arthroplasty promote reduced hospital length of stay: an analysis of 106 patients. Ochsner J 2017;17(3):233–8.
30. Scimia P, Giordano C, Ricci EB, et al. The ultrasound-guided iPACK block with continuous adductor canal block for total knee arthroplasty. Anaesthesia Cases 2017. Available at: https://www.anaesthesiacases.org/case-reports/2017-0117.

Pediatric Ambulatory Anesthesia Challenges

Steven F. Butz, MD[a,b,*]

KEYWORDS

- Pediatric ambulatory surgery • Preoperative evaluation • Discharge criteria
- Asthma • Sleep apnea • Postoperative nausea and vomiting (PONV)

KEY POINTS

- Preoperative evaluation is the lynch pin to have a successful ambulatory practice. Common pediatric issues to assess are asthma, respiratory infections, prematurity, congenital syndromes, sleep apnea, congenital heart disease, and obesity.
- Outcomes for an ambulatory practice can be maximized by looking at risk factors that are associated with worse outcomes and managing them effectively.
- Efficiency is a hallmark for ambulatory surgery centers. After surgery concludes, this must be continued into the recovery phase and evaluated for safe and timely execution.

Ambulatory surgery exploded in the 1990s. The most recent survey by the Center for Disease Control in 2009 indicated that there were 53,329,000 ambulatory surgeries in the United States. Of these, 3.266,000 were done on patients younger than 15 years. The cases were evenly split between freestanding and hospital-based facilities. The cases were largely adenotonsillectomy, myringotomy and tube placements, fracture reductions/fixations, circumcisions, and diagnostic procedures such as endoscopies.[1] Community providers performed most of these cases without specialty training in pediatric anesthesia.

Ambulatory surgery centers (ASC) are defined by the Centers for Medicare and Medicaid Services as any distinct entity that operates exclusively for the purpose of providing surgical services to patients not requiring hospitalization and in which the expected duration of services would not exceed 24 hours following an admission.[2] This limits some procedures, but much of what a pediatric anesthesia practice covers meets these rules. A robust ASC can accommodate subspecialty cases from otolaryngology, orthopedics, general surgery, urology, ophthalmology, plastic surgery, dermatology, dentistry, gastroenterology, and even neurology, radiology, and physiatry.

Disclosures: No disclosures.
[a] Medical College of Wisconsin, Milwaukee, WI, USA; [b] Children's Hospital of Wisconsin Surgicenter, 3223 South 103rd Street, Milwaukee, WI 53227, USA
* Children's Hospital of Wisconsin Surgicenter, 3223 South 103rd Street, Milwaukee, WI 53227.
E-mail address: SButz@mcw.edu

Anesthesiology Clin 37 (2019) 289–300
https://doi.org/10.1016/j.anclin.2019.01.002
anesthesiology.theclinics.com

The success of an ASC depends not only on being prepared for each case with proper staffing and equipment but also on careful patient selection. Ambulatory surgery depends on cases that are predictable with defined risks that can be accounted for. Predictability results not only from routine surgical and anesthesia care but also from patients with well-controlled medical issues. The common things seen in pediatric care that are capable of serious disruption to a surgical schedule are asthma, respiratory infections, congenital heart disease, congenital syndromes, sickle cell anemia, prematurity, and family history of malignant hyperthermia.

ASTHMA

Asthma is the number one chronic illness in children. Patients with reactive airway can certainly tolerate anesthesia, but screening for active disease is important. Asthma is marked by an inflammatory reaction of the airway leading to bronchoconstriction in response to triggers. Common triggers are respiratory infection, exercise, and allergies.

The history should elicit a baseline for treatments and control. Medication history can give an idea of how severe the disease is. Someone just using albuterol as needed has a milder disease than someone who is on maintenance steroids and leukotriene inhibitors with frequent beta agonist use. The medication history may better reflect the care by the caregivers than the disease severity. It is not uncommon to get a history of asthma triggered by respiratory infection in someone who shows up with an obvious respiratory illness. When asked about last inhaler use, the parents tell you it has been months!

A conservative approach to caring for these children begins with the planned surgical procedure and airway management. If the child is having airway surgery and/or planned intubation, giving a nebulizer treatment preoperatively can be beneficial. Patients who have been identified as having active disease on a preoperative phone call or have been recently canceled for illness may benefit from a 3-day course of steroid therapy preoperatively leading up to the day of surgery, but the evidence is not strong.[3] Otherwise, if the patient has an asthma plan with "sick day" care, they can follow that leading up to the day of surgery. If a child arrives ill or with active wheezing, a dose of intravenous (IV) steroids will not have effects until hours afterward and may be of little use in managing the patient in the recovery area after a short procedure.[4]

To get an idea of the spectrum of asthma treatments, a survey of pediatric pulmonologists in Israel demonstrated diversity in pediatric asthma treatment in the perioperative arena. When presented with a scenario of different ages and asthma severity/control, the recommendations varied, but themes emerged. The majority recommends rapid-acting beta agonists and an inhaled steroid course for a child with mild asthma on no long-term controller. A poorly controlled teen on intensive treatment (long-acting beta agonist and inhaled steroids) is surveyed most to receive an oral steroid course. A well-controlled toddler on low-dose inhaled steroids could receive a short-acting beta agonist preoperatively. A poorly controlled toddler on low-dose inhaled steroids was voted to receive an oral steroid course by the majority. The conclusion of the study was that the diversity of answers pointed to the need for an established guideline to be proposed. The overarching theme was that an increase in asthma treatment around the time of surgery was recommended.[5]

The patients should always be given a chance to improve before canceling them on the morning of a procedure. If a patient with asthma shows up with wheezing, they can proceed with surgery if it can be cleared with a nebulizer treatment. If they show up with a fever, unabated wheezing, and/or oxygen saturations below 95% on admission, they tend to be the patients who have desaturations in recovery and require aggressive respiratory therapy to get them stable enough to leave. These patients make up most of the patient transfers at a center.

Patients with asthma also have a disease that is manifestation of an inflammatory state. Thus, other atopic issues may manifest such as anaphylaxis to medications common in anesthesia such as muscle relaxants and antibiotics. Asthma patients with a frequent history of steroid use may require stress steroids. Counterintuitively, they are uniquely at risk for an anaphylactic reaction to IV steroids![3]

RESPIRATORY INFECTION

A practice controversy is what to tell the canceled patient about how soon they can return for surgery. A poll of anesthesiologists revealed that they wait 2 to 4 weeks with most at 4. Studies have supported the fact that the bronchiole tree remains irritated for 4 to 6 weeks after a respiratory illness and 6 weeks is a better choice to wait for a respiratory illness to completely resolve and of course, this all presumes that this is a single illness and that the patient will not get ill again immediately following. Otolaryngology patients have pathology inherent to their disease that puts them at risk for continued nasal congestion and respiratory illness.

The following is a guideline from Tait and Malviya[6] for the approach to a child with a respiratory illness. The first assessment is to see if surgery is emergent or if the rhinitis has a noninfectious cause. If either is yes, you proceed to the next step. Severe symptoms should be delayed. The need for general anesthesia requires a risk/benefit assessment. Things to consider are history of asthma, need for an endotracheal tube, time pressure, and experience of team caring for the child. If the risk assessment is poor for any reason, one should consider delaying the case until the patient's respiratory status returns to baseline. A low-risk assessment can indicate that it is safe to proceed, but the family (and patient when appropriate) needs to be aware of the increased risks for possible respiratory complications.

PREMATURITY

In 1983 the pediatric providers were made aware of the risks of anesthetizing infants with a history of prematurity. There were deaths among premature infants who experienced apnea postoperatively. A flurry of papers helped define what children were at risk, but they used small cohorts and inconsistent definitions of apnea. Postconceptual age (PCA) is an important concept and is defined by the weeks of gestation plus weeks in age. A newer, alternate concept is the postgestational age (PGA) or postmenstrual age (PMA) in which delivery is calculated in weeks from the date of the first day of the mothers last period before becoming pregnant. PGA and PMA are both 2 weeks longer than the PCA. Liu and colleagues[7] defined apnea as 15 to 20 seconds duration and found that the oldest infants to experience apnea had a PCA of 41 weeks. The group headed by Welborn found apnea in infants under 45 weeks PCA, and Kurth's group found apnea in an infant 55 weeks PCA.[8,9] In 1995, Dr Cote combined 8 studies to create a cohort of 255 premature infants. He determined that risk factors for apnea were related to gestational age, postconceptual age, and anemia (hematocrit <30%). He also found that most apnea occurred within 2 hours of an anesthetic but can be as long as 10 to 12 hours in some cases (**Table 1**).[10]

Fortunately, there is little that would be considered surgically appropriate on a premature infant to be done on an ambulatory basis. However, cases of ankyloglossia, extra digits, and eye examinations are possible. Using 60 weeks PCA as a minimum

Table 1
Summary of premature infant and apnea studies

Author and Year	Liu et al,[7] 1983	Welborn et al,[8] 1986	Kurth et al,[9] 1987	Gregory et al,[24] 1983
# of infants (preterm)	214 (41)	86 (38)	47 (49) (2 infants twice)	Editorial in same issue as Liu et al
Def. of apnea	20 s	15 s	15 s (less if bradycardia)	
Oldest with apnea	Under 41 wk PCA, under 4m old	PCA <45 wk	55 w PCA (in group 55–60 w PCA)	
Take home message	Anesthesia may unmask ventilatory defect in preterm infants 41–46 wk PCA	Only preterm infants less than PCA 45 w had postop apneic episodes. Full-term infants had none	Premies <45 w PCA need monitoring 36 h post-op, those 45–60 w PCA need 12–24 h	Monitor premies <45 wk PCA for 18 h. Delay surgery if possible. Be prepared with ventilator.

would exceed all recommendations in the literature for premature infants. Furthermore, using 45 weeks PCA for full-term infants would be prudent. For anyone doing cases on a population this young, it would be wise to have pediatric specialists available and evaluate the entire facility for appropriateness to care for patients this young.

CONGENITAL CARDIAC DISEASE

Children with cardiac disease can be approached in much the same way as adults. Pediatric cardiac patients with heart failure, poor general health (failure to thrive), cyanotic heart disease, or pulmonary hypertension have been shown to be at higher risk for postoperative mortality. Assessing a former cardiac patient can be a challenge in regard for fitness for ambulatory surgery. A strong rule of thumb is to not attempt to anesthetize a child with single-ventricle physiology as an ambulatory patient. These patients have complex physiology that does not tolerate positive-pressure ventilation well and once these patients begin to decompensate, it requires elements typically found in a high-level pediatric intensive care unit or advanced pediatric cardiology team to resuscitate them. Diagnoses that are associated with this type of physiology include hypoplastic left heart syndrome, tricuspid atresia, or pulmonary valve atresia. They also may have a history of a Norwood, Fontan, or hemi-Fontan (Glenn) procedure.[11]

A group at Washington University in St. Louis attempted to stratify risks for cardiac patients having noncardiac surgery. They grouped them to low-, moderate-, and high-risk patients. They looked at 100 consecutive patients but had no complications in any. However, the reasoning they used may be applicable to ambulatory surgery. This group used repaired atrial septal defects (ASDs) and ventricular septal defects (VSDs) or single, mild valvular disease as low risk. Conduction abnormalities, any pulmonary hypertension, heart or lung transplant, unrepaired ASD or VSD, and single-ventricle physiology were classified as moderate risk. High risk included complex, unrepaired lesions, severe valvular disease, New York Heart Association class III or IV, and heart failure. Although not stated, a logical conclusion could be that low-risk patients could tolerate outpatient surgery well, where those at high risk should have surgery where cardiac resources are immediately available. The moderate-risk patients tend to fall into a similar category but may deserve closer evaluation for comorbidities, age, and current illness to see if they would fit in an ambulatory setting. The comfort of the anesthesia and surgical team is also paramount to success.[12]

The rules for giving prophylactic antibiotics to prevent subacute bacterial endocarditis have been simplified as of 2009. They are required only in patients with unrepaired cyanotic lesions, completely repaired congenital heart defects (CHD) with prosthetic material or device during the first 6 months after the procedure, repaired CHD with residual defects at the site or adjacent to the site of a prosthetic patch or prosthetic device (which inhibit endothelialization), or patients with previous endocarditis.[13]

OBESITY

As in the adult population, obesity rates in children are increasing. Although absolute weight and body mass index have become criteria for exclusion from outpatient surgery in adults, the prospect of creating a management paradigm in pediatrics is a little more difficult. Heavy children do not run the same risks of breaking furniture or not fitting through doorways as a 300 or 400 kg adult does. However, a 40-kg toddler has issues to evaluate. Young, obese children are usually very tall for their age, which may be due to insulin acting as growth factor. So the morbidly obese 3-year-old, looks like a 7- or 8-year-old but needs to be treated psychologically like a 3-year-old. The larger height also mitigates some of the issues that just a higher weight may bring, such as positioning, airway management, and drug dosing.

Using the Michigan quality database, a study was done to assess for pediatric obesity-related issues. Obese pediatric patients have significantly more type 2 diabetes, asthma, and hypertension than their thinner cohort. They were also more likely to require 2-handed mask ventilation and need more than 1 direct laryngoscopy for intubation. However, cardiac arrest was not seen in either group. In the recovery room, obese pediatric patients had more airway obstruction, longer length of stay, and need for more than 2 antiemetics. Fortunately, even these issues did not lead to a higher need for unplanned admission.[14]

For the ambulatory surgery world, the risks do not necessarily mean that these patients are not appropriate. As with all ambulatory cases, a thorough preoperative evaluation needs to be done. Obesity has a significant association with obstructive sleep apnea (OSA).[15] Therefore, all obese patients should be screened for OSA as well as comorbidities of asthma, diabetes, and hypertension. OSA coupled with a narcotic-based analgesic plan and/or surgery on the airway is particularly concerning. Metabolic derangements are possible and may be associated with an underlying disease associated with the obesity, such as Cushing syndrome, Prader-Willi syndrome, trisomy 21, hormone therapy, and nephrotic syndrome.

CONGENITAL SYNDROMES

Congenital syndromes can be very troubling especially if they are rarely encountered. Fortunately, there are many sources either online or in print that detail congenital and genetic syndromes far too numerous to list here and their anesthetic implications. When teasing out the implications of a syndrome, it helps to determine if it has a genetic cause or is due to an error in development. For example, a patient with gastroschisis may be similar to one with an omphalocele. However, omphalocele occurs due to a problem with developmental steps; the gut fails to return to the abdominal cavity after rotating in the umbilical stalk. A gastroschisis occurs with the abdominal wall damaged or weakened such as during an ischemic event. Omphalocele can be associated with other genetic errors that are usually not seen in patients with gastroschisis. Examples of developmental issues that are typically in isolation are amniotic band syndrome, fetal alcohol syndrome, and intrauterine strokes.

The genetic syndromes are either inherited or from a spontaneous mutation. Many are quite familiar and represent classic cases in pediatric anesthesia, such as cystic fibrosis, tetralogy of Fallot, Down syndrome, CHARGE syndrome, and glycogen storage diseases. However, some patients with these syndromes may still be appropriate for ambulatory surgery. The key is to recognize the potential issues and assess if the facility is capable of handling them from a staffing and resource point of view. For instance, a tonsil patient with Down syndrome is a common occurrence. Airway obstruction may be multilevel and obstruction from a relatively large tongue may occur in recovery. A capable recovery nursing staff who can recognize and manage this issue is essential. These patients may have difficult IV access, atlantoaxial subluxation, cardiac disease, developmental delay, and perhaps sleep apnea. A competent surgeon and anesthesiologist are required, but the facility must be able to accommodate these patients and their special needs. As with all of ambulatory surgery, anticipating problems and being proactive will be the best practice to avoid poor patient outcomes.

MALIGNANT HYPERTHERMIA

Malignant hyperthermia (MH) is a topic that deserves some special attention. Children are no more at risk than adults except that they usually do not have a history of a prior anesthetic or may not be old enough to demonstrate some of the more subtle manifestations. The disease is autosomal dominant and has been mapped to the RYR1 and CACNA1S genes that code for skeletal muscle proteins involved in calcium transport. Although some mutations have been mapped, thanks to tissue donations from people diagnosed with malignant hyperthermia, there are many more possible. There are blood tests for some of the common genes, but not having a common gene does not mean a person does not have any gene making them susceptible.

Recently, a paper was released that detailed muscular dystrophies and their link to MH. The investigators concluded that 3 types of muscular dystrophy were definitely at risk for MH. The other types still were associated with hyperkalemic arrests and postoperative respiratory failure, but the risk of MH was considered similar to the general population. The 3 types of muscular dystrophy identified are rare and are King-Denborough syndrome, central core myopathy, and multiminicore disease with RYR1 mutation. Keep in mind that treatment of MH in the form of dantrolene has been available for many years, and yet, there are still deaths from this disease.[16]

The Malignant Hyperthermia Association of the United States has created teaching aids to assist in an MH crisis and staff a 24-hour hot line. They also have definite recommendations for equipment an ASC should have available and how susceptible patients should be managed. Part of those recommendations includes having complete treatment dose of dantrolene available (36 vials) or the newer formulations. Susceptible patients should be monitored for 12 hours following the anesthetic even if it is non-triggering. Susceptible patients are those who are at risk for MH either by personal history, genetic testing, or associated neuromuscular disorder, not just because they have a positive relative. With these thoughts in mind, it is easier to establish a policy for allowing MH-susceptible patients in a facility and being consistent with it. A single crisis in a freestanding ASC will quickly use all of the facility's resources (staff and supplies) and will have a large disruption in care given to other patients.

RISK ASSESSMENT

The risk of an adverse event is very real and needs to be actively prevented. As noted earlier, the best way to prevent an adverse event is to be able to predict it. In the adult world, some of these risks have been well studied. This has been just starting in the pediatric realm. One such article by Subramanian, and colleagues,[17] in 2016, used almost 9000 charts to develop risk criteria and then validated it in more than 10,000 more charts. This group was looking at adverse respiratory events including laryngospasm and bronchospasm in the operating room or recovery area, oxygen requirement postoperatively, and apnea. Respiratory adverse events are the leading cause of pediatric codes and deserve special attention when designing a system that limits risk and poor outcomes. A defined set of demographic data was searched. The overall risk of respiratory event was 2.8%. The risks identified on single and multivariate analysis were the following: younger than 3 years, ASA class II or III (no IV in study), preexisting pulmonary disease, morbid obesity, and having a surgical procedure (as opposed to radiologic procedure). Findings that were not significantly associated with a respiratory adverse event were gender and neurologic disease. A grading scale was also developed. A score of 4 or greater out of 8 possible was determined to have a strong negative predictive value and still retain a good specificity and sensitivity for positive finding of an adverse event. A point is assigned for being 3 years old or younger and having an ASA score of II. Two points are given for an ASA score of III, having preexisting pulmonary disease and morbid obesity. Three points are given for a surgical procedure as opposed to a radiology procedure. Because ambulatory surgical cases are all surgical, the focus of an ambulatory center should be on optimizing the other modifiable risk factors, which are summarized in **Table 2**.

Another study from 2016 by Whippey and colleagues[18] looked at risks for transferring pediatric patients from an ASC. The reasons were loosely grouped into anesthesia-related, surgical, social, and medical. The univariate risk factors included

Table 2
Summary of risk factors for adverse respiratory events and risk score assignment

Risk Factor	Significant Univariate Analysis	Significant Multivariate Analysis	Weighted Score
Age	Yes		
Age ≤3 y		No	0
Age >3 y		Yes	1
Gender	No	No	
ASA I	No	No	0
ASA II	Yes	Yes	1
ASA III	Yes	Yes	2
Morbid Obesity	Yes	Yes	2
Pulmonary Disease	Yes	Yes	2
Neurologic Disease	No	No	
Surgical Procedure	Yes	Yes	3
Radiologic Procedure	No	No	0

From Subramanyam R, Yeramaneni S, Hossain MM, et al. Perioperative respiratory adverse events in pediatric ambulatory anesthesia: development and validation of a risk prediction tool. Anesth Analg 2016;122(5):1582; with permission.

the following: age less than 2 years, prescription medication use, gastric reflux disease, OSA, and other comorbidities. On multivariate analysis age less than 2 years, ASA class III or IV, surgery greater than 1 hour, procedure complete after 1500 hours, OSA, orthopedic surgery, dental surgery, ENT surgery, or an intraoperative event all increased risk.

Some of these associated factors can be manipulated by creative scheduling and performing procedures on younger children earlier in the day. Consideration should be made going forward to limit the length of surgeries allowed in day surgery. Although an anesthesia provider cannot make a patient less obese, perhaps other factors can be optimized so that an obese patient who is noncompliant with CPAP use is not scheduled for a 3-hour orthopedic procedure late in the day (**Table 3**).

OBSTRUCTIVE SLEEP APNEA

OSA has been a large concern in the adult ambulatory world. The STOP-BANG grading system for OSA has become a regular part of preadmission screening for adult ambulatory surgery reflecting the work of Francis Chung's group in Toronto. Part of the irony with pediatric patients is that tonsil surgery with sleep-disordered breathing as a primary diagnosis accounts for one of the most frequent outpatient surgeries in children. In fact, data support that the more severe a child's OSA is, the more likely they are to be transferred to a higher level of care postoperatively. The leading diagnosis that precipitates transfer is hypoxia. To address this concern, Tait and colleagues developed a pediatric OSA scoring system known as STBUR.

The STBUR score asks about snoring, trouble breathing, and feeling unrefreshed after sleeping. The 5 questions are as follows:

1. Does the child snore more than half the time?
2. Can snoring be heard through a closed door?
3. Does the patient have pauses in his breathing at night?
4. Does the patient have gasps in her breathing at night?
5. Does the child find it difficult to wake up in the morning or fall asleep during school?

The maximum score is 5. Patients with a score of 3 have a 3-fold greater chance of respiratory complications. A score of 5 indicates a 10 times greater risk. Respiratory complications range widely and can be as mild as desaturations postoperatively so a score of 5/5 does not necessarily mean the patient will need to be admitted, but

Table 3 Summary of risk factors leading to transfer of pediatric patients from ambulatory surgery centers	
Univariate Analysis	**Multivariate Analysis**
• Age <2 y • Prescription medication use • GERD • OSA • Other comorbidities	• Age <2 y • ASA class III or IV • Surgery >1 h • Procedure complete after 1500 h • OSA • Orthopedics, dental, ENT surgery • Intraoperative event

Abbreviation: GERD, gastroesophageal reflux disease.

Data from Whippey A, Kostandoff G, Ma HK, et al. Predictors of unanticipated admission following ambulatory surgery in the pediatric population: a retrospective case-control study. Paediatr Anaesth 2016;26(8):831–7.

higher scores can focus on a provider's attention on the highest-risk patients. The author finds in his practice that the feeling of unrefreshing sleep is the one symptom that distinguishes the patients scoring a 5/5 versus 4/5. Finding a 5/5 score will generate a call from him to the surgeon for more details.[19]

EMERGENCE DELIRIUM

Following surgery, it is expected that excellent outcomes have occurred because the patients have been properly screened and everyone involved is a top pediatric provider. However, there are some things you can expect to see in any pediatric practice whether it is ambulatory or hospital based. Some of those are emergence delirium, postoperative nausea and vomiting, and readiness for recovery. Each episode of postoperative nausea and vomiting (PONV) can delay a discharge by 30 minutes. Likewise, emergence delirium can tie up nursing resources and delay patient discharge for an hour or more. Lastly, having solid criteria for going home can keep the path to leaving better defined and more regular.

Every pediatric anesthesia provider or recovery room nurse has likely experienced a patient with emergence delirium. It is defined as a motor agitation state without awareness of surroundings. Classically, children suffering this will not engage their favorite toy or television show. They also may alternate quickly between parents who are trying to comfort them. The pathology is poorly understood, but there are strong associations (**Box 1**). One of the minor issues is being able to explain this to the parents and what it means for going home and future anesthetics. Physicians tend to minimize these concerns, but they can be quite upsetting to a family.[20]

Somewhat related is the issue of developing posttraumatic stress disorder following an anesthetic. Taking a screaming child back to the operating room can have negative sequela. There can be bedwetting, temper tantrums, sleep disturbances, attention-seeking behaviors, or a new fear of loneliness. The risks are very similar to emergence delirium and may appear in a child who has suffered delirium postoperatively. Any of these risks may appear even months after the attributing anesthetic.

The next logical question is typically how to prevent emergence delirium. There is a frequent tendency to blame preoperative midazolam. However, there are about as many articles implicating midazolam as a cause as there are about exonerating it. Without a clear answer, anesthesia providers must weigh the benefit of the preoperative sedation and amnesia versus the possible risk of delirium. Patients should be screened for delirium risks including a history of delirium with previous anesthetics. Clinically, effective treatment is with a combination of propofol and dexmedetomidine. Take care to keep boluses of dexmedetomidine under 0.5 mcg/kg to avoid hemodynamic depression. The author has used 0.25 mcg/kg of dexmedetomidine IV and 0.5 mg/kg propofol IV with good results. The patient is sedated for 20 to 40 min

---

Box 1
Risk factors for pediatric emergence delirium

Preschool-aged patients

Sevoflurane or desflurane anesthetics

Patient preoperative anxiety

ENT surgery

May be unrelated to pain

with a patent airway. Afterward, the patient wakes much more clearly. Other drugs in the literature used singly in treatment are fentanyl, sufentanil, propofol, dexmedetomidine, ketamine, midazolam, and cloinidine.[20]

POSTOPERATIVE NAUSEA AND VOMITING

Pediatric PONV has a different set of risk factors than adult patients. It tends to be fairly rare in the very young and is associated more with a specific procedure. TJ Gan's group's published risk factor protocol from 2007 is still relevant today. This group identified 4 risk factors, which include surgery greater than 30 minutes, age 3 years or older, strabismus surgery, and personal or family history of PONV. The number of risk factors increases PONV risk nearly arithmetically. Three factors give a greater than 50% chance of PONV.[21]

The treatments follow a similar trend from the adult world. Patients with 2 or more risk factors should receive 2 drugs from different classes for prophylaxis. Treating everyone without regard to risk of PONV may only increase the incidence of side effects seen from the drugs without significantly altering the rate if PONV. As in adults, choices for antiemetics are based on appropriate receptor choice and not simply reusing the same type. In very young patients, the anticholinergic-based ones may be contraindicated. Propofol is still effective as a nonemetic anesthetic choice. However, the risk of narcotics triggering PONV does not seem to be as important in pediatrics as it is in adult patients.

DISCHARGE CRITERIA

Discharge times for patients can be highly variable. A couple of large studies shed some light on keeping them predictable and safe. A group in France led by Moncel looked at more than 1600 ASA class 1 and 2 patients aged 6 months to 16 years. They scored their patients at 1 and 2 hours postoperatively and found that more than 97% met discharge criteria at 1 hour and 99.8% at 2 hours. They used a scoring system that looked at hemodynamics, balance/ambulation, pain scores, PONV rating, respiratory status, and surgical bleeding. They also asked if the family had questions for anesthesia provider. The 2 scores most often associated with delay were respiratory status and questions for the anesthesia provider. Compared with historical control, they were able to consistently reduce discharge times by 69 minutes with less than 1% unexpected admission rate. The use of a scoring system helped them to focus on possible issues delaying discharge and gave an end point for patient care that was previously vague.[22]

Armstrong and colleagues[23] published a Canadian study that combined a scoring using postanesthetic discharge scoring system and Aldrete scores. The group found that physiologic-based criteria improved discharge times over simple, time-based criteria. Approximately 75% were discharged 15 to 45 minutes sooner. About 20% showed no difference. The scoring is similar to Apgar scores with values 0 to 2 assigned, but in this case using 7 domains. A score of 12 or greater indicates readiness for discharge. The domains include consciousness, respiratory status, oxygenation, hemodynamic stability, pain, nausea and vomiting, and incision site. A zero in any of the domains would likely be enough to prevent discharge, but a midscore of mild impairment in 1 or 2 domains would be acceptable for discharge.

Pediatric anesthesia certainly has a place in the ambulatory world. There are a great many cases that can be performed in a freestanding center with few risks of complications. As always, the secret to a successful pediatric ambulatory surgery center is based on wise patient selection, well-trained staff, and the ability to predict and treat complications. Personally speaking, it can be a rewarding practice but can be very labor-intensive and challenging even if patients are ASA class 1 or 2.

REFERENCES

1. Cullen KA, Hall MJ, Golosinskiy A. Ambulatory surgery in the United States, 2006. Natl Health Stat Report 2009;(11):1–25.
2. Federal register/monday/rules and regulations Vol. 76, No. 205, Washington, DC, 2011.
3. Doherty GM, Chisakuta A, Crean P, et al. Anesthesia and the child with asthma. Paediatr Anaesth 2005;15(6):446–54.
4. Maxwell LG, Yaster M. Perioperative management issues in pediatric patients. Anesthesiol Clin North America 2000;18(3):601–32.
5. Armoni-Domany K, Gut G, Soferman R, et al. Pediatric pulmonologists approach to the pre-operative management of the asthmatic child. J Asthma 2014;52(4): 391–7.
6. Tait AR, Malviya S. Anesthesia for the child with an upper respiratory tract infection: still a dilemma? Anesth Analg 2005;100(1):59–65.
7. Liu LM, Coté CJ, Goudsouzian NG, et al. Life-threatening apnea in infants recovering from anesthesia. Anesthesiology 1983;59(6):506–10.
8. Welborn LG, Ramirez N, Oh TH, et al. Postanesthetic apnea and periodic breathing in infants. Anesthesiology 1986;65(6):658–61.
9. Kurth CD, Spitzer AR, Broennie AM, et al. Postoperative apnea in preterm infants. Anesthesiology 1987;31(5):298.
10. Coté CJ, Zaslavsky A, Downes JJ, et al. Postoperative apnea in former preterm infants after inguinal herniorrhaphy. Surv Anesthesiology 1996;40(3):163.
11. Veyckemans F, Momeni M. The patient with a history of congenital heart disease who is to undergo ambulatory surgery. Curr Opin Anaesthesiol 2013;26(6): 685–91.
12. Saettele AK, Christensen JL, Chilson KL, et al. Children with heart disease: risk stratification for non-cardiac surgery. J Clin Anesth 2016;35:479–84.
13. Cannesson M, Earing MG, Collange V, et al. Anesthesia for noncardiac surgery in adults with congenital heart disease. Anesthesiology 2009;111(2):432–40.
14. Nafiu OO, Reynolds PI, Bamgbade OA, et al. Childhood body mass index and perioperative complications. Paediatr Anaesth 2007;17(5):426–30.
15. Mortensen A, Lenz K, Abildstrøm H, et al. Anesthetizing the obese child. Paediatr Anaesth 2011;21(6):623–9.
16. Gurnaney H, Brown A, Litman RS, et al. Malignant hyperthermia and muscular dystrophies. Anesth Analgesia 2009;109(4):1043–8.
17. Subramanyam R, Yeramaneni S, Hossain MM, et al. Perioperative respiratory adverse events in pediatric ambulatory anesthesia: development and validation of a risk prediction tool. Anesth Analgesia 2016;122(5):1570–85.
18. Whippey A, Kostandoff G, Ma HK, et al. Predictors of unanticipated admission following ambulatory surgery in the pediatric population: a retrospective case-control study. Paediatr Anaesth 2016;26(8):831–7.
19. Tait AR, Voepel-Lewis T, Christensen R, et al. The STBUR questionnaire for predicting perioperative respiratory adverse events in children at risk for sleep-disordered breathing. Paediatr Anaesth 2013;23(6):510–6.
20. Dahmani S, Delivet H, Hilly J. Emergence delirium in children: an update. Curr Opin Anaesthesiol 2014;27(3):309–15.

21. Gan TJ, Meyer TA, Apfel CC, et al. Society for ambulatory anesthesia guidelines for the management of postoperative nausea and vomiting. Anesth Analgesia 2007;105(6):1615–28.
22. Moncel JB, Nardi N, Wodey E, et al. Evaluation of the pediatric post anesthesia discharge scoring system in an ambulatory surgery unit. Paediatr Anaesth 2015;25(6):636–41.
23. Armstrong J, Forrest H, Crawford MW. A prospective observational study comparing a physiological scoring system with time-based discharge criteria in pediatric ambulatory surgical patients. Can J Anaesth 2015;62(10):1082–8.
24. Gregory GA, Steward DJ. Life-threatening perioperative apnea in the ex-"premie". Anesthesiology 1983;59(6):495–8.

Nonoperating Room Anesthesia

Anesthesia in the Gastrointestinal Suite

Sekar S. Bhavani, MD[a],*, Basem Abdelmalak, MD[b,c]

KEYWORDS

- NORA GI Suite • General anesthesia • MAC • NPO • DNR

KEY POINTS

- There is a pressing need for a careful and comprehensive preanesthetic clinical evaluation of the patient to develop an anesthetic plan that takes into consideration the facility, competence of the personnel involved, and the constraints of the system.
- Monitoring of ventilation (more so than oxygenation) during gastrointestinal endoscopy has been recognized as an area of extreme interest and patient safety focus.
- Airway management and monitoring may be challenging but the need for securing the airway with an endotracheal tube is not always essential.

The past decade has seen an increase in nonoperating room anesthesia (NORA) sites and services that have brought together the infrastructure, personnel, patients, and procedural requirements to facilitate efficient and safe patient care. Emphasis on cost reduction, efficiency, and expansion of subspecialties has contributed to this trend in the United States. Nagrebetsky and colleagues[1] showed that, in both hospital-based and nonhospital-based settings, of all analyzed procedures, the use of anesthesia services in the gastrointestinal (GI) suite increased from 10.8% to 17.3% between 2010 and 2014. At the same time, there was almost a 4-fold increase in volume and a higher number of older and sicker patients.[1] With the increasing number, complexity, and the acuity of the endoscopic procedures in the last decade, there has been an increased recognition of the need and the value for the use of anesthesia services in both diagnostic and therapeutic procedures. The aging population; presence of significant comorbidities; and the need to provide efficient, timely, and safe

Disclosure Statement: No conflict of interest.
[a] Department of General Anesthesiology, Cleveland Clinic, 9500 Euclid Avenue, Cleveland, OH 44195, USA; [b] Department of General Anesthesiology, Anesthesia for Bronchoscopic Surgery, Center for Sedation, Cleveland Clinic, 9500 Euclid Avenue, Cleveland, OH 44195, USA; [c] Department of Outcomes Research, Cleveland Clinic, 9500 Euclid Avenue, Cleveland, OH 44195, USA
* Corresponding author.
E-mail address: bhavans@ccf.org

Anesthesiology Clin 37 (2019) 301–316
https://doi.org/10.1016/j.anclin.2019.01.010
1932-2275/19/© 2019 Elsevier Inc. All rights reserved.

anesthesiology.theclinics.com

care have placed a large responsibility on the shoulders of the anesthesia team. In addition, in the last decade, there has been a significant shift from a mere diagnostic workup to therapeutic procedures.

PATIENT SELECTION

When determining if the GI NORA site is appropriate for a given patient, several factors need to be considered, not only those that affect patients' safety but also their convenience and satisfaction. Furthermore, procedural requirements, as well as the proceduralist and anesthesiologists' level of expertise and scheduling efficiencies, should be considered. Apfelbaum and Cutter[2] have emphasized the need to match the patient, procedure, and providers with the service setting.

A unique feature of most endoscopy units is that they often have open scheduling. The patients are referred to the proceduralist for an advanced endoscopy service and, more often than not, they have not had any physician–patient relationship with the endoscopist before this referral. Often, the referring service is not aware of the unique requirements for the procedure, particularly when a deep sedation or general anesthesia is warranted.[3] This imposes an added responsibility on the anesthesiologists to ensure that the patient is optimally prepared for the planned procedure (**Box 1**).

The anesthesiologist should obtain an informed consent for the anesthetic component of the procedure. At this time, it is important that the benefits, risks, limitations of the proposed anesthetic plan, and the alternatives be discussed. The final decision should address the level of sedation targeted commensurate with the patient's expectation and safety.

Do Not Resuscitate Status

Patients sometimes present to the endoscopy suite with a do not resuscitate (DNR) order in place. It is important to understand that the endoscopy procedure may provide significant benefit in terms of patient comfort even if there is no impact on the natural history of the underlying disease process. Anesthesia in patients with terminal disease is fraught with the danger of correctable cardiopulmonary instability in the perioperative period. The current thought is that disregarding or automatically canceling these orders does not support a patient's right to self-determination.[4,5] It

---

Box 1
Preanesthetic evaluation

The goals of the preanesthetic evaluation in the GI suite
1. Is the patient optimized for the procedure in relation to procedural and anesthetic requirements?
2. Are there any comorbidities that make it unsafe to perform the procedure in the NORA setting?
3. What is the depth of sedation or anesthesia that needs to be achieved?
4. Are there any allergies or intolerances that limit the use of the medications intended?
5. Is the position of the patient conducive to emergent access of the airway in case of a problem?
6. Is there a need for the airway to be protected by an endotracheal tube?
7. Is there adequate back-up (both infrastructure and personnel) available to address patient safety?
8. Will there be a need for blood or blood product transfusion?
9. Are there any final disposition problems that need to be addressed?
10. Is this the safest and most efficient way to address the care needs?

is important to have a discussion with the patient or his or her health power of attorney agent regarding the normal actions, such as use of vasoactive medications, intubation, and ventilation, that are an integral part of the intraoperative anesthetic care, and a care plan in line with the patient's wishes should be reached.[4,6] Any modifications to the DNR status should be documented in the patient's records and the plan for reinstatement should also be clarified and documented.[4,6] In case of a conflict, the help of the hospital's ethics and/or legal departments should be sought.[5]

Anesthetic Management

The anesthetic technique is dictated by the acuity of the problem, procedure planned, patient-related issues, nil per os (NPO) status, pregnancy status, and findings in the preanesthetic evaluation. The factors that often contribute to the authors' decision are listed in **Box 2**.

Fasting Before Gastrointestinal Procedures

NPO recommendations are meant to minimize the risk of aspiration, which is thought to have an incidence of about 1 in 2000 to 3000 anesthetics in adults, with a slightly higher risk of 1 in 1200 to 1 in 2600 in children. The most recent American Society of Anesthesiologists (ASA) NPO guidelines recommend a minimum of 2 and 8 hours of fasting for clear liquids and heavy meals, respectively, before anesthesia.[7] These recommendations are intended for healthy patients scheduled for elective procedures. It is controversial how to apply these recommendations to patients with coexisting conditions such as delayed gastric emptying and/or difficult airway.[7]

The diagnostic yield of a colonoscopy depends on a clean colon at the time of examination. In 2014, a large meta-analysis by Bucci and colleagues[8] demonstrated the clinical superiority and patient acceptability of splitting the total dose of the bowel cleansing solution into 2 doses, half given the day before and half on the day of the examination, and this has been borne out by other studies as well.[9–11] The efficacy of the split dosing is as high as 85% compared with 63% following a single large dose and is independent of the type of preparation method used.[8] This large meta-analysis also demonstrated that the advantage of split dosing is maintained for only 5 hours, the so-called 5 golden hours. A recent study by Tandon and colleagues[12] has shown that the residual gastric volume as measured by endoscopy direct suctioning did not differ between split dose and a single dose (the night before) preparation for colonoscopy. For more thorough discussion of this topic, the reader is referred to the original article and the accompanying editorial.[13]

MONITORING

The ASA guidelines for monitoring patients under moderate sedation emphasizes the need for monitoring patient level of consciousness, ventilation (using capnography), oxygenation (pulse oximetry), and hemodynamics (using a noninvasive blood pressure cuff and, when appropriate, an electrocardiogram). A continuous record of these parameters should be maintained and an individual should be available and responsible for patient monitoring.[14]

In 2009, Metzner and colleagues[15] investigated the risk and safety of administering anesthesia at NORA locations by querying the ASA closed claims between 2000 and 2009. Their analysis suggested that almost 50% of all claims involved the use of monitored anesthesia care. Adverse respiratory events were more common at the NORA locations (44% vs 20%) compared with the operating room (OR) claims.

Box 2
Factors that affect the choice of anesthetic technique in the gastrointestinal suite

- Emergent, urgent, or elective
- Allergies
- Pregnancy status
- Age and frailty
- NPO status
- Comorbidities
  - Morbid obesity
  - Cardiac
    - Hypertension or hypotension
    - Ischemic symptoms
    - Congestive heart failure
    - Rhythm disturbances
    - Presence of pacemakers and/or defibrillators
    - LVAD and ECMO
  - Respiratory
    - Restrictive or obstructive lung disease
    - Obstructive sleep apnea
    - COPD
    - Active smoking
  - Gastrointestinal
    - Reflux
    - GI bleeding
    - Gastroparesis
    - Abdominal surgery
    - Intestinal obstruction
  - Neurologic
    - Stroke
    - Seizures
    - Loss of consciousness
  - Renal and electrolyte imbalance
    - Need for renal replacement therapy
    - Last dialysis session and fluid balance
  - Diabetes
    - Degree of control
  - Hematological
    - Bleeding tendencies
    - Anticoagulation history
  - Substance abuse
    - Type, duration, and time interval from last exposure
- Prior anesthetic history
  - Airway issues
  - Complications

Abbreviations: COPD, chronic obstructive pulmonary disease; ECMO, extracorporeal membrane oxygenation; LVAD, left ventricular assist device.

Inadequate oxygenation and ventilation accounted for 22% versus 3% of all cases, respectively, and were judged to be preventable in 32% versus 8%, respectively, in the OR claims.

Thus, monitoring of ventilation and oxygenation during GI endoscopy has been recognized as an area of extreme interest and patient safety focus. Pulse oximetry has been shown to be a poor surrogate to monitor ventilation. The inherent lag time of pulse oximetry desaturation can lead to a significant delay in detection of hypoventilation, particularly when supplemental oxygen is used.[16,17]

Therefore, end tidal carbon monoxide ($EtCO_2$) monitoring of ventilation was mandated by the ASA in 2010 for all patients undergoing moderate and deep sedation unless precluded or invalidated by the nature of the patient, procedure, or equipment. Monitoring ventilation with $EtCO_2$ is more effective than physical visualization of chest excursions or pulse oximetry.[18] Upper endoscopies, however, do not lend themselves to a consistent, reliable, and accurate monitoring of $EtCO_2$ because the airway is shared. In addition, the use of carbon dioxide (CO_2) for insufflation also interferes with accuracy due to sampling error or contamination.[19] Moreover, the position of the patient, lack of direct visualization due to dimmed lights, and the positioning of the proceduralist and the endoscopy video monitors interfere with visual monitoring of chest wall movement and air exchange. Additional options to monitor ventilation include monitoring changes in the humidity with respiration[20] (respiR8 & Anaxsys Technology Ltd, Woking, UK), changes in temperature (Dymedix, Shoreview, MN, USA), apnea monitoring[21,22] (Masimo RRa, Irvine, CA), inductance plethysmography[23] (ExSpiron Respiratory Volume Monitor, Waltham, MA, USA), time of flight depth sensors, photoplethysmography, and transcutaneous CO_2 monitoring (SenTec Digital Monitoring System, Rostock, Germany).[19]

In 2017, Woodward and colleagues[24] revisited the incidence of NORA malpractice claims and concluded that the patients were older, had a higher ASA physical status (PS) class, and monitored anesthesia care was more commonly used at these sites (69% vs 9%). Adverse respiratory events were still the leading cause of injury (53% of claims). Inadequate oxygenation or ventilation and aspiration were proportionately higher in the NORA setting compared with the OR. Complications occurred more frequently at the cardiology and radiology locations compared with the GI suite.

Sedation Options

Most of the patients who present for a routine screening endoscopy are healthy and have very few comorbidities. A few of them may be able to undergo endoscopy without the use of any sedation or analgesia using topical anesthesia alone. Most patients request or require moderate (conscious) sedation with the use of an opioid and an anxiolytic, which is considered by many as the standard of care for screening and simple diagnostic endoscopy.[25,26] Mild to moderate sedation is used for patient comfort, amnesia, and to prevent untoward reactions such as gagging, retching, and chocking (in upper endoscopy), and thus facilitate completeness of the examination.

Sedation is a continuum: patients can slip into a deeper than intended plane and eventually to the stage of general anesthesia (**Table 1**).[27] The challenge is compounded because, not only are patients' responses to the medications unpredictable, they can be affected by preexisting comorbidities, prior exposure, and history of substance abuse. The depth of sedation requirement varies with the degree of stimulation during different stages of the procedure and these changes can be quite sudden. Therefore, when moderate sedation is used, careful titration of sedation medications is strongly recommended and specific antagonists of opiates (naloxone) and benzodiazepines (flumazenil) should be available for rescuing the patients.[26] Most advanced endoscopic procedures are carried out under deep sedation or general anesthesia. The ASA has also mandated that all patients under moderate and deep sedation should be monitored with an $EtCO_2$ to prevent ventilatory insufficiency and cardiovascular collapse,[14] a position not shared by the American Society for Gastrointestinal Endoscopies, the American College of Gastroenterology, and the American Gastroenterological Association.[28]

Table 1
Definition of general anesthesia and levels of sedation or analgesia

	Anxiolysis	Moderate Sedation	Deep Sedation	General Anesthesia
Response to Verbal and Tactile Stimulation	Normal	Purposeful	Purposeful after repeated stimulation	No response
Cognitive Function and Physical Coordination	May be impaired	Impaired	Absent	Absent
Airway	Maintained	Usually maintained	Intervention may be required	Needs to be supported
Ventilation	Unaffected	Adequate	May be inadequate	Frequently inadequate
Cardiovascular Function	Unaffected	Usually maintained	Usually maintained	May be impaired

Adapted from American Society of Anesthesiologists. Continuum of depth of sedation: definition of general anesthesia and levels of sedation/analgesia. Committee on Quality Management and Departmental Administration. 2014. Available at: https://www.asahq.org/standards-and-guidelines/continuum-of-depth-of-sedation-definition-of-general-anesthesia-and-levels-of-sedationanalgesia. Accessed January 9, 2019; with permission.

MEDICATIONS

Medications used for anesthesia and sedation in the endoscopy suite have to share some common features. They have to have a rapid onset and offset, should not cause any major cardiovascular instability, and should not increase the incidence of postoperative nausea and vomiting. It was a common practice to use a combination of benzodiazepine (midazolam), opioid (fentanyl), and an anticholinergic in the preoperative period as part of the premedication. With an increased realization that both benzodiazepines and opioids may increase the incidence of aspiration by interfering with the pharyngeal function, their routine use is now limited in upper endoscopies.[29]

The medications commonly used fall into 1 of the classes of drugs shown in **Table 2**.

The combination of the medications is often a personal preference based on experience. In most instances, when the moderate sedation is provided by the endoscopist, a combination of an anxiolytic (midazolam) with an opioid (meperidine or fentanyl) is commonly used.

AIRWAY MANAGEMENT

Because most of the patient's airway patency, reflexes, and ventilation drive are well preserved with anxiolysis or mild sedation, patients can usually be safely managed without any airway support. However, when a deeper plane of sedation or general anesthesia is reached, it may become necessary to support and protect the airway. Even under deep sedation, spontaneous ventilation may be preserved but may require some sort of airway support to maintain adequate gas exchange. Maneuvers used to maintain the patency of the airway include chin lift, jaw thrust, neck extension, or the use of a nasal airway when the patient is supine or in a lateral position. The prone position can help prevent airway obstruction by allowing the tongue to fall forward but access to the airway is limited (**Fig. 1**). Unlike in the main OR, it is possible to quickly abort the procedure and intubate the patient. However, the airway management in a nonintubated patient in a prone position can be more challenging.

Table 2
Medications commonly used in the gastrointestinal suite

Class	Medications	Characteristics
Anticholinergics	Glycopyrrolate	• Synthetic anticholinergic medication • Decreases salivary, tracheobronchial, and pharyngeal secretions • Usual dose of 0.2–0.4 mg • Usually produces xerostomia, mydriasis, photophobia, and tachycardia, and may produce mental confusion in older adults • Use with caution in the presence of uncorrected ischemic heart disease
Anxiolysis, Sedatives, or Hypnotics	Midazolam[30]	• Anxiolytic with antegrade amnesia • Preferred over diazepam due to its shorter duration of action • The usual dose varies from 0.5–2 mg bolus • May be repeated every 2–5 min • Onset is within 2–5 min and rapid offset to when patient is fully alert: 15.8 min[31] • Complete offset: 6.1 h[31] • It can cause respiratory depression when combined with an opioid • Paradoxic hyperactive or aggressive behavior may be seen in pediatric and geriatric patients and in patients with a history of alcohol abuse • Dose should be decreased in the elderly, obese, and in patients with deranged hepatic and renal function
Opioids	Meperidine[30]	• Analgesic sedative with no amnestic properties • Onset of action: 1–5 min, offset: 1–3 h • Usual starting dose is 25–50 mg intravenous (IV) • May be repeated with 25 mg every 2–5 min • Respiratory depression that is increased when combined with propofol, benzodiazepines, antihistaminics, MAO inhibitors, and phenothiazines • Can cause accumulation of normeperidine. which can induce seizures in patients with renal dysfunction
—	Fentanyl	• Analgesic and sedative with no amnestic properties • Onset of action: 2–5 min and offset: 30–60 min • Usually upper limit of 5mcg/kg should not be exceeded • Causes respiratory depression that is increased when combined with propofol or midazolam • May cause chest wall rigidity and interfere with ventilation in high doses • Does not cause histamine release
—	Remifentanil	• Analgesic and sedative with no amnestic properties • Used as a continuous infusion • Very quick onset and offset • No accumulation even after prolonged use • Can cause hyperalgesia

(continued on next page)

Table 2
(continued)

Class	Medications	Characteristics
Anesthetic Drugs	Propofol	• Most commonly used agent for deep sedation or general anesthesia • Very rapid onset (30–45 s) and offset (4–8 min) • Intermittent boluses titrated to effect, starting 20–60 mg bolus followed by 10–30 mg every minute • As an infusion (preferred) 100–150 mcg/kg/min and titrated to affect • Very strong antiemetic and antipruritic properties • Can cause pain on injection • Produces dose-dependent hypotension and respiratory depression • When used with benzodiazepines or opioids, respiratory depression may become profound • Interferes with swallowing and integrity of the upper airway • Dose should be adjusted in advanced age, presence of comorbidities, and hypovolemic patients
—	Fospropofol[32,33]	• Like propofol, shares the 2,6-diisopropyl phenol entity • Fospropofol is hydrolyzed by endothelial alkaline phosphatases and converted to propofol • Onset of action 4–8 min • Offset: 5–18 min • Produces transient perineal paresthesia and pruritus • Concern for oversedation approaching general anesthesia and respiratory depression when used for sedation due to dose-stacking secondary to its slow onset and cardiovascular effect seen with higher doses
—	Ketamine	• Is an NMDA agonist • More commonly used in the pediatric population • Produces dissociative anesthesia • Dose depends on route ○ IV: initial 1.5–2 mg/kg IV followed by 0.5–1 mg/kg ○ Intramuscular (IM): 3–5 mg/kg IM • Onset of action: 5 min • Effect lasts for: 20–30 min • Premedication with midazolam and an antisialagogue is recommended
—	Ketofol	• Introduced as a combination of propofol and ketamine • Considerable heterogeneity in the combination ratios • Stable when combined with each other • Rationale is to decrease the incidence of either drugs by using a smaller dose[34] • Onset is fast but offset may be slightly delayed • No clear-cut advantage in preventing respiratory or cardiovascular complications has been demonstrated
Newer Drugs	Remimazolam[35]	• Is in phase 3 trial • Midazolam is the parent compound • Properties are similar to benzodiazepines albeit with a much shorter duration of action • Rapid onset: 3 min[31] and rapid offset to when patient is fully alert: 7.35 min • Complete offset: 3.2 h

Abbreviations: MAO, monoamino oxidase; NMDA, N-methyl-D-aspartate.

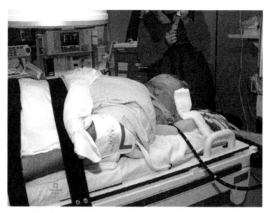

Fig. 1. Esophagogastroduodenoscopy in the prone position using propofol-induced deep sedation or general anesthesia, and maintaining capnography-monitored spontaneous ventilation. (*Courtesy of* Cleveland Clinic Center for Medical Art & Photography. All Rights Reserved. © 2018; with permission.)

AIRWAY ADJUNCTS

Airway adjuncts are occasionally required to facilitate monitoring of the $EtCO_2$ or for ventilation. These have included modified bite blocks with sampling ports in the mouth and the nose, face masks modified for allowing ventilation, $EtCO_2$ monitoring and the introduction of the endoscope, nasopharyngeal airway, nasal continuous positive airway pressure ventilator to stent the airways open, high-flow oxygen nasal cannulas, gastro-laryngeal tube (VBM Medical, Inc, Noblesville, IN, USA), and gastroLMA (Teleflex, Wayne, PA, USA). These can be used either for primary airway management in selected patients or as a rescue device in an emergency. Securing the airway for an endoscopy should not be thought of as a failure on the part of the anesthesiologist. Intubation is the safest way to ensure protection of the airway should regurgitation occur (**Fig. 2**). **Box 3** summarizes some of the most common indications for intubation in the GI endoscopy suite.

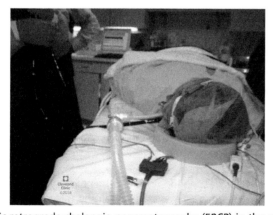

Fig. 2. Endoscopic retrograde cholangio-pancreatography (ERCP) in the prone position using propofol-induced general anesthesia with controlled ventilation through an endotracheal tube. (*Courtesy of* Cleveland Clinic Center for Medical Art & Photography. All Rights Reserved. © 2018; with permission.)

Box 3
Indications for intubation in gastrointestinal endoscopy

- Patient-related
  - Emergency
  - Significant cardiac or respiratory comorbidities
  - Sepsis
  - Intestinal obstruction (esophagus, stomach, duodenum, or small or large intestines)
  - Anatomic problems
    - Complex anatomy
    - Short gut syndrome
    - Zenker diverticulum
    - Short Roux-en-Y loop
    - Large hiatus hernia
  - Morbid obesity

- Procedure-related
  - Long duration of procedure (usually the arbitrary cutoff is >60 minutes)
  - Complex procedure
  - Drainage of a pancreatic pseudocyst
  - Use of large volume of fluid irrigant
  - Double balloon

- Anesthesia-related
  - Known difficult intubation
  - Inadequate NPO duration
  - Retained food
  - CO_2 use during the endoscopy

Use of Carbon Dioxide

One of the perquisites of safe completion of endoscopy is the distension of the bowel to prevent injury from the scope. There is an increased realization that the use of air is associated with pain, distension, and bloating because the insufflated air can be evacuated only by belching or flatus.[36,37] This discomfort sometimes persists for over 24 hours.[36] CO_2 is rapidly absorbed from the GI tract across the mucosa and excreted through the lungs. The absorption of CO_2 is much faster than the inert nitrogen (the major component of room air). However, because of the potential risk of hypercarbia, it has been suggested that some form of CO_2 monitoring should be considered. This is of particular importance when the airway is being shared, as in upper endoscopies.[36] Though it has been stated that "CO_2 insufflation appears to be well tolerated even in patients with underlying pulmonary disease,"[36] this has not been the authors' experience at our institution. Our patient population has been slower to wake up following the discontinuation of propofol sedation and, in a few instances, the patients have become drowsy and needed ventilatory support after return to the recovery area. Blood gas analysis in all these patients who needed active airway intervention has demonstrated significant hypercapnia (Pco_2 >60).

Carbon Dioxide and Gas Embolism

Gas embolism has been described most commonly after ERCP and endoscopic necrosectomy.[36] The systemic effects depend on the rate and volume of air that is entrained into the circulation.[38] This not uncommonly occurs at the end of the procedure when the patient is turned back to a supine position from prone. CO_2 embolism is thought to be better tolerated than air embolism due to its faster clearance from the blood.

Endoscopy in Patients on Anticoagulants

Some patients who present for an endoscopy may be on an anticoagulant or an antiplatelet agent for a comorbid condition. For diagnostic procedures it may not be essential to discontinue the anticoagulants. In contrast, continuing the oral anticoagulants in patients scheduled for a therapeutic endoscopy, such as polypectomy, ERCP with sphincterotomy, ampullectomy, endoscopic mucosal resection, stenting of the esophagus, small or large bowel, has been shown to be associated with a higher risk of GI bleeding.[39] However, discontinuation of the anticoagulant may place the patient at an increased risk of thromboembolism.[40] Hence, it is essential that the anesthesiologist, proceduralist, and the hematologist managing the anticoagulation have a plan in place before the procedure. The current practice for preoperative discontinuation of commonly encountered agents is shown in **Table 3**.

ENDOSCOPY IN PATIENTS WITH PERMANENT PACEMAKERS OR IMPLANTABLE CARDIOVERTER-DEFIBRILLATORS

It is not uncommon to undertake an endoscopy in a patient who has a permanent pacemaker, cardiac resynchronization device, or a defibrillator. It is important that, as part of the initial patient evaluation, the anesthesiologist determine the underlying rhythm, indication for, degree of dependence, programmed parameters, presence of rate responsiveness, and trigger and location of the device.[41] It is also essential

Table 3
Anticoagulants and management before the endoscopy

Agent Type	Agent	Discontinue before Elective Procedure	In Case of Emergency Consider Procedure
Antiplatelets	Aspirin	7 d	Hold, consider platelet transfusion
	Nonsteroidal antiinflammatory drugs	5–7 d	Hold
Thienopyridines	Clopidogrel	5–7 d	—
	Ticlopidine	10–14 d	—
GPIIb, IIIa inhibitors	Tirofiban	Hold	Hold
	Abciximab	24 h	Hold
	Eptifibatide	4 h	Hold
Anticoagulants	Coumadin	5 d	Vitamin K, FFP
	Heparin	4–6 h	Protamine
	Low-molecular-weight heparin	24 h from last dose	Protamine, rVIIa
Direct-acting Xa inhibitors	Xarelto and Eliquis	Hold 1–4 d depending on renal function	Charcoal-activated or nonactivated PCC
Direct-acting thrombin inhibitors	Pradaxa	Hold 1–3 d for procedures with moderate risk Hold 2–6 d for high-risk procedures	Charcoal-activated or nonactivated PCC, hemodialysis

Abbreviations: FFP, fresh frozen plasma; GPIIb, glycoprotein IIb; rVIIa, recombinant factor VIIa; Xa, factor Xa Stuart–Prower factor.

Adapted from ASGE Standards of Practice Committee, Acosta RD, Abraham NS, et al. The management of antithrombotic agents for patients undergoing GI endoscopy. Gastrointest Endosc 2016;83(1):4; with permission.

that the device be checked by the electrophysiology service at the site where the procedure is being carried out well in advance of the day of the procedure so that they can monitor, reprogram, or disable the device on the day of procedure if required.

In most instances when prolonged use of the cautery is not anticipated, it will not be necessary to change the parameters of a permanent pacemaker.[41,42] Intraoperative monitoring and vigilance would be the key to prevent any untoward event. To prevent electrical and electromagnetic interference when using an electrocautery tool, use of bipolar equipment set at the lowest possible energy level, used in short bursts lasting less than 5 seconds, and the placement of the grounding pad remote from the site of the implanted pacemaker is recommended.

In the presence of an implantable cardioverter-defibrillator (ICD), it may be prudent to involve the electrophysiology service to decide if there is a need for reprogramming the ICD to inactivate the tachyarrhythmia detection for the duration of the procedure. It is then necessary to have an external defibrillation pad attached to the patient for the duration of the procedure until the unit is reprogrammed. In case of an emergency, a magnet placed on the device could be helpful if that parameter has not been disabled.[41,42]

Postoperative Complications and Gastrointestinal Anesthesia Safety

Patients who undergo endoscopy are within a wide range of ASA PS classes. They include healthy adults coming for a screening endoscopy, patients with significant comorbidities, or patients on comfort care who are being offered the procedure as the last resort for relief of pain or suffering. There is evidence that patients presenting to remote locations have a higher acuity and a higher ASA PS class (37.6% and 33.0%, respectively) compared with those in the main OR.[1] Yet the overall complication rate is still very low.

Behrens and colleagues[43] reviewed 368,206 electronic charts from 39 GI centers (ProSed 2 Study) between 2011 and 2014. Of the 89% of patients who had some form of sedation for their endoscopy, the incidence of minor complications, major complications, and death were 0.3%, 0.01%, and 0.005%, respectively. ASA class, and type and duration of the procedure were significant factors for adverse outcome (**Box 4**).

More recently, reports in the GI literature suggest that proceduralist-directed sedation is safer than anesthesia services for GI procedures. Wernli and colleagues[44] examined 3,168,228 patients undergoing routine colonoscopies from 2008 through 2011 using the Truven Health Analytics Marketscan Research Databases and concluded that the overall risk of adverse outcome was higher in patients who had anesthesia personnel involved in their care. They also concluded that the incidence of bleeding and perforation were higher in anesthesia-assisted colonoscopies. A study from Bielawska and colleagues,[45] using data from a population-based cohort study, looked at outpatient colonoscopy in Ontario, Canada, between 2005 and 2012 and concluded that loss of feedback from the patient during colonoscopies was the primary cause of an increased incidence of perforation and splenic injury They also concluded that, given the challenge of controlling the depth of anesthesia in the continuum to sedation, the use of anesthesia personnel could be associated with a higher incidence of aspiration pneumonia due to a deeper plane of sedation than planned. These reports are database studies that suffer from many of the common shortcomings of retrospective studies (bias and uncontrolled confounding). The readers are reminded also that association (or correlation) is not causation. In 2017, Vargo and colleagues[46] analyzed 1,388,235 patients undergoing esophagogastroduodenoscopies and colonoscopies between 2002 and 2013 by querying the Clinical Outcomes Research Initiative National Endoscopic Database. They concluded that

---

Box 4
Postoperative complications

- Minor complications
  - PONV
  - Pain
  - Hemodynamic instability needing minimal intervention
    - Hypotension (drop in systolic BP >25%)
    - Bradycardia (drop of >20%)
    - Tachycardia (increase of >100 bpm)
  - Desaturation (SaO2 <90% for >10 seconds)
  - Irritability
  - Minor allergic reactions

- Major complications
  - Life-threatening allergic reactions
  - Airway issues
    - Airway edema
    - Laryngospasm
    - Aspiration and bronchospasm
    - Hypercarbia
  - Delayed awakening
  - Acute pancreatitis
  - Mucosal tears
  - Perforation

Abbreviations: BP, blood pressure; bpm, beats per minute; PONV, postoperative nausea and vomiting; SaO2, oxygen saturation.

---

anesthesiologist-directed sedation and endoscopist-directed sedation were associated with similar risks of significant adverse events following colonoscopies but higher risk in upper endoscopies. However, concluding that any technique is safer than another requires more rigorous research, such as a well-designed randomized trial of sufficient power.

SUMMARY

Endoscopic gastroenterology has exponentially advanced and grown in the last 2 decades. Simpler procedures continue to be performed in free-standing ambulatory surgery centers; however, the more complex ones are performed in NORA locations within the hospital because of the increasing complexity of the procedures and the comorbidities of the patients. Anesthesiologists are now involved more than ever in caring for these patients. Careful review and understanding of the inherent risks for patients and of procedures is extremely helpful to guide anesthesiologists to formulate and deliver a safe anesthetic plan and management.

REFERENCES

1. Nagrebetsky A, Gabriel RA, Dutton RP, et al. Growth of nonoperating room anesthesia care in the United States: a contemporary trends analysis. Anesth Analg 2017;124(4):1261–7.
2. Apfelbaum JL, Cutter TW. The four Ps: place, procedure, personnel, and patient. Anesthesiol Clin 2014;32(2). xvii–xxi.
3. Tetzlaff JE, Vargo JJ, Maurer W. Nonoperating room anesthesia for the gastrointestinal endoscopy suite. Anesthesiol Clin 2014;32(2):387–94.

4. ASA, Ethical guidelines for the anethesia care of patients with DO-NOT-RESUSCITATE orders or other directives that limit treatment. 2013. Guidelines available at: https://www.asahq.org/quality-and-practice-management/standards-guidelines-and-related-resources-search. Assessed September 09, 2018.

5. ACS, Statement on Advance Directives by Patients: "Do Not Resuscitate" in the Operating Room Assessed from the American College of Surgeons website. 2014. Available at: https://www.facs.org/about-acs/statements/19-advance-directives. Assessed September 09, 2018.

6. Sumrall WD, Mahanna E, Sabharwal V, et al. Do not resuscitate, anesthesia, and perioperative care: a not so clear order. Ochsner J 2016;16(2):176–9.

7. Practice guidelines for preoperative fasting and the use of pharmacologic agents to reduce the risk of pulmonary aspiration: application to healthy patients undergoing elective procedures: an updated report by the American Society of Anesthesiologists Task Force on Preoperative Fasting and the use of pharmacologic agents to reduce the risk of pulmonary aspiration. Anesthesiology 2017;126(3): 376–93.

8. Bucci C, Rotondano G, Hassan C, et al. Optimal bowel cleansing for colonoscopy: split the dose! A series of meta-analyses of controlled studies. Gastrointest Endosc 2014;80(4):566–76.e2.

9. Cohen LB. Split dosing of bowel preparations for colonoscopy: an analysis of its efficacy, safety, and tolerability. Gastrointest Endosc 2010;72(2):406–12.

10. Huffman M, Unger RZ, Thatikonda C, et al. Split-dose bowel preparation for colonoscopy and residual gastric fluid volume: an observational study. Gastrointest Endosc 2010;72(3):516–22.

11. Siddiqui AA, Yang K, Spechler SJ, et al. Duration of the interval between the completion of bowel preparation and the start of colonoscopy predicts bowel-preparation quality. Gastrointest Endosc 2009;69(3 Pt 2):700–6.

12. Tandon K, Khalil C, Castro F, et al. Safety of large-volume, same-day oral bowel preparations during deep sedation: a prospective observational study. Anesth Analg 2017;125(2):469–76.

13. Bhavani SS, Abdelmalak BB. Fasting before anesthesia: an unsettled dilemma. Anesth Analg 2017;125(2):369–71.

14. Practice Guidelines for Moderate Procedural Sedation and Analgesia 2018: A Report by the American Society of Anesthesiologists Task Force on Moderate Procedural Sedation and Analgesia, the American Association of Oral and Maxillofacial Surgeons, American College of Radiology, American Dental Association, American Society of Dentist Anesthesiologists, and Society of Interventional Radiology. Anesthesiology 2018;128(3):437–79.

15. Metzner J, Posner KL, Domino KB. The risk and safety of anesthesia at remote locations: the US closed claims analysis. Curr Opin Anaesthesiol 2009;22(4): 502–8.

16. Arakawa H, Kaise M, Sumiyama K, et al. Does pulse oximetry accurately monitor a patient's ventilation during sedated endoscopy under oxygen supplementation? Singapore Med J 2013;54(4):212–5.

17. Fu ES, Downs JB, Schweiger JW, et al. Supplemental oxygen impairs detection of hypoventilation by pulse oximetry. Chest 2004;126(5):1552–8.

18. Vargo JJ, Zuccaro G Jr, Dumot JA, et al. Automated graphic assessment of respiratory activity is superior to pulse oximetry and visual assessment for the detection of early respiratory depression during therapeutic upper endoscopy. Gastrointest Endosc 2002;55(7):826–31.

19. Mandel JE. Recent advances in respiratory monitory in nonoperating room anesthesia. Curr Opin Anaesthesiol 2018;31(4):448–52.
20. Anand GW, Heuss LT. Feasibility of breath monitoring in patients undergoing elective colonoscopy under propofol sedation: a single-center pilot study. World J Gastrointest Endosc 2014;6(3):82–7.
21. Mimoz O, Benard T, Gaucher A, et al. Accuracy of respiratory rate monitoring using a non-invasive acoustic method after general anaesthesia. Br J Anaesth 2012;108(5):872–5.
22. Tanaka PP, Tanaka M, Drover DR. Detection of respiratory compromise by acoustic monitoring, capnography, and brain function monitoring during monitored anesthesia care. J Clin Monit Comput 2014;28(6):561–6.
23. Voscopoulos C, Brayanov J, Ladd D, et al. Special article: evaluation of a novel noninvasive respiration monitor providing continuous measurement of minute ventilation in ambulatory subjects in a variety of clinical scenarios. Anesth Analg 2013;117(1):91–100.
24. Woodward ZG, Urman RD, Domino KB. Safety of non-operating room anesthesia: a closed claims update. Anesthesiol Clin 2017;35(4):569–81.
25. Al-Awabdy B, Wilcox CM. Use of anesthesia on the rise in gastrointestinal endoscopy. World J Gastrointest Endosc 2013;5(1):1–5.
26. ASGE Standards of Practice Committee, Early DS, Lightdale JR, Vargo JJ 2nd, et al. Guidelines for sedation and anesthesia in GI endoscopy. Gastrointest Endosc 2018;87(2):327–37.
27. ASA, Continuum of depth of sedation: Definition of general anesthesia and levels of sedation/analgesia* Committee of Origin: Quality Management and Departmental Administration (Approved by the ASA House of Delegates on October 13, 1999, and last amended on October 15, 2014). ASA, 2014. Available at: https://www.asahq.org/standards-and-guidelines/continuum-of-depth-of-sedation-definition-of-general-anesthesia-and-levels-of-sedationanalgesia.
28. ASGE. Statement - Universal adoption of capnography for moderate sedation in adults undergoing upper endoscopy and colonoscopy has not been shown to improve patient safety or clinical outcomes and significantly increases costs for moderate sedation. 2012 [cited 2018 20180928]. Available at: https://www.asge.org/docs/default-source/education/practice_guidelines/doc-90dc9b63-593d-48a9-bec1-9f0ab3ce946a.pdf?sfvrsn=6.
29. Hardemark Cedborg AI, Sundman E, Bodén K, et al. Effects of morphine and midazolam on pharyngeal function, airway protection, and coordination of breathing and swallowing in healthy adults. Anesthesiology 2015;122(6):1253–67.
30. Wiggins TF, Khan AS, Winstead NS. Sedation, analgesia, and monitoring. Clin Colon Rectal Surg 2010;23(1):14–20.
31. Rex DK, Bhandari R, Desta T, et al. A phase III study evaluating the efficacy and safety of remimazolam (CNS 7056) compared with placebo and midazolam in patients undergoing colonoscopy. Gastrointest Endosc 2018;88(3):427–437 e6.
32. Ilic RG. Fospropofol and remimazolam. Int Anesthesiol Clin 2015;53(2):76–90.
33. Abdelmalak B, Khanna A, Tetzlaff J. Fospropofol, a new sedative anesthetic, and its utility in the perioperative period. Curr Pharm Des 2012;18(38):6241–52.
34. Slavik VC, Zed PJ. Combination ketamine and propofol for procedural sedation and analgesia. Pharmacotherapy 2007;27(11):1588–98.
35. Daniel J, Pambiancoa BDC. New horizons for sedation: The ultra short acting benzodiazepine remimazolam. Tech Gastrointest Endosc 2016;18(1):22–8.

36. ASGE Technology Committee, Lo SK, Fujii-Lau LL, Enestvedt BK, et al. The use of carbon dioxide in gastrointestinal endoscopy. Gastrointest Endosc 2016;83(5): 857–65.

37. Lord AC, Riss S. Is the type of insufflation a key issue in gastro-intestinal endoscopy? World J Gastroenterol 2014;20(9):2193–9.

38. Donepudi S, Chavalitdhamrong D, Pu L, et al. Air embolism complicating gastrointestinal endoscopy: a systematic review. World J Gastrointest Endosc 2013; 5(8):359–65.

39. Veitch AM, Vanbiervliet G, Gershlick AH, et al. Endoscopy in patients on antiplatelet or anticoagulant therapy, including direct oral anticoagulants: British Society of Gastroenterology (BSG) and European Society of Gastrointestinal Endoscopy (ESGE) guidelines. Endoscopy 2016;48(4):c1.

40. Nagata N, Yasunaga H, Matsui H, et al. Therapeutic endoscopy-related GI bleeding and thromboembolic events in patients using warfarin or direct oral anticoagulants: results from a large nationwide database analysis. Gut 2018;67(10): 1805–12.

41. American Society of Anesthesiologists. Practice advisory for the perioperative management of patients with cardiac implantable electronic devices: pacemakers and implantable cardioverter-defibrillators: an updated report by the American Society of Anesthesiologists task force on perioperative management of patients with cardiac implantable electronic devices. Anesthesiology 2011; 114(2):247–61.

42. Parekh PJ, Buerlein RC, Shams R, et al. An update on the management of implanted cardiac devices during electrosurgical procedures. Gastrointest Endosc 2013;78(6):836–41.

43. Behrens A, Kreuzmayr A, Manner H, et al. Acute sedation-associated complications in GI endoscopy (ProSed 2 Study): results from the prospective multicentre electronic registry of sedation-associated complications. Gut 2018;68:575–6.

44. Wernli KJ, Brenner AT, Rutter CM, et al. Risks associated with anesthesia services during colonoscopy. Gastroenterology 2016;150(4):888–94.

45. Bielawska B, Hookey LC, Sutradhar R, et al. Anesthesia assistance in outpatient colonoscopy and risk of aspiration pneumonia, bowel perforation, and splenic injury. Gastroenterology 2018;154(1):77–85 e3.

46. Vargo JJ, Niklewski PJ, Williams JL, et al. Patient safety during sedation by anesthesia professionals during routine upper endoscopy and colonoscopy: an analysis of 1.38 million procedures. Gastrointest Endosc 2017;85(1):101–8.

Office-Based Anesthesia
A Comprehensive Review and 2019 Update

Brian M. Osman, MD[a],*, Fred E. Shapiro, DO[b]

KEYWORDS

- Office-based anesthesia • Patient safety • Safety checklists • Emergency manual
- Accreditation • Office-based practice legislation

KEY POINTS

- Key studies in office-based anesthesia are demonstrating a shift toward safer office practices over the last 25 years.
- Proper patient and procedure selection are crucial to patient safety in office-based anesthesia.
- Practice management to improve patient safety in office-based anesthesia includes the implementation of patient safety checklists and emergency manuals.
- Accreditation of office-based facilities allows a third party to monitor activities and provide external benchmarking, validation, and acknowledgment of a nationally recommended standard of care.
- New legislation involves quality and safety metrics specifically designed for office-based anesthesia and surgery.

INTRODUCTION AND HISTORY

Procedures that formerly took place within the walls of a hospital are increasingly being performed in the office setting. The proportion of outpatient and office-based surgeries has increased from a meager 10% to 15% in the early 1990s to closer to 60% in 2012.[1] According to the American Society of Anesthesiologists (ASA), the number of office-based procedures essentially doubled to 10 million cases per year from 1995 to 2005.[2] As of 2014, office procedures made up 11% of the estimated 885 million

Disclosure Statement: No Disclosures or Conflicts of Interest.
a Department of Anesthesiology, Perioperative Medicine and Pain Management, University Health Tower, University of Miami Miller School of Medicine, 1400 Northwest 12th Avenue, Suite 3075-H, Miami, FL 33136, USA; b Department of Anesthesia, Critical Care and Pain Medicine, Beth Israel Deaconess Medical Center, Harvard Medical School, 330 Brookline Avenue F-407, Boston, MA 02215, USA
* Corresponding author. Department of Anesthesiology, University of Miami, Miller School of Medicine, 1400 Northwest 12th Avenue, Suite 3075 Miami, FL 33136.
E-mail address: bosman@med.miami.edu

Anesthesiology Clin 37 (2019) 317–331
https://doi.org/10.1016/j.anclin.2019.01.004
1932-2275/19/© 2019 Elsevier Inc. All rights reserved.

anesthesiology.theclinics.com

office-based visits in the United States.[3] Some of the more common procedures include cosmetic surgeries such as liposuction and abdominoplasties, complex dental procedures, podiatry cases, gastrointestinal endoscopies and colonoscopies, radiologic procedures, and a variety of interventional vascular procedures. Over the past several decades, the advances of surgical and anesthetic techniques have drastically changed the landscape of the patient surgical experience and have allowed more invasive procedures to be safely performed in nonhospital settings.

Historically, office-based surgical suites have been less regulated in comparison with ambulatory surgical centers (ASCs) and hospitals. The increase in the number and complexity of office-based cases has raised some significant concerns in regard to patient safety. Specifically, private offices may not have the appropriate equipment, available resources, properly trained staff, or streamlined transfer policies in place should a medical or surgical emergency arise. In 2003, Vila and colleagues[4] raised issues of office anesthesia safety by comparing 2 years of reported adverse events in Florida offices and ASCs. They concluded that the relative risk of complications and death was 10 times greater in the office-based practices compared with ASCs. The possibility of an emergency occurring in the office has been highlighted by several recently documented, high-profile cases reported in the media.[5–10] The American Association for Accreditation of Ambulatory Surgery Facilities (AAAASF) performed a critical analysis of their mandatory quality assurance outcomes data in more than 5.5 million procedures performed in AAAASF-accredited facilities from 2001 to 2012. They found that the overall complication rate in all plastic surgery procedures was 1 in 251 procedures and 1 in 178 cases, and the risk of death for a patient having any plastic surgery was approximately 1 in 41,726 or 0.0024% of the total cases.[11] Soltani and colleagues[11] also discovered that not all procedures had equal risks. For example, the investigators stated that the most commonly reported adverse event associated with breast augmentation was postoperative bleeding; however, abdominoplasty was associated with more serious events, such as death from pulmonary embolism, especially when combined with additional procedures. These statistics are noteworthy considering that plastic surgery is only 1 of several specialties currently performing procedures in the office setting. Given these statistics, preparation and management of an office-based emergency is essential to improve patient safety and outcomes.

Considering the ever-changing complexity of patients, procedures, and specialties, maintaining the standards in accreditation is also challenging. In a comprehensive review of the literature, Shapiro and colleagues[12] concluded that there was a lack of randomized controlled trials to determine how office-based procedures and anesthesia affect patient morbidity and mortality, and that safety and outcome data analysis was performed retrospectively. They also asserted that improvements in patient safety outcomes can be made through nationwide standardization of care, proper provider credentialing, facility accreditation, the use of safety checklists, and adherence to professional practice guidelines.[12] A summary of these studies combined with recent updated data up to 2016 can be seen in **Table 1**.

SAFETY IN OFFICE-BASED ANESTHESIA

In 2010, the Society for Ambulatory Anesthesia (SAMBA) began focusing on office-based safety outcomes based on data reported to the SAMBA Clinical Outcomes Registry (SCOR). As of 2014, out of 37,669 cases performed in the office, major complications comprised less than 1%.[13] In 2010, the ASA also established the collection of patient outcome data through the National Anesthesia Clinical Outcomes Registry

Table 1
Key studies addressing safety in office-based anesthesia

Key Papers, Year	Method	Finding
Hoefflin et al, 2001	23,000 cases from single plastic surgery office	No significant complications
Vila et al,[4] 2003	2 y of adverse events reported to Florida board	10-fold relative risk in office compared with ASC
Perrot et al, 2003	>34,000 oral and maxillofacial surgeries	Complication rate of 0.4%–1.5% for all types of anesthesia
Byrd et al, 2003	5316 cases from single plastic surgery office	Complication rate 0.7% (mostly hematoma)
Coldiron et al, 2008	Self-reported data to Florida board from 2000 to 2007	174 adverse events; 31 deaths in this time frame
Soltani et al,[11] 2013	AAAASF data from 2000–2012; only reviewed plastic surgery offices	22,000 of 5.5 million cases; complication rate 0.4%; 94 deaths; 0.0017% death rate
Failey et al, 2013	2611 cases from single AAAASF facility under TIVA or conscious sedation	No deaths, cardiac events, transfers; 1 DVT
Shapiro et al,[12,13] 2014	Comprehensive literature review	Improvements in patient outcomes likely with credentialing, accreditation, safety checklists, state and federal regulation, and national societies
Gupta et al, 2016	Compared outcomes of 183,914 plastic surgery procedures in accredited facilities	Complication rates in OBSS, ASCs, and hospitals were 1.3%, 1.9%, and 2.4%, respectively. Multivariate analysis showed lower risk in OBSS when compared with ASCs or a hospital

Abbreviations: AAAASF, American Association for Accreditation of Ambulatory Surgery Facilities; ASC, Ambulatory Surgery Center; DVT, deep vein thrombosis; OBSS, office-based surgical suite; TIVA, total intravenous anesthesia.

Adapted from Shapiro FE, Punwani N, Rosenberg NM, et al. Office-based anesthesia: safety and outcomes. Anesth Analg 2014;119(2):276–85.

(NACOR). NACOR is the largest database of reported adverse anesthesia outcomes from more than 300 participating facilities performing office-based cases.[13] Despite the differences in specialties, type of cases performed, patient selection, anesthesia technique, and type of provider coverage, the NACOR database had only 17 adverse office-based anesthesia (OBA) outcomes as of 2014.[13] Although both database reporting systems have their merit and limitations, pervasive issues, including the lack of uniformity regarding state or federal regulations combined with voluntary reporting systems, could result in understating the risk of procedures performed in the office. By 2014, studies began to use the information in the NACOR database to scientifically evaluate office-based safety. Patient demographics and outcomes, procedure and anesthesia type, surgical duration, and case coverage by provider began to deliver vital information for continuous quality improvement, electronic health records, use of checklists, and outcomes data reporting.[13] An article by Jani and colleagues[14] examined the NACOR database and found that the office environment is unique and, although ambulatory office and ASCs are typically grouped together, the entities are not equivalent. The investigators verified that there was a significant increase in the number of office cases since 2010 and that there were significant differences in terms of patient age, comorbidities, and procedures performed.[14] In addition to the overall increase in cases from 2010 to 2014, the number of OBA patients between the ages of 19 and 49 years decreased (from 51% to 30%) as other age groups infiltrated the office setting.[14] ASCs saw a similar, albeit decreased, change, from 30% in 2010 to 25% in 2014.[14] These percentages highlight a shift to older patients in these settings.[14] The distribution of ASA physical status shifted as well. In the office, ASA physical statuses of 1, 2, 3, 4, and 5 were 37%, 44%, 19%, 0.3%, and 0%, respectively, in 2010. This changed to 35%, 32%, 32%, 0.8%, and 0.01%, respectively, in 2014.[14] Again, the shift for ASCs was similar but decreased: ASA physical statuses 1 to 5 of 54%, 30%, 16%, 0.6%, 0.02%, and 0.01% in 2010, with a change to 42%, 36%, 21%, 0.9%, and 0.01% in 2014.[14] The extremes have not changed much but these trends highlight a shift to sicker patients in these settings.

The office-based practice is a relatively isolated environment carrying the same potential risks regardless of the location where surgery and anesthesia is performed. The rapid proliferation of office practices and surgical procedures performed outside of hospitals, in addition to several recent high-profile incidents, has focused the attention of the ASA, multiple accreditation agencies, and other professional societies to implement a standardization of care for the improvement of patient safety and outcomes in offices, as well as ASCs and hospitals.[12] The ASA recently updated their guidelines involving office-based and ambulatory anesthesia, providers, and procedural sedation. Based on these guidelines, the ASA suggest that widespread accreditation would presumably create a more transparent process for assuring that office practices and their providers are operating within their scope of practice.[15] Starling and colleagues[16] reviewed cases from Florida and Alabama, examining the effect of mandatory physician board certification and credentialing standards on office-based safety and outcomes. Almost all of the reported adverse events in those 2 states involved board-certified physicians in accredited facilities. Shapiro and colleagues[12] noted a lack of uniformity and risk adjustment in the reporting of adverse outcomes.

In the past 25 years, has safety in the office-based surgical and anesthesia procedure setting improved? The simple answer is yes. Domino[17,18] examined the ASA Closed Claims database in 2001 and found that office-based claims were 3 times more severe than in the ASC (67% compared with 21%) with almost half of the adverse events deemed preventable by better monitoring. In 2003, an analysis by Vila and colleagues[4] asserted that the risk of death was 10 times greater in the office than the ASC. In 2014, with a 2018 update,[18] Shapiro and colleagues[12] performed a comprehensive literature review of office-based safety and outcomes and noted a vastly improved safety record. They concluded that the improvements seen in patient outcomes are likely due to proper credentialing of facilities and practitioners, accreditation, adherence to guidelines set forth by national societies such as the ASA, the incorporation of safety checklists, and the implementation of more oversight at both the state and federal levels.[19] In 2017, Gupta and colleagues[20] compared the outcomes of 183,914 aesthetic surgical procedures across different types of accredited facilities and demonstrated that the complication rates in the office-based setting compared with ASCs or hospitals were 1.3%, 1.9%, and 2.4%, respectively. Based on the current literature, it seems that safety in the office-based setting is improving.

ADVANTAGES AND DISADVANTAGES

The shift of practice into the office-based setting offers significant cost-savings with 60% to 75% lower costs. Value is further increased by maintaining or improving patient comfort and satisfaction.[20] One of the largest costs incurred in hospitals and ASCs is due to facilities fees. Their overhead costs are quite substantial and are passed on to the consumer. Conversely, in the office-based setting, the overhead expenses are less burdensome to office personnel and the patient. This allows patients to enjoy more personalized attention and privacy. Scheduling procedures and managing administrative issues may be easier and more efficient given a smaller more consistent staff roster. However, the administrative issues and patient safety concerns have increased commensurately with the increased number and complexity of patients and procedures. Therefore, appropriate patients and procedure selection is essential to improving safety and outcomes in office-based surgery and anesthesia.

PATIENT AND PROCEDURE SELECTION

More procedures are being performed in the office with older patients and sicker patients. This can present significant challenges for anesthesia providers in settings where personnel and resources are limited. Initially, more than 51% of OBA patients were 19 to 49 years old. That percentage has fallen to less than 30% as older age groups have entered the office setting.[14] An aging patient population also brings co-morbid conditions that may increase risk for complications and/or significantly change anesthetic management for procedures. Anesthesia providers must be vigilant regarding the presence of high-risk medical conditions such as morbid obesity, obstructive sleep apnea, chronic obstructive pulmonary disease, myocardial infarction in the last 6 months, stroke in the last 3 months, end-stage renal or liver disease, abnormalities of other major organ systems, poorly controlled diabetes mellitus, severe anemia, sickle-cell disease, personal or family history of malignant hyperthermia, known difficult airway, poorly controlled psychiatric problems, and acute or chronic substance abuse.[12]

The increasing complexity of cases performed in the office also poses new mounting concerns for patient safety. In addition to plastic surgery, other specialties have begun to address these concepts in the last few years. Ophthalmology, interventional radiology, gynecology, and interventional vascular surgery are just a few examples of specialties that are performing more complicated procedures in the office setting. A recent study by Lin and colleagues[21] in 2017 recognized that endovascular procedures, such as diagnostic arteriograms, arterial interventions, venous interventions, dialysis access interventions, and venous catheter management, all could be performed in an office-based facility with excellent outcomes. The best assessments in the process for determining patient selection are available through the ASA OBA guidelines updated in 2014 and the new 2018 practice guidelines for moderate procedural sedation and analgesia. The ASA office-based guidelines recognize the unique needs of this growing practice and have affirmed that the anesthesiologist should agree on the following:

1. The procedure undertaken is within the scope of practice of the health care practitioners and the capabilities of the facility
2. The procedure should be of a duration and degree of complexity that will allow the patient to recover and be discharged from the facility

3. The patient who may be at undue risk for complications because of a preexisting medical or other conditions should be referred to an appropriate facility for performance of the procedure and administration of anesthesia.[22]

The 2018 ASA practice guidelines for moderate procedural sedation address patient evaluation and preparation, and recommend the review of previous medical records for underlying medical problems, including sedation, anesthesia and surgical history, history of current problems pertaining to cooperation, pain tolerance, sensitivity to anesthesia or sedation, current medications, extremes of age, psychotropic drug use, use of supplements, and family history. The guidelines also stress the importance of performing a focused physical examination and any indicated preprocedure laboratory testing.[23] Surgery and anesthesia in the office is getting safer; however, as the complexity of procedures continue to increase, the door opens to greater risk and new areas of liability.[24]

REQUIREMENTS FOR OFFICE ANESTHESIA

The guidelines for OBA adopted by the ASA emphasize that the standard of anesthetic care in an office should be the same as the hospital or ASC. This includes qualified personnel being present for the entirety of the procedure until the patient has been discharged from anesthesia care, documentation of the discharge decision by a responsible physician, and immediate availability of personnel with training in advanced resuscitative techniques such as advanced cardiac life support (ACLS) and/or pediatric advanced life support (PALS).[22] The OBA setting should have enough space to accommodate all necessary equipment and allow for ample access to the patient; back-up power to ensure patient protection in case of a power outage; and a reliable source of oxygen, suction, resuscitation equipment, and emergency drugs.[22] Equipment should allow for standard ASA monitoring and all equipment should be maintained tested and inspected according to the manufacturer's specifications with the appropriate documentation.[22] If procedures are performed on children or infants, the required equipment, medication, and resuscitative capabilities for a pediatric population should be immediately available.[22]

The new practice guidelines for moderate procedural sedation and analgesia highlight continual monitoring of ventilatory function with capnography to supplement standard monitoring by observation and pulse oximetry.[23]

PRACTICE MANAGEMENT

Based on the assessment by Gupta and colleagues[20] of complications in 2016, complication rates were lowest in the office (1.3%) when compared with ASCs (1.9%) and hospitals (2.4%, $P<.01$). In addition, accreditation of office-based surgery suites seems to offer a safe alternative to ASCs and hospitals but standardizing accreditation activities across all different practice locations will be pivotal in improving patient safety.[19] Surgical checklists have also been introduced to further enhance patient safety in the office with promising results. Customizable preoperative checklists that target sources of error have already demonstrated some potential in avoiding serious medical errors and, with the modification of the World Health Organization (WHO) model, customized checklists can also be effective in the office-based practice.[25,26] Based on survey responses, ambulatory surgical checklists can also potentially facilitate patient education, increase patient satisfaction, and decrease anxiety.[27] An example of an office-based surgical safety checklist prepared by the Institute for Safety in Office-Based Surgery (ISOBS), adapted from the WHO Surgical Safety Checklist, can be viewed in **Fig. 1**. In 2017, the ISOBS Checklist for

Safety Checklist for Office–Based Surgery

from the Institute for Safety in Office-Based Surgery (ISOBS)

Introduction Preoperative encounter, with practitioner and patient	Setting Before patient in procedure room; with practitioner and personnel	Operation Before sedation/analgesia; with practitioner and personnel*	Before discharge On arrival to recovery area; with practitioner & personnel	Satisfaction Completed post-procedure; with practitioner and patient
Patient	Emergency equipment check complete (e.g. airway, AED, code cart, MH kit)? ☐ Yes	Patient identity, procedure, and consent confirmed? ☐ Yes	Assessment for pain? ☐ Yes	Unanticipated events documented? ☐ Yes
Patient medically optimized for the procedure? ☐ Yes ☐ No, and plan for optimization made.	EMS availability confirmed? ☐ Yes	Is the site marked and side identified? ☐ Yes ☐ N/A	Assessment for nausea/vomiting? ☐ Yes	Patient satisfaction assessed? ☐ Yes
Does patient have DVT risk factors: ☐ Yes, and prophylaxis plans arranged. ☐ No	Oxygen source and suction checked? ☐ Yes	DVT prophylaxis provided? ☐ Yes ☐ N/A	Recovery personnel available? ☐ Yes	Provider satisfaction assessed? ☐ Yes
Procedure	Anticipated duration ≤ 6 h? ☐ Yes ☐ No, but personnel, monitoring and equipment available	Antibiotic prophylaxis administered within 60 min prior to procedure? ☐ Yes ☐ N/A	*Prior to discharge:* *(with personnel and patient)*	
Procedure complexity and sedation/analgesia reviewed? ☐ Yes		Essential imaging displayed? ☐ Yes ☐ N/A	Discharge criteria achieved? ☐ Yes	
NPO instructions given? ☐ Yes		*Practitioner confirms verbally:* ☐ Local anesthetic toxicity precautions	Patient education and instructions provided? ☐ Yes	
Escort and post-procedure plans reviewed? ☐ Yes		☐ Patient monitoring (per institutional protocol).	Plan for post-discharge follow–up? ☐ Yes	
		☐ Anticipated critical events addressed with team.	Escort confirmed? ☐ Yes	
		☐ Each member of the team has been addressed by name and is ready to proceed.		

Fig. 1. Office-based surgical safety checklist. * Adapted from the WHO Surgical Safety Checklist. AED, automated external defribrillator; DVT, deep vein thrombosis; EMS, emergency medical services; MH, malignant hyperthermia. (*Courtesy of* Institute for Safety in Office-Based Surgery [ISOBS], Inc, Boston, MA; with permission.)

Office-Based Surgery was added to the American Academy of Healthcare Risk Management resource manual for office-based surgery and can be found at www.ahsrm. org.

The use of cognitive aids has historically improved people's knowledge and has proved to be effective in emergency situations. A tailored cognitive aid in the form of an emergency manual can also play a useful role for the anesthesiologist performing procedures in the office.[28] Given the continued growth of office-based surgery, practitioners and staff should have easy access to critical information when dealing with a crisis. ISOBS has customized an emergency manual, specifically for the office, after reviewing the most common emergencies in this unique setting and providing concise and user-friendly treatment algorithms. The purpose is to provide a quick and reliable safety resource for office practitioners and personnel, with limited resources in mind. As of 2018, this manual is available on Emergency Manuals Implementation Collaborative Web site (https://emergencymanuals.org/tools-resources/free-tools/) and includes easily accessible references for life-threatening unstable heart rhythms and cardiac arrest using ACLS or PALS protocols. It also deals with preparedness for facility emergencies, such as fire, fire or biohazards evacuation, and loss of oxygen or power; critical events, including severe allergic reactions, anaphylaxis, difficult airway, hemorrhage, hypoxia, hypercarbia, hypotension, local anesthetic systemic toxicity, loss of venous access, mental status changes, malignant hyperthermia, and general complications associated with spinal anesthesia; and office administrative issues, such as emergency transfer of care policies.[29]

The unique office-based surgical setting is conducive to the use of Enhanced Recovery After Surgery (ERAS) protocols. These are to enhance the patient perioperative experience by reducing postoperative pain, postoperative nausea, and vomiting; opioid pain medication use; and length of stay for inpatient procedures and same-day surgery.[30] When applied and customized to the office-based setting, ERAS can be used to enhance rapid discharge and recovery, increase patient satisfaction, and improve surgical outcomes. Multimodal therapies and nonopioid-based perioperative analgesia are some of the key components of ERAS. These include procedure-appropriate regional blocks, and oral and intravenous nonopioid adjuncts, such as steroids, pregabalin, nonsteroidal antiinflammatory drugs, acetaminophen, clonidine, intravenous lidocaine, and intraoperative injection of long-acting liposomal bupivacaine.[30] Improved pain control can be achieved while reducing the opioid-related side effects. Patient education regarding the anesthesia and surgery is another important aspect of ERAS that can be incorporated in the office. In addition, to engage the patient in shared decision-making, the ASA has preanesthesia patient education decision aids for spinal anesthesia, epidural anesthesia, peripheral nerve blocks, and is developing another for monitored anesthesia care, to guide patients through the process of making informed choices with their anesthetic management.[31]

ACCREDITATION

Currently, 33 states require offices performing medical and surgical procedures to obtain accreditation. The advantages of seeking accreditation include allowing for an objective third party to monitor the activities and practices of an office-based practice, offering validation, and providing a nationally established benchmark of quality and safety. Administrative issues include facility and equipment maintenance, medical records documentation, facility safety equipment, and credentialing of personnel. Clinical considerations include all aspects of perioperative patient care, infection control, approval of procedures in the office, nursing services, equipment, pharmacy, pathologic testing, diagnostic imaging, and disposal of hazardous waste. Examples of surgical issues include preoperative evaluation, testing requirements, medication administration, appropriate procedure selection, and risk management. Accreditation may also provide a competitive advantage.

There are currently 3 major nationally recognized accrediting organizations: Accreditation Association for Ambulatory Health Care (AAAHC), The Joint Commission (TJC), and AAAASF. All 3 agencies provide handbooks with their standards designed specifically for office-based surgery. The AAAHC Handbook has been developed to assist organizations seeking accreditation in the review and application of the standards for an office-based surgery practice with the intention of ensuring that the highest level of health care services is provided.[32] In 2001, the TJC introduced standards and a survey process for office-based surgery practices, currently providing accreditation for more than 400 office-based surgery practices.[33] The AAAASF, founded in 1980, provides accreditation for more than 2000 outpatient facilities, with the mission to standardize and improve the quality of medical and surgical care while assuring high standards of patient care.[34]

All 3 agencies have similar requirements for accreditation but there are some subtle differences. An office-based practice will need to take into consideration the minor differences between the 3 organizations and apply for the accreditation that best suits the setting and providers. TJC published revised survey eligibility criteria in 2018 for office-based surgery to ensure that they are current and relevant for organizations seeking accreditation or reaccreditation.[35] An office-based practice must be proactive and keep up to date in the application process.

To facilitate this, all 3 agencies publish yearly top-10 lists of standard deficiencies. In 2017, the common thread with the AAAHC, TJC, and the AAAASF included deficiencies in credentialing and privileging, documentation, quality improvement, benchmarking, patient safety, infection control, and emergency preparedness.[36–38] Consistent with the 2018 ASA practice guidelines for procedural sedation, the AAAHC updated their standards regarding continual monitoring of ventilation and the authors suspect that other accreditation agencies will follow.[23]

QUALITY IMPROVEMENT PROGRAMS

Quality improvement programs are another important objective of the accrediting organizations for validation, and internal and external benchmarking. A unique characteristic of the AAAASF is the requirement to document quality improvement measures and adverse events, which are crucial in identifying and eliminating vulnerabilities in safety. Lapses in quality and patient safety can range from lesser issues, such as patient wait times or procedure room turnaround times, to more pressing issues, such as antibiotic administration, complication rates, and serious adverse events. Effective January 2018, TJC published a set of national patient safety goals to complement the office-based surgery accreditation program. These goals include improving the accuracy of patient identification and effectiveness of communication, improving medication safety, reducing harm associated with clinical alarm systems, reducing the risk of infections, identifying inherent demographic risks, and addressing the universal protocol for preventing wrong site, wrong procedure, and wrong person surgery.[39]

LEGISLATION AND REGULATIONS

As of 2017, 24 states and the District of Columbia have laws to regulate facilities that perform office-based surgery, whereas an additional 8 states are regulated by their state medical board–issued guidelines, policies, or position statements regarding office-based surgery.[40] Because of the lack of uniform regulation of office-based practices, adverse event reporting varies from state to state making it difficult to obtain robust outcome data. As an example, **Table 2** displays some of the office-based statues, regulations, and policies related to office-based surgery outcomes reporting by 5 different states.[13] Currently, multiple states are proposing legislation that would affect OBA practices and the reporting of anesthesia-related adverse events. Florida introduced a bill in early 2018 that would define the term adverse incident and would require dentists practicing in the state to notify the board of any mortality or other adverse incident that occurs in the outpatient facility as a direct result of the use of general anesthesia, deep sedation, or conscious sedation. In 2017, New Hampshire proposed to require adverse event reporting and also regulate the use of general anesthesia, deep sedation, or moderate sedation by dentists. Specifically, a licensed dentist, anesthesiologist, or certified registered nurse anesthetist (CRNA) would be required to be physically present while general anesthesia, deep sedation, or moderate sedation is in effect. For patients under the age of 13 years, additional rules include the completion of an informed consent statement and a requirement for additional staff trained in the monitoring and resuscitation of pediatric patients to be present. Pending legislation in New York would require certification of nurse anesthetists and define office-based surgery. It would also add the following language: "administration of anesthesia in office based surgery venues means the anesthesia component of the medical or dental procedure must be supervised by an anesthesiologist, physician, dentist or podiatrist qualified to supervise the administration of anesthesia who is physically present and available to immediately diagnose and treat the patient for anesthesia complications or emergencies. Nurse anesthetists with the appropriate training and experience may be permitted to administer unconscious or deep sedation, and/or general anesthesia, regional anesthesia, and/or monitor the patient."

States such as Alabama, Alaska, Texas, and Utah have implemented new regulatory activity in 2018 regarding anesthesia in dental facilities. Utah recently adopted regulation in 2017 that establishes reporting requirements for anesthesia-related adverse events that occur in outpatient settings. It further defines what constitutes an adverse event, the levels of sedation, and describes a level-of-harm scale (UT 42332 2017). Recently adopted regulations in Oregon relate to in-office anesthesia administration and amend current rules to require a documented ASA physical status evaluation when performing level II or III office-based procedures. It also prohibits level II or III procedures from being performed on patients with an ASA physical status of 4 or greater (OR 39594 2017). An additional adopted amendment (OR 39586 2017) prohibits CRNAs from providing moderate sedation, deep sedation, or general anesthesia for even level I office-based procedures if the patient is assigned an ASA classification of 4 or greater.

In the state of New York, the New York Department of Health (NYDOH) made changes to office-based surgery law, effective April 13, 2016, that introduced 2 new requirements to existing adverse event reporting. In addition to adverse events such as unplanned transfer to a hospital or emergency department, unscheduled admission to the hospital, patient death within 30 days, suspected transmission of the blood-borne pathogens to patients, and any other serious or life-threatening event, office-based surgery practitioners must now report unplanned emergency department visits or unscheduled assignments to observation services within a hospital within 72 hours of an office surgery.[41] Second, based on the practice guidelines for moderate procedural sedation and analgesia published by the ASA in 2018, the NYDOH mandated

Table 2
Office-based surgery outcomes reporting requirements by 5 states

State	Statutes, Regulations, and Policies
Alabama	540-X-10-.11. Reporting Requirement. Reporting to the Alabama Board of Medical Examiners is required within 3 business days of the occurrence and will include all surgical-related deaths and all events related to a procedure that resulted in an emergency transfer of the surgical patient to the hospital, anesthetic or surgical events, cardiopulmonary resuscitation, unscheduled hospitalization related to the surgery, and surgical site deep wound infection
Kansas	K.A.R. 100-25-3. Each physician who performs any office-based surgery or special procedure that results in any of the following quality indicators shall notify the board in writing within 15 calendar days following discovery of the event: 1. The death of a patient during any office-based surgery or special procedure, or within 72 h thereafter 2. The transport of a patient to a hospital emergency department 3. The unscheduled admission of a patient to a hospital within 72 h of discharge, if the admission is related to the office-based surgery or special procedure 4. The unplanned extension of the office-based surgery or special procedure >4 h beyond the planned duration of the surgery or procedure being performed 5. The discovery of a foreign object erroneously remaining in a patient from an office-based surgery or special procedure at that office 6. The performance of the wrong surgical procedure, surgery on the wrong site, or surgery on the wrong patient
Kentucky	Guidelines for Office Based Surgery. Emergency Transfer and Reporting. In the event of anesthetic, medical, or surgical complication or emergency, all office personnel should be familiar with a documented plan for the timely and safe transfer of patients to a nearby hospital. This plan should include arrangements for emergency services and appropriate escort of the patient to the hospital. Anesthetic or surgical mishaps requiring resuscitation, emergency transfer, or death should be reported to the medical board within 3 business days using a specified form.
Louisiana	Chapter 73. Office-Based Surgery § 7313. Reports to the Board A. A physician performing office-based surgery shall notify the board in writing within 15 d of the occurrence or receipt of information that an office-based surgery resulted in the following: 1. An unanticipated and unplanned transport of the patient from the facility to a hospital emergency department 2. An unplanned readmission to the office-based surgery setting within 72 h of discharge from the facility 3. An unscheduled hospital admission of the patient within 72 h of discharge from the facility 4. The death of the patient within 30 d of surgery in an office-based facility
New Jersey	Subchapter 4a. Surgery. Special Procedures, and Anesthesia Services Performed in an Office Setting 3:35-4A.5. Duty to report incidents related to surgery, special procedures, or anesthesia in an office. Any incident related to surgery, special procedures, or the administration of anesthesia within the office that results in a patient death, transport of the patient to the hospital for observation or treatment for a period in excess of 24 h, or a complication or untoward event as defined in N.J.A.C. 13:35-4A.3, shall be reported to the Executive Director of the Board within 7 d, in writing, and on such forms as shall be required by the Board. Such reports shall be investigated by the Board and will be deemed confidential pursuant to N.J.S.A. 45:9-19.3

From Shapiro FE, Punwani N, Rosenberg NM, et al. Office-based anesthesia: safety and outcomes. Anesth Analg 2014;119(2):280; with permission.

(effective January 31, 2018) office-based surgery practices must provide continual monitoring of end-tidal carbon dioxide using capnography during moderate sedation, deep sedation, and general anesthesia.[42]

However, despite the numerous legislative and regulatory changes taking place, as of 2018, there are still 17 states that do not require adverse event reporting. Certain high-profile cases of adverse events or mortality have caught the attention of the media and the lack of uniform reporting has come to light as an issue for patient safety.[5–10,43]

SUMMARY

The migrating from inpatient hospitals and ASCs to the office-based setting has evolved for a variety of reasons: advances in technology and innovation in both anesthetic and surgical techniques, increased importance for convenience and privacy, and providing a more cost-effective solution to surgical care. The numerous advantages for medical providers and patients are not void of risk. Due to the lack of uniformity of OBA regulations combined with the high-profile cases of morbidity and mortality in the media, there is more attention being drawn to the safety concerns of performing surgical procedures in an office suite. Most OBA data to date are retrospective in nature, with a paucity of randomized controlled trials to aid in determining how office-based procedures and anesthesia affect morbidity and mortality. Recent data suggest that safety in the office-based setting is improving and may be due to the use of proper selection of procedures and patients, incorporating patient safety checklists and cognitive aids, following professional society guidelines, and maintaining accreditation. In addition, the advancement of state and federal governmental agencies exercising regulatory authority over practice management, adverse event reporting, and outcomes analyses, will enable the development of an evidence-based standard of care in the office-based surgery and anesthesia setting.

REFERENCES

1. Kutscher G. Outpatient care takes the inside track: ambulatory services continue to account for a growing share of systems' revenue, as they work to bring care closer to the customer. Mod Healthc 2012;42(32):24–6.

2. Koenig L, Doherty J, Dreyfus J, et al. An analysis of recent growth of Ambulatory surgery centers: final report. KNG Health Consulting. Available at: http://citeseerx.ist.psu.edu/viewdoc/download?doi=10.1.1.512.4498&rep=rep1&type=pdf. Accessed May 31, 2018.

3. Ashman JJ, Rui P, Okeyode T. Characteristics of office-based physician visits, 2014. NCHS Data Brief, no. 292. Hyattscille (MD): National; Center for Health Statistics; 2017.

4. Vila H Jr, Soto R, Cantor AB, et al. Comparative outcomes analysis of procedures performed in physician offices and ambulatory surgery centers. Arch Surg 2003; 138:991–5.

5. Messer L, Katersky. Joan Rivers' cause of death revealed. ABC News 2014. Available at: https://abcnews.go.com/Entertainment/joan-rivers-death-revealed/story?id=25264318. Accessed November 2, 2018.

6. Phillips S. Dental patient's sudden death raises questions. FOX 5 San Diego 2013. Available at: https://fox5sandiego.com/2013/04/02/dental-patients-sudden-death-raises-questions/. Accessed November 2, 2018.

7. Dental visit deaths spark push for political action. CBS News 2016. Available at: https://www.cbsnews.com/news/todder-dental-visit-dead-anesthesia-dangers/. Accessed November 2, 2018.

8. Raven Maria Blanco Foundation Inc. Crowdrise. 2007. Available at: https://www.crowdrise.com/rmbf. Accessed November 2, 2018.

9. Healy M. After child surgery deaths, experts discuss the risks. USA Today 2014. Available at: https://www.usatoday.com/story/news/nation/2014/01/11/children-dental-tonsils/4405525/. Accessed November 2, 2018.

10. Diaz M. Teen's parents speak out. Deerfield Beach (FL): South Florida Sun Sentinel; 2009. Available at: https://www.sun-sentinel.com/news/fl-xpm-2009-09-24-0909230487-story.html. Accessed November 2, 2018.

11. Soltani AM, Keyes GR, Singer R, et al. Outpatient surgery and sequelae: an analysis of the AAAASF internet quality assurance and peer review database. Clin Plast Surg 2013;40(3):465–73.

12. Shapiro FE, Punwani N, Rosenberg NM, et al. Office-based anesthesia: safety and outcomes. Anesth Analg 2014;119(2):276–85.

13. Shapiro FE, Samir RJ, Xiaoxia K, et al. Initial results from the National Anesthesia Clinical Outcomes Registry and overview of office-based anesthesia. Anesthesiol Clin 2014;21:431–44.

14. Jani S, Shapiro FE, Kordylewski H, et al. A comparison between office and other ambulatory practices: analysis from the National Anesthesia Clinical Outcomes Registry. J Healthc Risk Manag 2016;35(4):38–47.

15. Osman BM, Shapiro FE. Safe anesthesia in the office-based setting. ASA Monitor 2014;78(9):14–7.

16. Starling J 3rd, Thosani MK, Coldiron BM. Determining the safety of office-based surgery: what 10 years of Florida data and 6 years of Alabama data reveal. Dermatol Surg 2012;38:171–7.

17. Domino KB. Office-based anesthesia: lessons learned from the closed claims project. ASA Newsl 2001;65(6):9–11, 15.

18. Young S, Shapiro FE, Urman RD. Office-based surgery and patient outcomes. Curr Opin Anaesthesiol 2018;31(6):707–12.

19. Vila H. Commentary on: Is office-based surgery safe? Comparing outcomes of 183,914 aesthetic surgical procedures across different types of accredited facilities. Aesthet Surg J 2017;37(2):236–8.

20. Gupta V, Parikh R, Nguyen L, et al. Is office-based surgery safe? Comparing outcomes of 183,914 aesthetic surgical procedures across different types of accredited facilities. Aesthet Surg J 2017;37(2):226–35.

21. Lin PH, Yang KH, Kollmeyer KR, et al. Treatment outcomes and lessons learned from 5134 cases of outpatient office-based endovascular procedures in a vascular surgical practice. Vascular 2017;25(2):115–22.

22. American Society of Anesthesiologists. Guidelines for office-based anesthesia. Available at: http://www.asahq.org/quality-and-practice-management/standards-guidelines-and-related-resources/guidelines-for-office-based-anesthesia. Accessed July 11, 2018.

23. Practice guidelines for moderate procedural sedation and analgesia 2018: a report by the American Society of Anesthesiologists Task Force on moderate procedural sedation and analgesia, the American Association of oral and Maxillofacial Surgeons, American College of Radiology, American Dental Association, American Society of Dentist Anesthesiologists, and Society of Interventional Radiology. Anesthesiology 2018;128(3):437–79.

24. Metzner J, Kent CD. Ambulatory surgery: is the liability risk lower? Curr Opin Anaesthesiol 2012;25:654–8.

25. Rosenberg NM, Urman RD, Gallagher S, et al. Effect of an office-based surgical safety system on patient outcomes. Eplasty 2012;12:e59.

26. Robert MC, Choi CJ, Shapiro FE, et al. Avoidance of serious medical errors in refractive surgery using a custom preoperative checklist. J Cataract Refract Surg 2015;41:2171–8.

27. Fernando RJ, Shapiro FE, Urman RD. Survey analysis of an ambulatory surgical checklist for patient use. AORN J 2015;102(3):290e1–10.

28. Young S, Shapiro FE, Urman RD, et al. Customizing an emergency manual. ASA Monitor 2018;82(2):10–3.

29. The ISOBS emergency manual for office-based surgery. Available at: https://emergencymanuals.org/tools-resources/free-tools/. Accessed July 16, 2018.

30. Hughes CD, Urits I, Fukudome E, et al. Safe anesthesia for outpatient cosmetic surgery. Intern Med Rev (Wash D C) 2018;4(1):1–20.

31. Resources from ASA Committees. American Society of Anesthesiologists. Available at: https://www.asahq.org/resources/resources-from-asa-committees. Accessed August 6, 2018.

32. Accreditation handbook for office-based surgery including review guidelines. Skokie (IL): Accreditation Association for Ambulatory Health Care (AAAHC); 2017.

33. The Joint Commission. Facts about Office-Based Surgery Accreditation. 2018. Available at: https://www.jointcommission.org/accreditation/accreditation_main.aspx. Accessed August 6, 2018.

34. The American Association for Accreditation of Ambulatory Surgery Facilities, Inc. Inspecting and accrediting for over 30 years. Available at: http://www.aaaasf.org/aboutus.html. Accessed July 16, 2018.

35. Revised eligibility criteria for office-based surgery. The Joint Commission. Available at: https://www.jointcommission.org/assets/1/18/OBS_Eligibility_flyer_2018.pdf. Accessed August 6, 2018.

36. AAAHC Quality Roadmap 2017: a report on accreditation survey results. The Accreditation Association for Ambulatory Health Care, Inc.; 2017. Available at: http://www.aaahc.org/Global/AAAHC%20Institute_Quality%20Roadmap/AAAHC_Quality_Roadmap_2017_FINAL.pdf. Accessed September 24, 2018.

37. Oliver E. Common deficiencies cited by AAAASF and how to fix them. Becker's Review ASC 2017. Available at: https://www.beckersasc.com/asc-quality-infection-control/10-deficiencies-aaaasf-cites-most-and-how-to-correct-them-no-1-the-life-safety-code-standard.html. Accessed July 16, 2018.

38. Top standards compliance data announced for 2016. The Joint Commission perspectives. Available at: https://www.jointcommission.org/assets/1/6/Perspectives-ambuzz-17AHC_2016_chall_stds.pdf. Accessed August 6, 2018.

39. National Patient Safety Goals Effective January 2018. The Joint Commission. Available at: https://www.jointcommission.org/assets/1/6/NPSG_Chapter_HAP_Jan2018.pdf. Accessed July 16, 2018.

40. Office-Based Surgery Laws. The Policy Surveillance Program: a LawAtlas Project 2018. Available at: http://lawatlas.org/datasets/office-based-surgery-laws. Accessed October 31, 2018.

41. Changes to Office-Based Surgery Law Effective April 13, 2016. New York State Department of Health. Available at: https://www.health.ny.gov/professionals/office-based_surgery/. Accessed Septermber 24, 2018.

42. Use of capnography/end tidal CO2 monitoring in patients receiving moderate sedation, deep sedation & general anesthesia. NYS DOH Office-Based Surgery.

Available at: https://www.health.ny.gov/professionals/office-based_surgery/docs/use_of_capnography.pdf. Accessed July 16, 2018.

43. Jewett C, Alesia M. When routine surgery results in death: Memphis center cited for lack of accurate reporting. Commercial Appeal (Memphis, TN) Westlaw New Room 2018;24601282:1–8.

Advancing the Safe Delivery of Office-Based Dental Anesthesia and Sedation
A Comprehensive and Critical Compendium

Mark A. Saxen, DDS, PhD[a,b,*], James W. Tom, DDS, MS[c,d],
Keira P. Mason, MD[e]

KEYWORDS

- Anesthesia • Capnography • Dental • *NFPA 99* • Office-based • Precordial
- Pediatric

KEY POINTS

- Anesthesiologists asked to perform dental office-based anesthesia should anticipate a population of preschool-aged children undergoing treatment by a pediatric dental specialist.
- The average dental operatory is one-third to one-fourth the size of the average hospital or surgery center operating room. Anesthesia providers must be prepared to manage this environment and anticipate emergency routines in an environment that is, very different from the operating room.
- In addition to standard anesthetic monitors, simultaneous use of pretracheal stethoscopy and capnography provides a more reliable and real-time method of monitoring than using any of these modalities alone.
- The 2018 edition of the *National Health Care Facilities Code* contains explicit standards for dental office anesthetics.

[a] Anesthesia, Oral Surgery and Hospital Dentistry, Indiana University School of Dentistry, Indianapolis, IN, USA; [b] Private Practice, Indiana Office-Based Anesthesia, 3750 Guion Road, Suite 225, Indianapolis, IN 46222, USA; [c] Section on Dental Anesthesiology, Herman Ostrow School of Dentistry, University of Southern California, Los Angeles, CA, USA; [d] Divisions 1 & 3, Herman Ostrow School of Dentistry, University of Southern California, 925 West 34th Street, Los Angeles, CA 90089, USA; [e] Department of Anesthesiology, Critical Care and Pain Medicine, Bader 3, Boston Children's Hospital, Harvard Medical School, 300 Longwood Avenue, Boston, MA 02115, USA
* Corresponding author. 3750 Guion Road, Suite 225, Indianapolis, IN 46222.
E-mail address: msaxen93@gmail.com

Anesthesiology Clin 37 (2019) 333–348
https://doi.org/10.1016/j.anclin.2019.01.003
1932-2275/19/© 2019 Elsevier Inc. All rights reserved.

INTRODUCTION

The provision for and administration of dental office-based sedation and anesthesia requires considerations and preparations that are unique to dentistry and unlike that of any other office-based and nonoperating room procedures. Anesthesia services in dental office-based settings pose challenges and considerations that can be unpredictable, as reflected in the recently published American Society of Anesthesiologists (ASA) *Statement on Sedation & Anesthesia Administration in Dental Office-Based Settings*.[1] This article explores in depth the idiosyncrasies and risks of dental office-based anesthesia (OBA) and sedation, both of which are often underappreciated by operating room–based anesthesia providers.

All providers, regardless of the venue, must be familiar with and prepared for emergencies, including malignant hyperthermia, a difficult (recognized and unrecognized) airway, anaphylaxis, local anesthesia toxicity, respiratory depression and apnea, aspiration, and acute cardiovascular emergencies. Specialty guidelines, statements, and recommendations should be followed, with deviations carefully documented and supported. Dentistry is unique in that it spans multiple areas of medicine: surgery, medicine, pediatrics, geriatrics, and anesthesia. There are multiple societies and organizations with an interest in anesthesia for dental procedures including the American Society of Dentist Anesthesiologists (ASDA), the American Academy of Pediatrics (AAP), the ASA, the American Academy of Pediatric Dentistry (AAPD), and the American Dental Association. This article presents a comprehensive compendium of current clinical practice and knowledge.

PATIENT DEMOGRAPHICS AND CHARACTERISTICS

A review of 5,929,953 nonoperating room anesthesia cases in the National Anesthesia Clinical Outcomes Registry (NACOR) between 2010 and 2014, describes the average patient as 53.8 ($\pm$ 20.8) years old. The most common procedures were short (mean 40 minutes) and included colonoscopy, esophagogastroduodenoscopy, electroconvulsive therapy, endoscopic retrograde cholangiopancreatography, and elective cardioversion.[2] In contrast, an examination of 7041 office-based dental anesthesia cases from the Society for Ambulatory Anesthesia (SAMBA) Clinical Outcomes Registry over the same time period revealed a significantly younger patient population (mean 4.7 $\pm$ 2.9 years), and slightly longer procedure duration (mean 58 minutes). Almost all procedures involved comprehensive dental restoration of early childhood caries, an aggressive form of dental caries. Of these dental office-based anesthesia (OBA) cases, 39% were performed under general anesthesia, either with oral or nasal endotracheal intubation.[3] Office-based dental procedures were shorter in duration compared with equivalent procedures in the hospital operating room setting.[4]

Although the NACOR and SAMBA data suggest that most dental anesthesia involves children, these databases do not include the estimated 2.8 million annual deep sedations and general anesthetics delivered by oral and maxillofacial surgeons in their offices.[5] A 2003 outcomes study of 34,191 patients undergoing anesthesia or sedation in oral surgery offices revealed the average age was 28 ($\pm$ 16.1) years. Generally, oral surgery cases are much shorter than pediatric dental rehabilitation cases, 59.1% being completed within 10 to 30 minutes and 95.7% completed within 60 minutes. Of these, 99% involve third molar removal or other dentoalveolar surgery, with 97% having an ASA physical status of ASA I or ASA II. Deep sedation and general anesthetics in oral surgery offices are almost always directed and administered by the operating oral surgeon with his or her team of dental assistants. Physician anesthesiologists and dentist anesthesiologists are used in less than 1% of oral and maxillofacial cases and certified registered nurse anesthetists in 2.5%.[6] Based on these data, anesthesiologists asked to perform dental OBA should anticipate a population of preschool-age children undergoing treatment by a pediatric dental specialist. **Fig. 1** shows the relative distribution of dental providers in a typical dentist anesthesiologist's practice.

RISK FACTORS AND PREDICTABLE ADVERSE EVENTS

In an analysis of 98 dentistry-related adverse events drawn from the ASA Closed Claims Project, Domino[7] identified 6 damaging events underlying the claims: difficult intubation, accidental extubation, premature extubation, aspiration, preexisting cardiovascular abnormalities, and the application of an external heat source. This analysis did not discriminate among cases performed in hospitals, surgery centers, and offices. The prominence of airway issues in Domino's report is consistent with an earlier analysis that cites airway complications, inadequate ventilation, and underlying disease as important factors in pediatric adverse events.[8] Although these studies provide observations drawn from anesthesia-related sources, other publications examining dental office morbidity and mortality repeat the themes of failed airway management, inadequate monitoring, and failed rescue as consistent precursors to morbidity and mortality in dental office sedation and anesthesia.[9,10]

THE DENTAL OFFICE ENVIRONMENT
Patient Selection, Preoperative Evaluation, Anesthesia or Sedation Planning, and Strategies to Minimize Risk for Dental Office-Based Anesthesia

Establishing a policy mandating a preoperative history and physical examination and documenting a preanesthetic evaluation, decreases the chances of unanticipated medical issues on the day of service and associated case delays or cancellations. In general terms, the lowest risk patients to treat in the remote dental office-based setting are ASA 1 and 2 patients who do not require extensive postoperative medical management or recovery. Under exceptional circumstances, the authors will consider office-based management of ASA 3 patients who require urgent or emergent dental procedures (eg, extraction of painful and infected dentition, incision and drainage of an intraoral or extraoral space infection, intraoral laceration suturing) that may provide

Type of Office Served

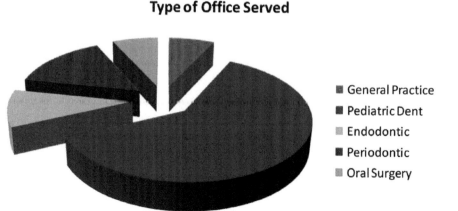

- General Practice
- Pediatric Dent
- Endodontic
- Periodontic
- Oral Surgery

Fig. 1. Distribution of the type of dentist served in typical dentist anesthesiologist practice.

substantial benefit to a patient. Providers for pediatric dental patients should be familiar with preexisting medical conditions and risk factors that have been shown to carry a greater likelihood of postanesthesia or sedation morbidity. A review of dental anesthesia and sedation-related closed claims from 1993 to 2007, revealed that 76% of the claims were sedation-related.[9] In 2013, a review of trends in death associated with pediatric dental anesthesia and sedation searched media reports from 1980 to 2011. A total of 44 deaths were reported in patients younger than the age of 21 years, with half of the deaths being in children 2 to 5 years of age undergoing relatively simple procedures of fillings, crowns, and extractions. Of these deaths, 45% were reported as occurring while the patient was under moderate sedation. A higher percentage of deaths occurred in office-based settings.[11] Airway and respiratory-related events make up most sedation-related and anesthesia-related cases of morbidity and mortality.[12] A 2017 retrospective review of 83,491 airway adverse events from the Pediatric Sedation Research Consortium by Mallory and colleagues[13] examined children with and without an upper respiratory infection undergoing procedural sedation in a hospital for a wide variety of procedures. Their analysis suggests that the presence of an upper respiratory tract infection within the preceding 2 weeks, increases the risk of airway events from 6.3% to 9.1%. The risk escalates with clear (14.6%) and thick (22.2%) secretions.

Although a causal relationship between asthma and dental caries has not been demonstrated, there are investigators who suggest children with severe caries are at increased risk of reactive airway disease.[14,15] In summary, it is advisable to restrict most dental OBA only to those who are ASA 1 and 2, without airway anomalies or craniofacial malformations that could pose airway risks, without risk factors for aspiration, who are not at the extremes of age or size (high body mass index), and who present without upper respiratory tract symptoms for a minimum of 2 weeks.

Patients with significant behavioral and cognitive challenges (autism spectrum disorder) that could pose a risk for the patient, family, or providers, should be carefully considered for alternative methods and places of treatment. Notably, in regard to premedication, that the AAPD "Guidelines for Monitoring and Management of Pediatric Patients Before, During, and After Sedation for Diagnostic and Therapeutic Procedures: Update 2016"[16] specifically states that the administration of sedating medications at home poses an unacceptable risk, particularly for infants and pre-school aged children traveling in car safety seats because deaths as a result of this practice have been reported. Furthermore, protective stabilization (papoose boards) should be reserved for special circumstances and should follow the 2013 and 2015 AAPD "Guideline on Protective Stabilization and Behavior Guidance for the Pediatric Dental Patient."[17] The AAPD considers protective stabilization to be an advanced behavior guidance technique and defines it as "Any manual method, physical or mechanical device, material, or equipment that immobilizes or reduces the ability of a patient to move his or her arms, legs, body or head freely." It requires informed consent and parental presence (unless an exception is noted and documented).

Part of sedation and anesthesia preoperative planning should include a patient's appropriateness for undergoing an OBA with same-day discharge home. Strict discharge criteria should be followed and it is important that the meeting of discharge criteria be clearly documented in the medical record. A parental questionnaire of post-discharge events (first 24 hours) occurring in pediatric dental patients after deep sedation reported the following: incidence of sleepiness in 62%, lack of appetite in 29%, insomnia in 13% and nausea, and in vomiting 11%.[18] Patients with symptoms or a diagnosis of apnea (central, obstructive, sleep) should be carefully screened and the authors suggest, deferred to care in a hospital setting.

Specific Dental Preoperative Evaluation

In addition to the patient medical history and physical examination, careful consideration should be given to the anticipated procedure along with any concomitant risks. Of particular concern is the fear of aspiration of loose dentition and subsequent foreign object obstruction during airway instrumentation, visualization, or positioning (supine, semisupine). For adults, close consultation with the dental provider may indicate problematic mobility or risk of tooth fracture in dentition from moderate to severe periodontal disease, previous trauma, or advanced dental decay.[19] In children, primary (deciduous) dentition generally follows a predictable eruption table in healthy individuals with uncomplicated development, therefore facilitating the ability of anesthesia providers to predict risk of shedding teeth. Typically, around age 6 years, children will begin to lose primary upper and lower incisors, followed by first primary molars around age 9 to 11 years, then canines around 9 to 12 years, and finally second primary molars. The placement of dental appliances and dental devices must be noted before sedation and anesthetic treatment planning (**Fig. 2**). Adults may have removable appliances (complete or partial dentures, implant retained dentures, orthodontic retainers, and/or other devices) that should be removed before the induction of sedation or anesthesia because these may pose significant foreign object airway obstruction or aspiration risks. Smaller devices, such as dental implant devices and implant tissue healing abutments (small screws or other fixtures) may be removed by dentists before sedation or anesthesia as well. With children and adolescents, semipermanent

Primary Teeth

Upper Teeth	Erupt	Shed
Central Incisor	8–12 Mo	6–7 Y
Lateral Incisor	9–13 Mo	7–8 Y
Canine (Cuspid)	16–22 Mo	10–12 Y
First Molar	13–19 Mo	9–11 Y
Second Molar	25–33 Mo	10–12 Y

Lower Teeth	Erupt	Shed
Second Molar	23–31 Mo	10–12 Y
First Molar	14–18 Mo	9–11 Y
Canine (Cuspid)	17–23 Mo	9–12 Y
Lateral Incisor	10–16 Mo	7–8 Y
Central Incisor	6–10 Mo	6–7 Y

Fig. 2. Eruption and exfoliation chart of the primary dentition. Although wide variety exists among individuals, a general knowledge of when to expect the shedding of primary teeth can alert anesthesia providers to the potential for inadvertent tooth loss and possible aspiration during laryngoscopy. (*From* ADA Division of Communications; Journal of the American Dental Association; ADA Council on Scientific Affairs. For the dental patient. Tooth eruption: the primary teeth. J Am Dental Assoc 2005;136:1619; with permission.)

fixtures, such as orthodontic brackets, wires, and even palatal expanders (**Fig. 3**) affixed directly in the palatal vault, may pose significant problems when inserting a laryngoscope, supraglottic airway, oropharyngeal airway, or endotracheal tube. Different strategies should be discussed before the induction of anesthesia, including emergent removal, if patient safety is compromised with problematic hardware.

Intermaxillary fixation is often used to stabilize the maxillomandibular complex following a fracture of the mandible. This technique uses wires and rubber bands, affixed to interdigitating teeth, to achieve semipermanent closure of the mouth. It is imperative that the anesthesia provider has immediate access to and is adept at using a wire cutter (**Fig. 4**) or a similar device, should there be a need for emergent airway access.

Strict nil per os (NPO) guidelines should be followed. For elective procedures, the protocols outlined in the most recent ASA "Practice Guidelines for Preoperative Fasting and the Use of Pharmacologic Agents to Reduce the Risk of Pulmonary Aspiration: Application to Healthy Patients Undergoing Elective Procedures"[20] should be followed. Anesthesia providers, caretakers and parents, and office staff must be particularly aware of easy access to drinking fountains and other sources of food that are commonly offered in many dental waiting rooms. Dental operatories can inadvertently lend themselves to risk of NPO violations if cups of water used to rinse or drink are easily accessible. The typical air-water syringe found on most dental chair units can readily dispense water for drinking as well. Efforts should be made to ensure all sources of drinking water and food are removed from patient waiting areas and treatment areas to minimize NPO violations. Dentistry and oral and maxillofacial procedures impart a greater potential for intraoral bleeding, and a strategy to minimize postoperative nausea and vomiting should be strongly considered.

Operatory Size and Emergency Response Planning

The size and layout of the dental operatory is an important factor in crisis planning for office-based general anesthesia. Most dental operatories are much smaller than the operating rooms found in hospitals or surgery centers. If anesthesia services are being provided in an office-based setting, it is important to be familiar with and follow the *ASA Statement on Sedation & Anesthesia Administration in Dental Office-Based Settings*,[1] "American Society of Dentist Anesthesiologists Parameters of Care,"[21] and the

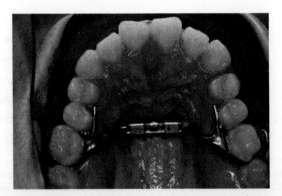

Fig. 3. Semipermanent pediatric palatal expansion device cemented onto the molars of the maxilla. The device has an expansion screw in the vault of the palate and can interfere with laryngoscopy and airway devices. (*Courtesy of* K. McClure, DDS, Los Angeles, CA.)

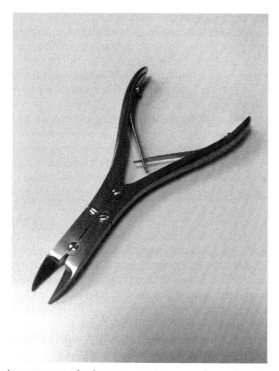

Fig. 4. Intraoral wire cutters to obtain emergent access to the oral cavity and permit mouth opening if a patient is placed into intermaxillary fixation or has multiple elastic ligatures to temporarily stabilize the mandible. (*Courtesy of* J. Tom, DDS, MS, Los Angeles, CA.)

AAP-AAPD "Guidelines for Monitoring and Management of Pediatric Patients Before, During, and After Sedation for Diagnostic and Therapeutic Procedures: Update 2016."[19]

The ideal dental operatory has been described as a 10.5 ft by 11.5 ft a space,[22] which is approximately one-fourth to one-third of the average hospital or surgery center operating room,[23] and 33% less than the minimum space standard for endoscopy suites.[24] Many dental operatory designs include fixed cabinetry in the space immediately behind the head of the chair, requiring the anesthesiologist to rotate and reposition the chair to perform airway management. Space for portable anesthesia machines and ventilators is often at a premium, and most often the space is shared with the operating dentist and dental assistant seated in very close proximity to the patient's head, anesthesia circuit (if used), and direct visual monitoring. The placement of monitors, drugs, and instruments will likely vary with every location because few operatories contain enough space to accommodate the average hospital-sized anesthesia cart.

The stability of the dental chair in a fully extended position should also be verified before beginning the case, as many dental chairs are not conducive to conducting chest compressions during cardiopulmonary resuscitation. Most modern dental chairs can be moved with assistance, despite the common assumption that they are fixed to the floor. If resuscitation needs to be provided, it is important to consider that CPR compression boards or similar support should be immediately available. Also, the placement of an available dental assistant's chair under the headrest of a dental chair aids in the stability of the resuscitation platform when vigorous chest compressions are delivered. It should be noted that moving the patient from the dental chair to the floor to perform resuscitation may cause further injury and delay timely care. The "ASA Statement on Nonoperating Room Anesthetizing Locations"[25] requires that the room have enough space available to accommodate equipment, monitors, and personnel needed to perform anesthesia and respond to emergencies.

Mock resuscitation drills, with appropriate office personnel, are part of essential emergency training for dental OBA. Simulation has been shown to play an important role even for dental trainees and assistants. A medical crisis management simulation activity was given to dental assistants and first-year and second-year dental residents. Common emergency scenarios were presented that included anaphylaxis, laryngospasm, sedative medication overdoes, and multiple drug interaction with cardiac arrhythmias. Of all participants, 91.7% acknowledged that this simulation activity is a good tool for crisis management skill development. Strategies for effective simulation training for OBA have also been comprehensively presented in an oral maxillofacial journal.[26] The simulation should involve all members of the team, with each member being given clearly defined tasks. The team members include the proceduralist, anesthesia and surgical assistant, and the front office clerk. Scenarios include airway management; vascular access; drug preparation; drug administration; and use of defibrillator, cardioversion, or pacer.

The ASA "Practice Guidelines for Moderate Procedural Sedation and Analgesia 2018"[27] clearly delineate the expectations regarding emergency preparedness and management. These include the availability of pharmacologic antagonists to benzodiazepines and opioids, and the presence of at least 1 skilled individual to provide positive pressure ventilation and establish intravenous access. They recommend team training, simulation drills, and the development and implementation of checklists. The creation and implementation of a quality improvement process is expected. The World Health Organization supports the use of checklists in improving safety and has created a comprehensive pediatric procedural sedation checklist covering everything from presedation evaluation to recovery room and discharge.[28] This checklist can be adopted and modified for adult sedation and tailored, when necessary, to different procedures and environs.

Oxygen and Suction in the Dental Office

A great deal of variability exists in the oxygen supply systems for dental operatories. Central oxygen and nitrous oxide delivery systems using H-sized tanks secured in a remote location are relatively common; however, some offices may only use portable E-sized cylinders. Pressure gauges will be found in the manifold above the tanks in the central tank storage space as well as on the cabinet in the operatory. In addition to checking capacity and pressures at the tank itself, both pressure gauges on the low-pressure side (patient delivery circuit) should read near or at 50 psi, assuring no leak exists within the system before the start of the case. A minimum backup of 2 functional E-sized cylinders should be available with a functioning regulator and self-inflating hand resuscitator (Bag-Valve-Mask or BVM) in the case of a central oxygen system failure or depletion.

Most gas delivery systems allow the anesthesiologist to manually control oxygen and nitrous oxide concentrations and inspired fresh gas flows by means of a rotary knob; useful in the event of a system malfunction. Some newer digital units are controlled solely with electronic control panel buttons, without immediate and direct access to oxygen and nitrous supply valves. Anesthesia providers should be aware and have a backup oxygen supply immediately available in the room before the start of anesthesia. Often, dental settings will incorporate E-sized oxygen tanks into a nitrous-oxide inhalation sedation unit that also uses E-sized cylinders of liquid nitrous oxide. Notably, most dental nitrous-oxide inhalation sedation units do not have provisions to provide positive pressure oxygen sources such as found in a typical volatile anesthesia gas delivery machines. The Porter 2210K Directional Y Valve (Porter, Hatfield, PA) (**Fig. 5**) is a useful device for OBA because it allows immediate, rapid switching from a supplemental oxygen or nitrous oxide delivery system to an anesthesia breathing circuit with positive pressure capabilities.

Two types of surgical suctions are typically available on dental units: a low-volume evacuator and a high-volume evacuator. The low-volume evacuator, also commonly referred to as a saliva ejector, is designed to be seated in a dental patient's mouth and passively evacuate saliva over several minutes. In contrast, the high-volume evacuator removes fluid at a rate similar to systems found in operating rooms. Anesthesia providers should use the high-volume evacuator system because it has the capacity to rapidly remove fluid and debris from the airway in the event of laryngospasm or obstruction. This may require planning, because the high-volume evacuator is almost always used by the operating dentist, and many offices have only 1 high-volume line per operatory. High-volume suction tips seldom have multiple orifices found in standard tissue suction tips and may be easily be occluded by the tongue, buccal tissue, or pharyngeal tissue during most routine dental procedures. A standard Yankauer suction tip can be made to attach and detach from the system in a few seconds using an adaptor, should sharing the system with the operating dentist be required. In contrast, the low-speed system uses a smaller diameter orifice, may take several seconds to evacuate mouth obstructed with blood and fluids, and is more easily clogged by viscous fluids and particulate debris. Notably, most dental operatory systems do not use the surgical suction canisters or standard surgical suction lines commonly found in operating room settings, so length of reach and adaptability to suction tips and catheters must be considered before the procedure.

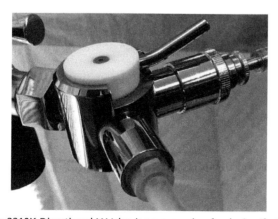

Fig. 5. The Porter 2210K Directional Y Valve is an example of a device that can be fitted to a common Porter portable nitrous oxide delivery system and allows immediate conversion from a small-bore supplemental oxygen supply to a large-bore system capable of delivering positive pressure ventilation using a modified Jackson-Rees circuit. (*Courtesy of* Porter MXR Flowmeter and Directional Y Valve Image. Porter Instrument, Parker Hannifin Corporation.)

VENTILATORY MONITORING

In addition to the standard anesthetic monitors, the authors have found that the simultaneous use of pretracheal stethoscopy complements capnography to provide a more reliable and real-time method of ventilatory monitoring during dental sedation and general anesthesia than using capnography alone.

The "American Society of Anesthesiologists Standards for Basic Anesthetic Monitoring"[29] mandate continual monitoring for the presence of exhaled carbon dioxide unless invalidated by the nature of the patient, procedure, or equipment. The 2018 ASA "Guidelines for Moderate Procedural sedation and Analgesia"[27] also require that a separate, designated individual, who is not the proceduralist, be responsible for monitoring capnography and physiologic monitoring. This person should be able to recognize apnea and airway obstruction and be authorized to call for help. This individual may assist with minor, interruptible tasks (suctioning, light curing, tissue and cheek retraction) if the level of sedation and vital signs are stable. The guidelines recommend that capnography be instituted, ideally before initiating sedation (may be applied as moderate sedation is being achieved in uncooperative patient) and monitored continually unless precluded or invalidated by nature of patient, procedure or equipment. For deep sedation and general anesthesia in a dental setting, the ASA, AAP-AAPD, and the ASDA require the presence of a separate anesthesia provider, such as a dentist or physician anesthesiologist, a certified registered nurse anesthetist, or a separate oral and maxillofacial surgeon, who is not involved in the procedure.[1,30,31] The important role of capnography in reducing risk of respiratory-related events is supported by a recent meta-analysis of 13 randomized controlled trials published since 2006 that involve capnography in procedural sedation.[21] Capnography was found to increase the likelihood of detecting adverse events, possibly reducing the need for airway interventions. The combination of capnography, visual assessment, and pulse oximeter decreased the occurrence of mild and severe oxygen desaturations and the need for assisted ventilation.

Capnography is especially valuable for confirming the ventilatory status during times of high ambient noise levels such as the use of the dental handpiece, which often diminishes or eliminates the ability to monitor breath sounds. In addition to handpieces, high-speed suction, which is used extensively throughout most dental procedures, also obscures breath sounds, making stethoscopy less useful during the intraoperative phase compared with induction and emergence. Furthermore, when positive pressure ventilation is required for rescue from apnea in a patient with a nonprotected airway, capnography remains the most valuable monitor to determine the adequacy of successful ventilation. Taken together, the simultaneous use of both techniques provides the anesthesiologist with the benefit of continuous ventilatory monitoring, whereas the use of either technique alone is associated with a high likelihood of interruption.

Several routinely-performed dental maneuvers have the potential to alter or obstruct ventilation. These include full-mouth dental radiographs, the extraction of mandibular teeth, full-mouth dental impressions, the seating of mandibular stainless-steel crowns, the placement of rubber dams or isolation devices, and other commonly performed, dentistry-related tasks. The capacity of stethoscopy to immediately alert the anesthesiologist to changes in ventilation during these maneuvers makes it a very useful adjunct to capnography, which is associated with an event-to-signal lag time of a few to several seconds. Some investigators claim direct patient observation make the capnographic lag time clinically insignificant; however, in anesthesia performed in dental settings, the anesthesia provider is typically located several feet away from the airway and direct observation of the patient's head and thorax is hindered by the oral barrier or isolation devices, drapes, lights, and instrumentation used by dental operators.

Modern pretracheal stethoscopes possess the sensitivity to detect qualitative changes in breath sounds, such as increased resonance and early wheezing, that cannot be appreciated with a visual monitor (**Fig. 6**). In a well-known study of the breathing periods in asthmatics after intravenous induction, Pisov and colleagues[32] found wheezing to occur in 25% of asthmatics compared with 6% in nonasthmatics. Given the high rate of reactive airways and asthma in children with early childhood caries, perioperative auscultation usually provides valuable information to dental anesthesia providers.

STABILIZATION OF THE HEAD

In both dental and oral surgical procedures, the operator can be expected to move the head and mandible throughout the course of the procedure or surgery, particularly when performing the previously mentioned procedures. If the head is left unsecured, operator-induced movement may be sufficient to dislodge the intended position of an endotracheal tube or laryngeal mask airway. For this reason, it is highly desirable to fix the position of the head before the start of the surgery or procedure. This relatively simple maneuver can become complicated when performing anesthesia in a dental chair, given the wide variety of dental chairs in use.

Most dental chairs are contoured, none provide patient straps, and most are not constructed to accommodate small children in a position desirable for general anesthesia. This is overcome with the use of a stabilization board, which serves the dual purposes of securing the patient and allowing the head to be taped into position with the aid of neck and shoulder supports. Protective stabilization must follow the guidelines of the AAPD, as previously cited. When secured in this way, airway obstruction is much less likely to occur. Although some operators may be unaccustomed to keeping the patient's head in a fixed position and initially find it restrictive with limited vision and mobility, adjusting the dental chair to reverse Trendelenburg can circumvent these concerns.

INTRAOPERATIVE FIRE SAFETY

Surgical fires during dental surgery are a rare but devastating event that has only recently become appreciated on a large scale. The same conditions that promote operating room fires exist in the dental operatory: oxygen pooling, the proximity of an ignition source, and the presence of flammable substrates. Supplemental oxygen from a nasal cannula has been shown to result in concentrated pools of oxygen

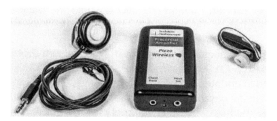

Fig. 6. A wireless pretracheal stethoscope can provide continuous auscultation of breath sounds within a range of several feet. (*Courtesy of* Sedation Resources Inc, Lone Oak, TX.)

around the face ranging from 24.9% to 53.5%, with highest concentrations occurring at the corners of the mouth and beneath the lower lip.[33–35] Ignition sources include electrocautery devices and occasional sparking that may occur during certain cutting procedures in operative dentistry.[36] Flammable materials and solvents are also commonplace in dental procedures, however in the presence of enriched oxygen, even normally nonflammable materials can combust.[37–39] Especially in an office-based setting, it is prudent to locate and contact the local emergency services (emergency medical facilities and paramedic-level responders, including the fire department) to make them aware of the office-based practice and its location.

The use of supplemental oxygen during deep sedation for pediatric dental procedures is an accepted component of safe procedural sedation.[19,40] Supplemental oxygen before a respiratory collapse has been shown to provide increased time until oxygen desaturation. A head up or reverse Trendelenburg position can also prolong time to desaturation.[41] Several strategies have been proposed to balance the value of having a reserve of enriched oxygen for pediatric patients with the risk of potential surgical fire. The Anesthesia Patient Safety Foundation recommends practitioners restrict supplemental oxygen to concentrations lower than 30% fraction of inspired oxygen (Fio_2).[42] Oxygen-air blenders, devices capable of delivering precision Fio_2 mixtures between 21% and 100% with a 3% error, have been proposed as a way of achieving this.[43] Although such blenders are easily attached to standard anesthesia machines, the use of blenders with dental oxygen-nitrous oxide delivery systems typically used in dental offices is not straightforward.

The ASA operating room fires algorithm[44] recommends providers consider general anesthesia with an endotracheal tube or laryngeal mask instead of moderate or deep sedation when anticipating the need for high Fio_2 during surgery of the head, neck, or face.[45] A simpler but equally important strategy is the conscientious use of high-speed intraoral suction to evacuate pooled oxygen in the vicinity of electrocautery and other potential ignition sources. VanCleave and colleagues[46] observed combustion in only 10% of in vitro trials compared with 52% of trials performed without suction. Finally, excellent communication between the dental operator and anesthesia provider maximizes fire safety because the use of electrocautery is typically planned, and dentists are typically aware of conditions that may produce the required conditions for intraoral fires.

INHALATIONAL ANESTHESIA IN THE DENTAL OFFICE

By virtue of their training, anesthesiologists are fully aware of the operation and use of the front end of an inhalational anesthetic system; that is, the components that include the anesthesia machine, the circuit, and the patient. Very few have equal familiarity with the back end of the system, which includes the medical gas piping, vacuum, and scavenging system of the facility. Anesthesia providers who visit dental offices to perform anesthesia typically assume the back end of an inhalational anesthesia system to be fully functional and safe, however this might not be true.

All dental offices are expected to comply with National Fire Protection Association (NFPA) code, entitled *NFPA 99: Health Care Facilities Code*.[47] This code, which was created in 1999 and is updated every 3 years, specifies the minimum safe standards for all medical and dental gas installations in the United States.[23] Although some dentists mistakenly assume this code does not apply to their offices, the NFPA has actually become increasingly concerned over the years about structural defects in dental office gas piping systems that have resulted in injury or death.

Table 1
Categories of medical or dental gas systems

Category Type	Type 3	Type 2	Type 1
Permissible Depth of Anesthesia	Anxiolysis and minimal sedation	Moderate sedation	Deep sedation and general anesthesia
Zone Valves Required	No	Yes	Yes
Zone Alarms Required	No	Yes	Yes
Master Alarm Panel	Yes	Single	Dual
Line-Pressure Control	Per Manufacturer	Plus flow for peak demand	Plus flow for peak demand
Vacuum System	Dental Vacuum	Simplex	Separate waste anesthetic gas and medical vacuum from dental vacuum
Testing and Verification	Local code and manufacturer specs	ASSE 6030 3rd party verifier	ASSE 6030 3rd party verifier
Reserve Gas Supply	Minimum not required	1-day reserve supply	1-day reserve supply

Comparison of *NFPA 99* Medical and dental gas system requirements. The requirements are based on the level of anesthesia being administered in the facility.

Reproduced and modified with permission from the APSF. Wong JL, Gschwandtner G. Safe Gas Systems and Office-Based Anesthesia. Anesthesia Patient Safety Foundation Newsletter 2018;33(1):18.

The 2018 edition of the *NFPA 99* contains explicit standards for dental offices in chapter 15: "Dental Gas and Vacuum Systems." Dental offices belong in 1 of 3 categories: category 1 includes offices that provide deep sedation and general anesthesia, category 2 are facilities that provide moderate sedation; and category 3 facilities provide only nitrous oxide anxiolysis and minimal sedation. Each of the 3 levels contains a unique set of standards for its medical gas supplies (**Table 1**). Offices with built in nitrous oxide analgesia systems using category 3 specifications may not have the type of safety features and redundancy that are intended for category 1 systems. Insidious consequences may result from this mismatch. For example, anesthesia machines connected, with adaptors, to the gas and vacuum supply of category 3 system could result in fluctuations in fresh gas and vacuum flows to the anesthesia machine. To ensure compliance with *NFPA 99*, an independent American Society of Safety Engineers (ASSE) 6030 medical gas verifier should check any new facility or when adding additional sedation and anesthesia services to an office or facility.[48]

SUMMARY

Providing OBA or sedation for dental patients creates a unique set of challenges and limitations. A thorough knowledge of the policies, guidelines, statements, and recommendations of the various dental societies, as well as the most recent ASA and AAP positions specifically pertaining to dental settings, is important to ensure safe and compliant practice. The limitations of the office-based floor plan and anesthetizing or sedation location should elicit creative planning and resourcefulness. Emergency preparedness, simulation drills, and emergency checklists should be rehearsed regularly and involve all members of the office team, from the front desk staff to the assistants to the physician or dentist. Physiologic monitoring must meet the standard of care and include capnography for all but minimal sedation and anxiolysis.

Supplemental oxygen can provide some extra valuable minutes before severe oxygen desaturation, in the event of apnea, respiratory compromise, or cardiovascular arrest. Fire safety should be carefully followed and safety drills performed in the event of fire. Local emergency services, including the fire department, emergency medical, and paramedical services, should be notified of the exact location of the office-based setting. Should the office be difficult to locate, drills should include routine walk-through visits from these respective services. Maximizing safety and optimizing dental care requires a comprehensive team approach and a thorough knowledge of and commitment to following and keeping up with relevant guidelines and statements.

REFERENCES

1. Available at: https://www.asahq.org/standards-and-guidelines/statement-on-sedation–anesthesia-administration-in-dental-officebased-settings. Accessed February 26, 2019.
2. Nagrebetsky A, Gabriel RA, Dutton RP, et al. Growth of nonoperating room anesthesia care in the United States: a contemporary trends analysis. Anesth Analg 2017;124(4):1261–7.
3. Spera AL, Saxen MA. Office-based anesthesia: safety and outcomes in pediatric dental patients. Anesth Prog 2017;64:144–52.
4. Saxen MA, Urman RD. Comparison of anesthesia for dental/oral surgery by office-based anesthesiologists versus operating room-based physician anesthesiologists. Anesth Prog 2017;65:212–20.
5. Bennett JD, Kramer KA, Bosack RC. How safe is deep sedation or general anesthesia while providing dental care? J Am Dent Assoc 2015;146(9):705–8.
6. Perrott DH, Yuen JP, Andresen RV, et al. Office-based anesthesia: outcomes of clinical practice of oral and maxillofacial surgeons. J Oral Maxillofac Surg 2003;61:983–95.
7. Domino K Anesthesia outside the operating room: a look at the ASA closed claims experience presented at the American Society of Dentist Anesthesiologist's Annual Scientific Session. Seattle, WA, April 16, 2010.
8. Morray JP1, Geiduschek JM, Caplan RA, et al. A comparison of pediatric and adult anesthesia closed malpractice claims. Anesthesiology 1993;78(3):461–7.
9. Chicka MC, Dembo JB, Mathu-Muju KR, et al. Adverse events during pediatric dental anesthesia and sedation: a review of closed malpractice claims pediatric dentistry. Pediatr Dent 2012;34(3):231–8.
10. Cote C, Notterman D, Karl HW, et al. Adverse sedation events in pediatrics: a critical incident analysis of contributing factors. Pediatrics 2000;105(4):805–14.
11. Lee HH, Milgrom P, Starks H, et al. Trends in death associated with pediatric dental sedation and general anesthesia. Paediatr Anaesth 2013;23(8):741–6.
12. Metzner J, Posner KL, Domino KB. The risk and safety of anesthesia at remote locations: the US closed claims analysis. Curr Opin Anaesthesiol 2009;22(4):502–8.
13. Mallory MD, Travers C, McCracken CE, et al. Upper respiratory infections and airway adverse events in pediatric procedural sedation. Pediatrics 2017;140(1) [pii:e20170009].
14. Turkistani JM, Farsi N, Almushayt A, et al. Caries experience in asthmatic children: a review of literature. J Clin Pediatr Dent 2010;35(1):1–8.
15. Milano M1, Lee JY, Donovan K, et al. A cross-sectional study of medication-related factors and caries experience in asthmatic children. Pediatr Dent 2006;28(5):415–9.

16. Cote CJ, Wilson S. Guidelines for monitoring and management of pediatric patients before, during, and after sedation for diagnostic and therapeutic procedures: update 2016. Pediatrics 2016;138(1) [pii:e20161212].
17. Office of the Federal Register. Code of Federal Regulations. 42 Public Health, 482.13; 2010.
18. Davidovich E, Meltzer L, Efrat J, et al. Post-discharge events occurring after dental treatment under deep sedation in pediatric patients. J Clin Pediatr Dent 2017;41(3):232–5.
19. Warner ME, Benenfeld SM, Warner MA, et al. Perianesthetic dental injuries : frequency, outcomes, and risk factors. Anesthesiology 1999;90(5):1302–5.
20. Practice guidelines for preoperative fasting and the use of pharmacologic agents to reduce the risk of pulmonary aspiration: application to healthy patients undergoing elective procedures: an updated report by the American Society of Anesthesiologists task force on preoperative fasting and the use of pharmacologic agents to reduce the risk of pulmonary aspiration*. Anesthesiology 2017; 126(3):376–93.
21. Saunders R, Struys M, Pollock RF, et al. Patient safety during procedural sedation using capnography monitoring: a systematic review and meta-analysis. BMJ Open 2017;7(6):e013402.
22. Amos J. Dental operatory design – 9 tips you need to know. Available at: http://howtoopenadentaloffice.com/dental-operatory-design/. Accessed February 26, 2019.
23. Trends in surgery suite design 2007 healthcare design magazine. Available at: www.healthcaredesignmagazine.com/architecture/treands-surgery-suite-design-art-one/. Accessed February 26, 2019.
24. Guidelines for the design and construction of hospitals and healthcare facilities. Washington, DC: American Institute of Architecture; 2010.
25. Available at: www.asahq.org/standards-and-guidelines/statement-on-nonoperating-room-anesthetizing-locations. Accessed February 26, 2019.
26. Ritt RM, Bennett JD, Todd DW. Simulation training for the office-based anesthesia team. Oral Maxillofac Surg Clin North Am 2017;29(2):169–78.
27. Practice guidelines for moderate procedural sedation and analgesia 2018: a report by the American Society of Anesthesiologists Task Force on Moderate Procedural Sedation and Analgesia, the American Association of Oral and Maxillofacial Surgeons, American College of Radiology, American Dental Association, American Society of Dentist Anesthesiologists, and Society of Interventional Radiology*. Anesthesiology 2018;128(3):437–79.
28. Kahlenberg L, Harsey L, Patterson M, et al. Implementation of a modified WHO pediatric procedural sedation safety checklist and its impact on risk reduction. Hosp Pediatr 2017;7(4):225–31.
29. Available at: www.asahq.org/standards-and-guidelines/standards-for-basic-anesthetic-monitoring. Accessed February 26, 2019.
30. American Society of Dentist Anesthesiologists parameters of care. Anesth Prog 2018;65:197–203.
31. American Academy of Pediatric Dentistry. Use of anesthesia providers in the administration of office-based deep sedation/general anesthesia to the pediatric dental patient. 2018. Available at: http://www.aapd.org/media/Policies_Guidelines/BP_AnesthesiaPersonnel.pdf. Accessed February 26, 2019.
32. Pisov R, Brown RH, Weiss YS, et al. Wheezing during induction of general anesthesia in patients with and without asthma. Anesthesiol 1995;82:1111–6.

33. Orhan-Sunger M, Komatsu R, Sherman A, et al. Effect of nasal cannula oxygen administration on oxygen concentration at facial and adjacent landmarks. Anaesthesia 2009;54(5):521–6.
34. Greco RJ, Gonzalez R, Johnson P, et al. Potential dangers of oxygen supplementation of facial surgery. Plast Reconstr Surg 1995;95(6):978–84.
35. Reyes RJ, Smith AA, Mascaro JR, et al. Supplemental oxygen; ensuring its safe delivery during facial surgery. Plast Reconstr Surg 1995;95(5):924–8.
36. Joint Commission on Accreditation of Healthcare Organizations Sentinel Event Alert: preventing surgical fires. 2003. Available at: https://www.jointcommission.org/assets/1/18/SEA_29.PDF. Accessed February 26, 2019.
37. Wolf GL, Sidebotham GW, Lazard JL, et al. Laser ignition of surgical drape materials in are, 50% oxygen and 95% oxygen. Anesthesiol 2004;100(5):1167–71.
38. Goldberg J. Brief laboratory report: surgical drape flammability. AANA J 2006; 74(5):352–4.
39. Muchatuta NA, Sale SM. Fires and explosions. Anaesthesia & Intensive Care Medicine 2007;8(11):457–60.
40. Practice guidelines for sedation and analgesia by non-anesthesiologists. Anesthesiol 2002;96(4):1004–17.
41. Weingart SD, Levitan RM. Preoxygenation and prevention of desaturation during emergency airway management. Ann Emerg Med 2012;59(3):165–75.e1.
42. Anesthesia patient safety foundation prevention and management of operating room fires. 2010. Available at: https://www.apsf.org/videos/or-fire-safety-video/. Accessed February 26, 2019.
43. Ahmed OI, Sanchez G, McAllister K, et al. Fire safety in the operating room. Anesthesia Patient Safety Foundation Newsletter 2013;28(1):2013.
44. Apfelbaum JL, Caplan RA, Barker SJ, et al. Practice advisory for the prevention and management of operating room fires: an updated report by the American Society of Anesthesiologists Task Force on Operating Room Fires. Anesthesiology 2013;118(2):271–90.
45. Practice advisory for the prevention and management of operating room fires. Anesthesiology 2013;118:271–90.
46. VanCleave AM, Jones JE, McGlothlin JD, et al. The effect of intraoral suction on oxygen-enriched surgical environments: a mechanism for reducing surgical fires. Anesth Prog 2014;61(4):155–61.
47. Available at: https://www.csemag.com/articles/applying-nfpa-99-to-health-care-facilities/. Accessed 2018.
48. Wong JL, Gschwandtner G. Safe gas systems and office-based anesthesia. Anesth Patient Saf Found Newsl 2018;33(1):17–9.

Quality Improvement in Ambulatory Anesthesia
Making Changes that Work for You

Christopher J. Jankowski, MD, MBOE*, Michael T. Walsh, MD

KEYWORDS

- Quality • Lean management • Continuous improvement • Waste

KEY POINTS

- Quality improvement efforts should focus on creating value for patients.
- Lean is an improvement methodology that seeks to create value for customers by eliminating waste and developing the problem-solving skills of employees.
- Lean is rooted in the scientific method.

INTRODUCTION

Perfection is not attainable. But if we chase perfection, we can catch excellence.
—Vince Lombardi

Every system is perfectly designed to get the results it gets.
—Paul Baltaden, MD[1]

It is not the strongest of the species that survives, nor the most intelligent, but the one most responsive to change.
—Charles Darwin

Health care in the United States is expensive. In 2016, US health care expenditures were $3.3 trillion, amounting for 17.9% of the gross domestic product (GDP).[2] Other industrialized countries only spend between 9.6% and 12.4% of the GDP and, despite that, perform better on a variety of health outcomes.[3] In addition, between one-quarter and one-half of US health care expenditures are wasteful[4–9] and medical errors may be the third-leading cause of death.[10,11] Errors are common in surgery and contribute to burnout,[12] as do many of the processes by which care is delivered.[13] Thus, there is

Disclosure: Drs C.J. Jankowski and M.T. Walsh have no relevant financial or commercial relationships.
Mayo Clinic College of Medicine and Science, Charlton 1-145, 200 First Street, Southwest, Rochester, MN 55905, USA
* Corresponding author.
E-mail address: jankowski.christopher@mayo.edu

ample opportunity for quality improvement within the health care system and its processes, and these improvements will benefit providers, health care institutions, and payers, as well as patients.[14] As reimbursement becomes increasingly tied to quality measures[15] and as health care consumers are becoming more sophisticated, with expectations of exceptional value, the incentive for providing high quality care and continuously improving it only increases.

Outpatient surgery may be an ideal setting for quality improvement work. First, it is common. More than 23 million operations are performed annually in ambulatory surgery centers (ASCs) in the United States,[16] a number that will continue to increase as ASCs take on increasingly complex procedures. So, improvements in ambulatory surgery have the potential to make a significant impact on public health and the health care economy. In addition, the rapid turnover and patient-centeredness concerning timeliness, pain control, nausea, and vomiting prophylaxis, and so forth inherent in ambulatory surgery provide ample opportunities for quality work. Finally, cross-disciplinary cooperation between anesthesia providers, surgeons, nurses, and other personnel is the norm rather than the exception. Such teamwork is essential for making meaningful improvements in quality.

This article briefly reviews measures of quality, the difference between quality improvement and quality assurance, and discusses using lean as a methodology for improving quality in ambulatory surgery.

WHAT IS QUALITY?

Value is classically described as $V = Q/C$, where V is value, Q is quality, and C is cost (Fig. 1). Cost is defined as the amount of resources (financial and otherwise) required to achieve a given level of quality and calculating it is relatively straightforward. However, defining quality is more challenging. Thus, the first step in developing a quality program is coming to agreement on what defines quality. This is a necessary prelude to deciding which key performance indicators form the basis for improvement work within a model cell (see later discussion).

One approach is to use quality measures developed by various regulatory agencies, accreditation organizations, or medical societies.[17] These predefined determinants of quality have the advantage of being ready to use off the shelf. In addition, a practice may already be tracking them because of reporting requirements. However, when deciding on which metrics to track, it is important to choose either outcome measures that are meaningful to patients or process measures that are tightly correlated to those outcomes.

$$\text{Value} = \frac{\text{Quality}}{\text{Cost}}$$

$$\text{Value} = \frac{\text{Health Outcomes that Matter to Patients}}{\text{Cost}}$$

Fig. 1. The value equation. A variation on the classic value equation. In the classic equation, Value = Quality/Cost, where Cost is defined as the amount of resources, financial and otherwise, required to achieve a given level of quality. However, Quality is often difficult to characterize. In this variation, the numerator is Health Outcomes that Matter to Patients, and Cost is defined as the amount of resources, financial and otherwise, required to achieve a given outcome. (*Data from* Porter ME, Lee TH. The strategy that will fix health care. Harvard Business Review 2013;91(10):50–70.)

Another approach is to choose metrics that belong in broader categories of quality measures. This will encompass the more specific measures noted previously but will also allow for work on improvement in metrics that are meaningful locally but not included in published quality measures. The National Academy of Medicine (formerly the Institute of Medicine) defines quality as "the degree to which health care services for individuals and populations increase the likelihood of desired health outcomes and consistent with current professional knowledge."[18]

Six domains of quality are identified[18]:

- Effectiveness: providing care processes and achieving outcomes as supported by scientific evidence
- Efficiency: maximizing the quality of units of health care delivered or health benefits achieved per unit of resources used
- Equity: providing care of equal quality to those who may differ in personal characteristics other than their clinical condition or preferences for care
- Patient-centeredness: meeting patients' needs and preferences, and providing education and support
- Safety: minimizing actual or potential bodily harm
- Timeliness: obtaining needed care while minimizing delays.

Regardless of the quality schema a practice adopts, the overarching goal for providers and other stakeholders must be to improve value for patients, where value is defined as the health outcomes achieved that matter to patients relative to the cost achieving those outcomes[19] (see **Fig. 1**).

QUALITY ASSURANCE VERSUS IMPROVEMENT

Though both are essential, it is important to distinguish quality improvement from quality assurance. In health care, quality has traditionally been approached from an assurance, rather than improvement, perspective. Quality assurance is an effort to find and overcome problems to improve quality.[20] The aim is to achieve benchmarks for outcomes (often arbitrarily defined), adherence to process measures, costs, or all three.[21,22] Thus, the focus is on addressing outliers or the statistical tail, to be "good enough." The result is a dichotomous judgment of whether a practice or individual meets standards of acceptable performance or compliance. The assumption is that by meeting those standards, excellence will be achieved. However as noted previously, many benchmarks, especially those for process measures, may not be associated with improved outcomes or value for patients. In addition, merely aiming for benchmarks places an artificial ceiling on quality.

In contrast, quality improvement methodologies are data-driven, and focus on process and the entire sample (rather than statistical outliers) to achieve the best possible outcome. The approach is inquisitive (What does perfect look like? How can our processes to be improved to move us closer to perfection?) and scientific (see later discussion).

LEAN

Lean is a quality improvement methodology whose primary focus is "the endless transformation of waste into value from the customer's perspective."[23] Classically, waste is divided into 7 categories: transportation, inventory, motion, waiting, overprocessing, overproduction, and defects. Examples of each can be found in ambulatory surgical settings (**Table 1**). An eighth waste, underutilizing people's talent, skills, and knowledge, is common in health care settings, whether it is employees

Table 1		
The 7 wastes of lean		
Type of Waste	**Description**	**Ambulatory Surgical Example**
Transportation	The movement of people, products, or information from place to place	Patients moving from admissions to a preoperative holding area to the operating room.
Inventory	Work-in-progress or materials or information on hand beyond what is required to serve the customer	Overstocked consumables
Motion	Excessive movement within the workspace	Supplies not stored where needed
Waiting	1. People waiting for a service, product, or equipment 2. Idle equipment	1. Patients are told to arrive at 6:30 AM for an operation that will not begin until 2:00 PM 2. A surgical robot that is only used once per week
Overprocessing	Doing more work, adding more components, or having more steps in a product or service than what is required by the customer	Follow-up appointments that do not improve outcome
Overproduction	Making more product than is necessary	Unnecessary preoperative diagnostic testing
Defects	Mistakes or errors that need to be reworked	Medication errors

not performing tasks commensurate with their level training or leaders not using the knowledge of frontline staff in identifying and remedying opportunities for improvement. Given the high level of training and motivation of health care providers, this may be the most important waste of all.

Though fully developed by the Toyota Motor Company through the Toyota Production System (TPS), the origins of lean date back centuries. During the Punic Wars, the Venetian Arsenal was producing ships at the rate of 1 per hour via the use of interchangeable parts, standardization, and an early assembly line.[24] The modern history of lean begins with Henry Ford and the Highland Park assembly line. In 1913, Ford opened the Highland Park, Michigan plant at which the moving assembly line and other innovations allowed for mass production of the Model T. Later, representatives from Toyota studied the Ford manufacturing process and improved on it by seeking advice and input from workers and having them take ownership of processes. In addition, it began to use statistical process control and other principles introduced by Deming and Shewhart.[25] The term lean was introduced by Womack, Jones, and Ross[26] in their 1990 book describing the TPS, *The Machine That Changed the World*. Since then, lean principles and the TPS have been adopted throughout a variety of industries.

Lean has its roots in manufacturing. However, although the health care system has a unique history, culture, set of technologies, and complex processes, the managerial practices involved in deciding what works, and what does not, are the same across industries, including health care.[27,28] Beginning in the early 2000s, several health systems in the United States embraced lean, including ThedaCare in northeastern Wisconsin and Virginia, and Mason Medical Center in Seattle, Washington.[29,30] Since then, lean has been adopted by health systems world-wide and is the most commonly reported-on improvement methodology in the health care literature.[31,32] Lean can be applied to improve all processes within an ambulatory surgical setting: scheduling, operating room and other resource utilization, supply chain, pharmacy, laboratory, clinical care, pharmacy, and so forth.[33,34] When successfully implemented, it results in improved integration of care, higher staff and patient satisfaction, better scheduling, increased profit margins, fewer patient deaths, significant reduction in waiting time for laboratory tests results, marked increases in productivity, and reduced inventory costs.[34–37] Most importantly, it is an approach that can transform the culture of an organization to one focused on improving value and seeking perfection in a way that is respectful to patients and health care workers.

Cultural transformation is the key to making changes that last. Transformation can begin with a single improvement project. Having a specific problem to focus on is an excellent place to start. However, organizations must guard against approaching quality improvement from a purely project-oriented perspective. In those instances, individual projects frequently show great initial promise because intensity is high and well-focused. Early results may be encouraging but backslide quickly as energy and attention are shifted to newer projects or different priorities.[38] Research examining lean projects in the banking industry has identified both the scope of the fade problem, as well as its contributing factors.[39] In a 5-year review of hundreds of lean projects, 27% regressed to baseline after the first year, and more than half did at 2 years. Moreover, only 36% of successful projects were sustained 2 years after launch. Thus, taking a project-only approach is not likely to lead to long-term success. Further, factors associated with the inability to sustain improvements were different from those typically linked to initial success (eg, experience of local leaders, level of lean training, how long a team has worked together). The most important driver for sustained success was strong continued support of senior leadership. Improvements focused on the organization's core purpose or those easing employee so-called pain points were also more likely to last over the long haul.[40] A lean transformation requires commitment from the entire organization.

STARTING THE LEAN JOURNEY

A full description of how to implement lean within the ambulatory surgical setting is beyond the scope of this article. What follows is a description of some of the salient features that predict a successful lean transformation. Many resources and books are available for more in-depth reading on lean tools and philosophy (see Further Reading). However, organizations contemplating beginning a lean journey should seek an experienced coach.

The A3

A3 refers to an international-size piece of paper that is approximately 11 by 17 inches in dimension. However, within organizations that use lean, the A3 is a method for capturing issues confronting an organization on a single piece of paper.[41] The design of the A3 can vary according to the needs of a particular problem or organization. An example of an A3 form is seen in **Fig. 2**. The format can be adapted to a specific problem or needs of an organization. However, the A3 format and goals should be guided by the following questions[41]:

1. What is the problem or issue?
2. Who owns or is responsible for the problem?
3. What are the root causes of the problem?

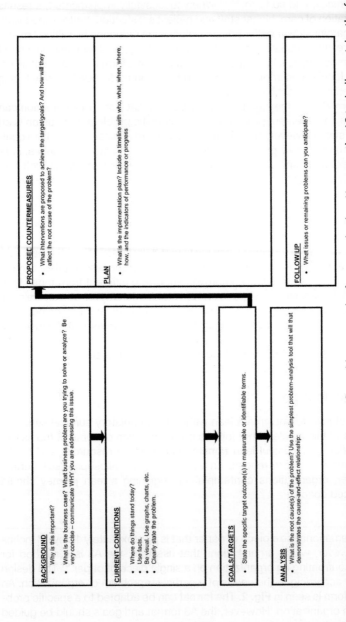

Fig. 2. An A3 form. The format can be adapted to a specific problem or needs of an organization. However, the A3 typically contains the following: (1) title, names the problem or issue being addressed; (2) owner, identifies who owns the problem; (3) date, the date of the latest revision of the A3 form; (4) background, establishes the importance of the issue; (5) current conditions, describes what is currently known about the problem; (6) goals, identifies the desired outcome; (7) analysis, identifies the causes for the gap between the current conditions and desired outcome; (8) proposed countermeasures, potential interventions to address the problem or reach a goal; (9) plan, the plan for testing and implementing countermeasures; and (10) follow-up, describes the plan for reviewing the results and anticipates remaining issues. (*Adapted from* Shook J. Managing to learn: Using the A3 management process to solve problems, gain agreement, mentor and lead. Boston: Lean Enterprise Institute, Inc.; 2008; with permission.)

4. What are the proposed countermeasures to solve the problem?
5. Which countermeasures should be tried?
6. What is the plan for obtaining buy-in from all stakeholders?
7. What is the plan to implement the countermeasures?
8. What problems can be anticipated during implementation?
9. What metrics will determine whether a countermeasure is successful?
10. How will the results be shared?

The A3 is a living document that is meant to be revised as a project progresses and a given problem is better understood. It visually captures the problem-solving thought process. Its use is foundational to encouraging and enabling rational problem-solving and learning using the scientific method.[41]

Plan-Do-Study-Act

Our own attitude is that we are charged with discovering the best way of doing everything, and that we must regard every process employed in manufacturing as purely experimental.[42]

—*Henry Ford*

A plan-do-study-act (PDSA) cycle is a simple, powerful method for systematically assessing small tests of change. It was introduced by Shewhart and Deming in the in the 1920s,[43] are commonly used in business, and are an important part of a lean approach to quality improvement. To health care providers, the concept initially may seem foreign. However, it is analogous to the scientific method: (1) observe, (2) hypothesize, (3) perform an experiment to test the hypothesis, and (4) draw conclusions from the results of the experiment and refine the hypothesis (**Fig. 3**). Thus, PDSA cycles are an intrinsically familiar approach to problem-solving and improvement to those with health care or scientific backgrounds.

The most important characteristic of PDSA cycles is that they are meant to be performed iteratively, with the results and analysis of the previous cycle forming the basis for the hypothesis being tested in the next. The goal is to use each cycle as an opportunity to test an individual hypothesis about a potential intervention for improvement. As each cycle is performed, knowledge about the effectiveness of various countermeasures is gained. A PDSA cycle that does not lead to improvement is not a failure. Rather, t provides information about which improvement interventions or countermeasures

Scientific Method

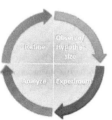

PDSA Cycle

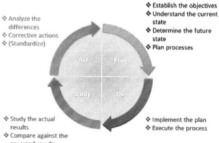

Fig. 3. The PDSA cycle is analogous to the scientific method. Thus, this approach to testing improvements will be familiar to health care providers. (Deming, W. Edwards, The New Economics for Industry, Government, Education, second edition, PDSA Cycle, p. 132, © 2000 Massachusetts Institute of Technology, by permission of The MIT Press.)

may not be effective for given situation or problem. The effectiveness of PDSA cycles to yield improvements has been questioned.[43] However, failure of a PDSA approach to improvement is often due to only using the Plan-Do portion of the cycle without studying the results, adjusting the hypothesis, and subsequently testing a new hypothesis rooted in the results of the previous experiment in a cyclic fashion.[43]

CUSTOMIZING STANDARDIZED WORK

There is no harm in repeating a good thing.
— *Plato, 428/427 to 328/327 BCE*

We are what we repeatedly do. Excellence, then, is not an act, but a habit.
— *Aristotle, 384 to 322 BCE*

Standardized work is a powerful tool to improve quality. It is the starting point, and improvement is impossible without it.[44,45] Standardized work is defined as the current best way to safely achieve the highest value outcome.[44] In the clinical setting, standardized work involves consistently applying best practices to patient care. Despite physician resistance[46] and concerns that it constitutes cookbook medicine,[47] its use has been common in medicine and surgery for decades. Examples include advanced cardiac life support algorithms, enhanced recovery after surgery pathways, cancer chemotherapy protocols, and immunization schedules. In ambulatory surgery, standardized work might include Society for Ambulatory Anesthesia clinical practice guidelines.[48,49]

It is essential to realize that application of standardized work to clinical practice assumes that there will be deviations from usual practice when circumstances dictate. In fact, standardized clinical care can be used as an indicator of patient problems. For example, failure to meet recovery milestones should prompt a search for the cause. Another key feature of standardized work is that it evolves over time based on current understanding of best practices. As new knowledge is generated, it is incorporated into standardized work.

Finally, and most importantly, standardized work is foundational to quality improvement, because it stabilizes a system, allows it to be analyzed, and opportunities for improvement to be identified.

THE MODEL CELL

A model cell is vital to successfully implementing lean. Model cells are discrete areas within an organization where lean thinking is initially applied. Having a discrete group work as a model cell allows them to become well-versed in lean, its approach to problem-solving, and tools. The cliché is that a model cell should be "an inch wide and a mile deep."

The model cell can be a department, a service line, or even a single operating room. Beginning with a discrete model cell, rather than an entire organization, has several advantages. First, it reduces the resources and time needed for transformation, and is less risky than attempting a simultaneous transformation across an entire organization.[50] It also provides an opportunity for team members to test new ideas and concepts, and to use failure as a path for learning.[51] Finally, it becomes a showcase within the organization, demonstrating what good looks like and gaining buy-in for the effort and approach from others groups and leaders.[51]

Several factors influence the choice of model cell. There may be a specific, high-priority problem that needs to be addressed or waste to be eliminated. The readiness of team members within a proposed model cell to begin the journey should be considered. Managers, staff, and physicians should agree that improvement is necessary and possible.

To be successful, the model cell must be focused on a problem that is meaningful to the enterprise. All team members should be able to clearly state the business case for doing the improvement work, and having a discrete focus will improve the likelihood of success.

The aim could be to address a safety issue or patient-focused outcome measure such as postoperative pain. However, efforts centered on issues such as improving operating room scheduling are appropriate as well. There is evidence that the early stages of lean implementation should focus on nonclinical problems.[34]

Equally important is that the scope work of the cell be aligned with the strategic goals or key performance indicators of the organization. If these have not been identified, that should be the first goal. Moving forward, all improvement work should center on an organization's handful of key metrics.

The new processes developed by the model cell should be rooted in standardized work; that is, the current best way to do the process (see previous discussion). Team members should follow the standardized work. However, the standardized work can be altered based on PDSA cycles (see previous discussion).

Finally, the model cell must have the backing of senior leadership. Change and improvement are challenging, especially when the goal is to develop a culture of patient-centered improvement that focuses on process improvement. These efforts are less likely to be successful without explicit support from the executive team. One method to engage senior leadership is to make initial improvement efforts cost-neutral. If support from senior leadership is lacking, the decision to use a model cell should be reconsidered.

DEVELOPING LEAN LEADERSHIP

By far, the most important predictor of a successful lean transformation is leadership. Leadership sets the direction for an organization, and without its commitment, a lean transformation will fail. Implementing lean requires a new approach to leadership. The traditional approach to health care management is autocratic and involves management by objectives, wherein leadership sets objectives and management does whatever is necessary to achieve them.[52] By contrast, lean involves management by process.[53] With this approach, management's goal is to teach front-line staff to identify and solve problems on their own.[52] Especially for physicians, this may require learning a set of competencies and attitudes that are unfamiliar[54] (**Table 2**). However,

Table 2	
White coat versus improvement leadership	
White Coat Leadership	**Improvement Leadership**
• All-knowing	• Patient
• Captain of the ship	• Knowledgeable
• Autocratic	• Facilitator
• The buck stops here	• Teacher
• Impatient	• Student
• Blaming	• Helper
• Controlling	• Communicator

Comparison of the characteristics of traditional, white coat leadership and improvement leadership styles.

Adapted from Toussaint J. A management, leadership, and board road map to transforming care for patients. Front Health Serv Manage 2013;29(3):12; with permission.

an improvement approach to leadership will facilitate development of staff and allow an organization to leverage their knowledge, skill, and enthusiasm.

SUMMARY

Ambulatory surgery will take on an increasingly important role in a health care system that is increasingly focused on creating value for patients. Lean is a well-developed improvement methodology for eliminating waste, increasing value for patients, and improving staff satisfaction.

REFERENCES

1. Proctor L. Editor's notebook: a quotation with a life of its own. Middleton (MA): Patient Safety & Quality Healthcare Blog; 2008. Available at: https://www.psqh.com/analysis/editor-s-notebook-a-quotation-with-a-life-of-its-own/. Accessed November 1, 2018.
2. Center for Medicare & Medicaid Services National Health Expenditure Fact Sheet. Available at: https://www.cms.gov/research-statistics-data-and-systems/statistics-trends-and-reports/nationalhealthexpenddata/nhe-fact-sheet.html. Accessed November 2, 2018.
3. Papanicolas I, Woskie LR, Jha AK. Health care spending in the United States and other high-income countries. JAMA 2018;319(10):1024–39.
4. Bentley TG, Effros RM, Palar K, et al. Waste in the U.S. health care system: a conceptual framework. Milbank Q 2008;86(4):629–59.
5. Farrell D, Jenson E, Kocher B, et al. Accounting for the cost of US health care: a new look at why Americans spend more. New York: McKinsey and Company; 2008. Available at: https://healthcare.mckinsey.com/sites/default/files/MGI_Accounting_for_cost_of_US_health_care_full_report.pdf. Accessed January 11, 2018.
6. New England Healthcare Institute, How many more studies will it take? A collection of evidence that our health care system can do better. Boston (MA): NEHI. Available at: https://www.nehi.net/writable/publication_files/file/how_many_more_studies_will_it_take_introduction.pdf, Accessed January 11, 2018.
7. PricewaterhouseCoopers' Health Research Institute. The price of excess: identifying waste in healthcare spending. New York: PricewaterhouseCoopers; 2008.
8. Berwick DM, Hackbarth AD. Eliminating waste in US health care. JAMA 2012; 307(14):1513–6.
9. Cutler DM. What is the US health spending problem? Health Aff 2018;37(No. 3): 493–7.
10. Makary MA, Daniel M. Medical error – the third leading cause of death in the US. BMJ 2016;353:i2139.
11. Shojania KG, Dixon-Woods M. Estimating deaths due to medical error: the ongoing controversy and why it matters. BMJ Qual Saf 2017;26:423–8.
12. Shanafelt TD, Balch CM, Bechamps GJ, et al. Burnout and career satisfaction among American surgeons. Ann Surg 2009;250(3):463–71.
13. West CP, Dyrbye LN, Shanafelt TD. Physician burnout: contributors, consequences and solutions. J Intern Med 2018;283(6):516–29.
14. Dimick JB, Weeks WB, Karia RJ, et al. Who pays for poor surgical quality? building a business case for quality improvement. J Am Coll Surg 2006;202(6):933–7.
15. Centers for Medicare & Medicaid Services. Hospital value-based purchasing 2015. Available at: https://www.cms.gov/Outreach-and-Education/Medicare-Learning-Network-MLN/MLNProducts/Downloads/Hospital-VBPurchasing-Fact-Sheet-ICN907664TextOnly.pdf. Accessed October 31, 2018.

16. Castro GM, Miller M. Making ambulatory surgery safer. Oakbrook Terrace (IL): The Joint Commission blog; 2018. Available at: https://www.jointcommission. org/ambulatory_buzz/making_ambulatory_surgery_safer/. Accessed October 19, 2018.

17. 2018 QCDR Measure Specifications: Anesthesia Quality Institute, National Anesthesia Clinical Outcomes Registry, Available at: https://www.aqihq.org/files/MIPS/ 2018/2018_QCDR_Measure_Book.pdf, Accessed November 2, 2018.

18. Committee on Quality Health Care in America, Institute of Medicine. Crossing the quality chasm: a new health system for the 21st century. Washington, DC: National Academy Press; 2001.

19. Porter ME, Lee TH. The strategy that will fix health care. Harvard Business Review 2013;91(10):50–70.

20. Goldstone J. Sony, Porsche and vascular surgery in the 21st century. J Vasc Surg 1997;201–10.

21. Lohr KN. Quality of health care: an introduction to critical definitions, concepts, principles, and practicalities. In: Palmer RH, Donabedian A, Povar G, editors. Striving for quality in health care; an inquiry into policy and practice. Ann Arbor (MI): Health Administration Press; 1991. p. xi–xvi.

22. Laffel GL, Berwick DM. Quality health care. JAMA 1993;270:254–5.

23. Womack JP, Jones DT. Lean thinking: banish waste and create wealth in your corporation. New York: CRC Press; 2003.

24. Davis RC. Shipbuilders of the Venetian Arsenal: workers and work place in the preindustrial city. Baltimore (MD): Johns Hopkins University Press; 1991.

25. Best M, Neuhauser D. Walter A Shewhart, 1924, and the Hawthorne factory. Qual Saf Health Care 2006;15(2):142–3.

26. Womack JP, Jones DT, Ross D. The machine that changed the world. New York: Rawson Associates; 1990. p. 323.

27. Manos A, Sattler M, Alukal G. Make healthcare lean. Qual Prog 2006;39:24.

28. Teich ST, Faddoul FF. Lean management-the journey from toyota to healthcare. Rambam Maimonides Med J 2013;4(2):e0007.

29. Barnas K. Theda Care's business performance system: sustaining continuous daily improvement through hospital management in a lean environment. Jt Comm J Qual Patient Saf 2011;37(9):387–99.

30. Kenney C. Transforming health care: Virginia Mason medical center's pursuit of the perfect patient experience. Boca Raton (FL): CRC Press; 2011.

31. Black J, Miller D. The Toyota way to healthcare excellence: increase efficiency and improve quality with lean. Chicago: Health Administration Press; 2008.

32. Mazzocato P, Thor J, Bäckman U, et al. Complexity complicates lean: lessons from seven emergency services. J Health Organ Manag 2014;28(2):266–88.

33. Simon RW, Canacari EG. Surgical scheduling: a lean approach to process improvement. AORN J 2014;99:147–59.

34. Martin LD, et al. Mejoramiento de los procesos en el quirófano mediante la aplicación de la metodología Lean de Toyota. Rev Colomb Anestesiol 2014;42(3): 220–8.

35. Weber D. Toyota-style management drives Virginia Mason. Physician Exec 2006; 32:12.

36. Toussaint JS, Gerald RA. On the mend: on the mend: revolutionizing healthcare to save lives and transform the industry. Boston: Lean Enterprise Institute, Inc; 2010.

37. Barnas K, Adams E. Beyond heroes: a lean management system for healthcare. Appleton (WI): ThedaCare Center for Healthcare Value; 2014.

38. Anonymous. Making Process Improvements Stick: Early excitement usually leads to backsliding. Harvard Business Review 2018;16–9.

39. Holweg M, Staats BR, Upton DM. Making process improvements stick. 2018. Kenan Institute of Private Enterprise Research Paper No. 18-22. Available at: SSRN: https://ssrn.com/abstract=3240097 or https://doi.org/10.21.39/ssrn.3240097.

40. Anonymous. Making Process Improvements Stick: Early excitement usually leads to backsliding. Harvard Business Review 2018;16–9.

41. Shook J. Managing to learn: using the A3 process to solve problems, gain agreement, mentor and lead. Cambridge (MA): Lean Enterprise Institute; 2010.

42. Zarbo R, Tuthill JM, D'Angelo R, et al. The Henry Ford Production System: reduction of surgical pathology in-process misidentification defects by bar code–specified work process standardization. Am J Clin Pathol 2009;131:468–77.

43. Taylor MJ, McNicholas C, Nicolay C, et al. Systematic review of the application of the plan-do-study-act method to improve quality in healthcare. BMJ Qual Saf 2014;23:290–8.

44. Liker JK, Meier D. The Toyota way fieldbook: a practical guide for implementing Toyota's 4Ps. New York: McGraw-Hill; 2006.

45. Imai M. Kaizen: the key to Japan's competitive success. New York: McGraw-Hill/Irwin; 1986.

46. Hung D. Implementing a lean management system in primary care: facilitators and barriers from the front lines. Qual Manag Health Care 2015;24(3):103–8.

47. Hartzbrand P, Groopman J. Medical taylorism. N Engl J Med 2016;074:100–8.

48. Gan TJ. Society for ambulatory anesthesia consensus statement on perioperative blood glucose management in diabetic patients undergoing ambulatory surgery. Anesth Analg 2010;111:1378–87.

49. Gan TJ. Consensus Guidelines for the Management of postoperative nausea and vomiting. Anesth Analg 2014;118(1):85–113.

50. Graban M. Lean hospitals: improving quality, patient safety, and employee engagement, Third Edition. Boca Raton (FL): CRC Press; 2016.

51. Toussaint J. The Model Cell. Becker's Hospital Review. 2015. Available at: https://www.beckershospitalreview.com/hospital-management-administration/the-model-cell.html. Accessed October 20, 2018.

52. Toussaint J, Conway PH, Shortell SM. The Toyota production system: what does it mean, and what does it mean for healthcare?. 2016. Available at: https://www.healthaffairs.org/do/10.1377/hblog20160406.054094/full/. Health Affairs Blog. Accessed November 2, 2018.

53. Deming WE. Out of the crisis. Cambridge (MA): MIT Press; 1986.

54. Toussaint J. A management, leadership, and board road map to transforming care for patients. Front Health Serv Manage 2013;29(3):3–15.

FURTHER READINGS

The Lean Enterprise Institute. Available at: www.lean.org. Accessed January 1, 2019.
Toussaint JS. The promise of lean in healthcare. Mayo Clin Proc 2013;88(1):74–82.

Outcomes in Ambulatory Anesthesia
Measuring What Matters

Leopoldo V. Rodriguez, MD[a],*,
Joshua A. Bloomstone, MD, MSc[b,c,d],
Gerald A. Maccioli, MD, MBA, FCCM[b]

KEYWORDS

- Outcome • Performance • Measure • MIPS • Unintended consequences
- Patient-reported experience measure (PREM)
- Patient-reported outcome measure (PROM) • Quality Payment Program (QPP)

KEY POINTS

- What matters in health care depends on the perspective: patient, provider, facility, payer, or government regulator. Thus, measuring what matters differs depending on the stakeholder. This article reviews key measures relative to each.
- Providing high-quality, patient-centered health care demands that the strategic focus remains squarely on patient concerns, desires, experience, and outcomes.
- The Quality Payment Program (QPP) was designed to help patients choose a provider based on quality reports, reward high-quality performing clinicians, and change practice patterns to achieve high-quality care at lower cost.
- The QPP has unintended consequences and pitfalls: adverse selection, increase of providers' nonclinical time to report quality, costly process, and removal of topped-out measures may decrease quality as incentives are removed.
- Future quality measures will include multidisciplinary team shared measures, patient-reported experience measures, and patient-reported outcome measures, and will require the development of a national health information network by payers and the Federal government.

Disclosure: The authors have no financial interest in the subject matter or materials discussed in this article.
[a] Society for Ambulatory Anesthesiology (SAMBA), ASA Committee on Performance and Outcome Measures, Surgery Center of Aventura, Envision Physician Services, 7700 West Sunrise Boulevard, Plantation, FL 33322, USA; [b] Envision Physician Services, 7700 West Sunrise Boulevard, Plantation, FL 33322, USA; [c] Department of Anesthesiology, University of Arizona College of Medicine-Phoenix, 550 E. Van Buren Street, Phoenix, AZ 85004, USA; [d] University College London, Centre for Perioperative Medicine Division of Surgery and Interventional Science, UCL 2nd Floor Charles Bell House, 43-45 Foley Street, London W1W 7TS, UK
* Corresponding author. 1199 South Federal Hwy # 392, Boca Raton, FL 33432.
E-mail address: Leopoldo.Rodriguez@shcr.com

Not everything that counts can be counted, and not everything that can be counted counts.

William Bruce Cameron

What matters in health care depends on the perspective: patient, provider, facility, payer, or government regulator. Thus, measuring what matters differs depending on the stakeholder. This article reviews key measures relative to each.

PATIENTS

Providing high-quality, patient-centered health care demands that the strategic focus remain squarely on patient concerns, desires, experience, and outcomes.[1] Traditional clinical outcome measures, such as hospital length of stay or readmissions, do not represent outcomes that are of import to patients.[2] Similarly, metrics focused on adherence to process, such as timely antibiotic administration, are also of little import to patients.[3] In the manufacturing industries, quality is defined by the customer, not the company. Furthermore, customers buy solutions to their problems, not products.[4] To these points, the quality of clinicians' product can only be determined via patient feedback that focuses on the degree to which the clinicians have solved their presenting problems.

Patient-centeredness resides at the epicenter of the Institute for Healthcare Improvement's Triple Aim: improving population health, enhancing the patient experience and outcomes, and reducing the cost of care. To this point, both patient experience and outcomes, from the patient's perspective, must be considered key measures of quality health care. After all, only patients can truly define the quality of their experience. Patient-reported experience measures (PREMs) and patient-reported outcome measures (PROMs) thus form the basis for measuring what matters most to patients. Regardless of patient care location, all patients desire an experience defined by the same elements (**Table 1**).

Of importance is the relationship between patient experience and patient outcomes. In 2014, Black and colleagues[5] studied the relationship between PREMs and PROMs in patients undergoing hip, knee, and groin surgery within UK National Health Service (NHS) hospitals. The results are summarized in **Box 1**. Although a weak overall positive association exists between PREMs and PROMs, the evidence

Table 1	
Sample patient-reported experience measures and patient-reported outcome measures	
Measure	**Measure Type**
Clean environment	PREM
Clear Instructions	PREM
Complication free	PREM/PROM
Cost of care	PREM
Feel Safe	PREM
Pain and symptom management	PREM/PROM
Quiet environment	PREM
Respectful treatment	PREM
Return to function	PREM/PROM

Box 1
Relationship between patient-reported experience measures and patient-reported outcome measures

1. A significant positive association between a patient's overall PREM score and their PROM change score was noted for all 3 procedures.

2. The 1 aspect of patients' experiences that was most strongly associated with the reporting of better outcomes was the level of communication and trust in their physicians.

3. Of interest, (1) men reported positive experiences more often than women; (2) older patients (>60 years) were more likely to report a good experience compared with younger patients; (3) there was no significant association between PREM and PROM scores as a function of socioeconomic status.

4. One of the striking features of this article was the proportion of patients reporting complications following surgery (hip, 31%; knee, 34%; hernia, 23%). The key finding was that there was a significant negative association between patient experience and reporting complications.

5. This study confirms the notion that the patient experience cannot be used as a proxy for outcomes.

Data from Black N, Varaganum M, Hutchings A. Relationship between patient reported experience (PREMs) and patient reported outcomes (PROMs) in elective surgery. BMJ Qual Saf 2014;23(7):534–42.

---

suggests that physicians wanting to optimize PROM scores should ensure optimal patient experience.

Although a detailed discussion of PREM and PROM tools is beyond the scope of this article, those with interest are urged to review the publication by Kingsley and Patel.[6] In addition, and specifically related to the perioperative experience, tools have been designed to assess the quality of recovery, such as the QoR40, which is a 40-element questionnaire that describes the many components of a quality recovery from the patient perspective. Tools like this allow not only for an assessment of the recovery experience but also for comparisons between anesthetic techniques, providers, facilities, and so forth.[7]

PROVIDERS AND PAYERS

In 1999, the Institute of Medicine (IOM) authored *To Err is Human: Building a Safer Health System*,[8] which revealed that as many as 98,000 people die in hospitals each year as a result of preventable medical errors. Following this publication, the 100,000 Lives Campaign began, which set goals and deadlines for improving health care quality within the United States.[9] The investigators proposed the creation of a nationwide voluntary error reporting system of adverse events and encouraged health care practitioners and organizations to participate. The goal was to improve patient safety by learning from reported errors. The IOM also recommended enhanced oversight of health care organizations, and that professional groups and purchasers of health care should lead the process, create benchmarks, and monitor changes. In response to the IOM, accreditation bodies, payers, nonprofit organizations, governments, and health care systems launched major initiatives and invested considerable resources to improve patient safety,[10–12] The Medicare Access and Children's Health Insurance Program Reauthorization Act (MACRA) of 2015 required the Centers for Medicare and Medicaid Serves (CMS) to implement a quality payment incentive program, referred to as the Quality Payment Program (QPP), which rewards value and achieving specific process and outcome measures in one of 2 ways:

1. Merit-based incentive payment system (MIPS)
2. Advanced alternative payment models (APMs)

In general, the QPP was designed to accomplish 3 issues:

1. Help patients choose a provider based on quality reports (Physician Compare)
2. Reward high-performing clinicians based on value and change the practice patterns of low-performing clinicians to improve value
3. Achieve high-quality care at lower cost

CMS and professional organizations, such as the American Society of Anesthesiologists (ASA), have been developing performance and outcome measures that facilitate objective data collection. Organizations that are federally listed as patient safety organizations, such as the Anesthesia Quality Institute (AQI) and the Envision patient safety organization, have been collecting data from group practices and individual anesthesia providers, analyzing it, and creating benchmarks using these specific measures. The goal is to improve the quality of perioperative patient care and provide objective data on which pay for performance may be based.[13] The AQI uses the National Anesthesia Clinical Outcomes Registry (NACOR), which has been approved by CMS as a Qualified Clinical Data Registry (QCDR), as well as a Qualified Registry, as the measuring tool for anesthesiologists to review their performance, identify gaps, and compare themselves with other physicians or practices. NACOR is able to identify performance trends and physician outliers, and provides practice improvement tools to assist members with their performance. In addition, NACOR also meets CMS's regulatory requirements to submit practice data to both the Physician Quality Reporting System and the Value Modifier program. In addition, groups and facilities can use NACOR-generated reports to meet Joint Commission maintenance of certification requirements.

The IOM and health care consumers have called for government payers to increase payments to health care providers who deliver high-quality care. Improving the quality of care requires change in practice, attitude, and behavior.[14] Health plans and purchasers are therefore moving to payment models that focus on physicians' behavior.[15] In 2004, Epstein and colleagues'[16] "Paying Physicians for High-quality Care" proposed the need to substantially increase pay-for-performance incentives. They noted that physicians were more likely to respond to financial incentives if the dollar figures were large enough. The impact of such incentives depends on the efforts of large purchasers. Cleverly, Epstein and colleagues[16] point out that a small number of individual measures would be unlikely to yield a broad-scale improvement. They proposed tying financial payments to rotating measures and expanding performance indicators over time as a more successful long-term strategy. In addition, the investigators point out the need to continue investing in systems for measuring and tracking quality in affordable ways and of the continued need for investments in information technology to facilitate change.

Presently, US health care spending exceeds $3 trillion a year, more than 17% of its gross domestic product.[17] In an effort to curb the growth in health care spending, MACRA was signed into law by Congress on April 16, 2015. MACRA ended the flawed and unpopular sustainable growth rate formula and by law required CMS to implement the QPP.[18] Led by Medicare, third-party payers are increasingly reimbursing physicians and hospitals according to the quality of care they provide or the value they produce instead of, or in addition to, the volume of services they generate. CMS views the fee-for-service model as a major problem underscoring the cost of American health care, because, in their eyes, the model leads to highly fractionated and thus expensive care without demonstrable clinical outcomes benefit. Thus, CMS has been enticing physicians to move away from the fee-for-service model with financial incentives.

Under the QPP, there are 2 tracks:

1. MIPS.
2. APM. Under the APMs, there are 2 subgroups:
   - Advanced APMs
   - MIPS APMs

Physicians who receive Medicare payments will be required to choose participation in one of these 2 tracks beginning in 2019. Although the purpose of the 2 tracks is to enhance quality while ensuring cost control, there are significant differences that physicians should be familiar with. Although a detailed explanation of these 2 programs is beyond the scope of this article, the major differences between the programs are highlighted here:

1. MIPS: in this track, physician performance in 4 categories (the use of an electronic health record [EHR], clinical practice improvement, quality, and cost) is measured and scored. The score is used to adjust Medicare payments. Over time, the percentage allotted to each category changes.
2. APMs include participation in programs such as the Medicare Shared Savings Program, CMS Innovation Center programs, and accountable care organizations. Unlike MIPS, participating clinicians must accept financial risk for underperformance; that is, inability to deliver enhanced quality while maintaining cost or reduced cost without affecting the quality of delivered care. Although participating physicians are at financial risk, there is the potential for physicians to realize greater financial reward for success.

UNINTENDED CONSEQUENCES OF THE QUALITY PAYMENT PROGRAM

Shen[19] studied the effect of performance-based contracting on access to care among severely ill patients being treated for substance abuse. This study highlighted the risk of adverse selection (ie, the financial incentive to treat less severely ill patients in order to improve overall performance) as an unintended consequence of a pay-for-performance system. adverse selection may also affect care within the ambulatory surgery space when healthy, insured patients are preferentially cared for relative to patients who are either higher risk or uninsured.

QUALITY MEASURES

There are at 4 types of quality measures for physicians:

1. *Process measures*: these measure the adherence to specific steps in a process that are thought to enhance outcomes. Although it is not always true, it is hoped that adherence to process measures leads to better outcomes, as shown by surgical care improvement project (SCIP) antibiotic prophylaxis.[20]
2. *Balance measures*: these relate to health system metrics, which ensure that an improvement in one area does not adversely affect another. For example, if length of stay in recovery is being measured after implementing multimodal analgesia, but the patient feels rushed, this may affect patient satisfaction.

3. *Outcome measures*: these are defined by the World Health Organization as the change in the health of an individual, group of people, or population that is attributable to an intervention or series of interventions. Examples include mortalities, readmission rates, or surgical site infection (SSI) rates. Outcome measures require risk adjustment to avoid penalizing physicians who treat high-risk patients. Risk adjustment based on clinical data is difficult and costly to perform. In contrast, if based on administrative data, it is less costly but can fail to distinguish a preexisting condition from a complication.

4. *Structural measures*: these are structural measures that provide patients a sense of a health care provider's capacity, systems, and processes to provide high-quality care. Examples of structural measures include use of an electronic medical record, patient portal, medication order entry and reconciliation, the proportion of board-certified physicians, or the ratio of providers to patients.[21]

PITFALLS

- *Process measures are more sensitive* to differences in quality of care than are outcome measures. They involve *taking measurements at 2 times*, and they require that all other factors that might affect outcomes remain unchanged during the interval between measurements. In addition, strict adherence to process metrics do not guarantee enhanced patient outcomes, as shown by the aforementioned failure of SCIP antibiotic prophylaxis to reduce SSI rates in specific surgical procedures.[22]

- *Poor outcome does not necessarily imply poor quality of care*, because other factors influence outcomes, including complex comorbidities. One way to change physician behavior is to create incentives that are based on a combination of adherence to process, outcome, and structural measures.

- *Time spent on quality efforts*: Casalino and colleagues[23] found that, on average, physicians and staff spent a total of 15.1 hours per physician per week dealing with quality measures. The average physician spent 2.6 h/wk, whereas other staff spent 12.5 hours. Ironically, most of this time was spent on entering information into the medical record only for the purpose of reporting for quality measures from external entities. Assuming that physicians work 48 weeks annually. 2.6 h/wk equates to about 5% of physician time, or about 2.25 weeks out of the year. Therefore, the result of the requirement to document quality measures is the de facto removal of about 5% of physicians' time from the clinical workforce of approximately 800,000 full-time-equivalent (FTE) physicians, or about 40,000 FTEs. The current system is far from efficient and contributes to negative physician attitudes toward quality measures.

- *Practice guidelines are intended to offer guidance* by providing information to clinicians to help them decide how best to care for patients, allowing for clinical judgment and patient preferences. In contrast, *performance measures are quantitative tools*, such as rates or percentages, used to set standards that, if not met, almost certainly identify poor-quality care.[24,25]

- *Several pitfalls have been found to occur when converting practice guidelines into performance measures.* Creating performance measures based on guidelines requires the guideline to be based on high-quality evidence and not just on expert opinion. Other issues include problems selecting the appropriate target population, determining target screening rates, and measuring screening performance. Such problems seem particularly important to understand given the recent recommendation by the IOM to apply the Veterans Affairs health care system's performance measurement and reporting practices to the US health care system as a whole.[26]

The scope of this article is not to explain the QPP. However, readers can obtain more information about this topic from the following sources:

- Overview of the MIPS program: https://qpp.cms.gov/mips/overview
- 2018 list of approved improvement activities for MIPS: https://qpp.cms.gov/mips/explore-measures/improvement-activities?py=2018 #measures
- CMS Ambulatory Surgery Care (ASC) payment system ICN 006819 December 2017: https://www.cms.gov/Outreach-and-Education/Medicare-Learning-Network-MLN/MLNProducts/downloads/AmbSurgCtrFeepymtfctsht508-09.pdf (accessed on September 1, 2018)[27]
- MIPS: 2018 CMS-approved QCDRs measures link: https://www.cms.gov/Medicare/Quality-Payment-Program/Resource-Library/2018-Qualified-Clinical-Data-Registry-QCDR-Measure-Specifications.xlsx (accessed on September 1, 2018)
- Blueprint for the CMS Measurement Management System: https://www.cms.gov/Medicare/Quality-Initiatives-Patient-Assessment-Instruments/MMS/Downloads/Blueprint-130.pdf
- 2018 CMS Quality Measure Development plan: https://www.cms.gov/Medicare/Quality-Payment-Program/Measure-Development/2018-MDP-annual-report.PDF
- The ASA: http://www.asahq.org/macra

HOW ARE QUALITY MEASURES CREATED?

Quality measures are developed and validated relative to existing evidence-based medicine. Environmental scans and gap analyses are performed. Seeking the help of stakeholders, expert panels are created. Concept measures are then developed and approved by the ASA Committee on Performance and Outcome Measures (CPOM). The preliminary measures are submitted to the ASA Web site for public review (opinion by ASA members), after which CPOM finalizes the measure. Once the final measure is approved by the House of Delegates, it is then submitted to CMS for approval. If CMS does not approve the measure, it may still be used in the QCDR registry for testing, gathering data, and/or resubmitted to CMS for further consideration.

A list of items considered during measure development includes:

- Use of expert input about the measures needed by ASA committees and other organizations, such as the Society for Ambulatory Anesthesiology (SAMBA).
- Prioritize which measures to develop.
- Evaluate existing quality measures.
- Reduce the reporting cost and burden for clinicians.
- Meet the goal of person-centered, value-based measures to support the QPP.
- CMS puts patients first in every endeavor, including in the development of measures to support the QPP.

FACILITY

CMS publishes a consumer-oriented Hospital Compare Web site. The Joint Commission also publishes Quality Check, a Web site that lists a facility accreditation status and a report of key quality measures. Similarly, the ASC Quality Collaboration (QC) is a cooperative effort of organizations and companies interested in ensuring that

ASC quality data are measured and reported in a meaningful way. The ASC QC was formed in 2006 to initiate the process of developing standardized ASC quality measures. The organization's stakeholders include ASC corporations, ASC associations, professional societies, and accrediting bodies with a focus on health care quality and safety. The ASC QC publishes ASC facility quality data, measured and presented in a meaningful way. ASCs are obligated to report these quality data, and anesthesiologists play a key role in the implementation of ASC quality measures. CMS implemented the Ambulatory Surgical Care Quality Reporting Program (ASCQR) in 2012. Examples of ASCQR measures include patient burns, patient falls, wrong-site procedures, and all cause hospital transfer.[28] To learn more about the ASC payment system visit: https://www.cms.gov/Outreach-and-Education/Medicare-Learning-Network-MLN/MLNProducts/downloads/AmbSurgCtrFeepymtfctsht508-09.pdf (accessed on September 1, 2018).

TRANSPARENCY IN THE INTERNET AGE

When patients, reporters, and health care leaders review quality data and Hospital Compare Web sites, the score they view is an overall reflection of a wide array of measures compiled into a single score. The weight of each of those measures has been determined by CMS based on their policies and priorities. But what if the CMS priorities are not aligned with what a patient wants? In 2018, Rumball-Smith and colleagues[29] published a perspective in the *New England Journal of Medicine*, titled "Personalized Hospital Ratings – Transparency for the Internet Age." The investigators suggest the creation of a scoring system that can be modified by patients based on their personal preferences. They cite several examples, such as a patient that requires a knee arthroscopy after having a bicycle accident. This young, healthy man is comparing 2 different hospitals, a local community hospital and a regional referral medical center. The CMS Hospital Compare Web site scores the local hospital as a 4-star hospital, but the regional medical center as 5 stars. However, when the patient is able to modify scores based on his fears, wants, and needs, he ranks effectiveness, safety, and avoiding readmission as most important, and ranks other aspects of his care at a lower level. After these changes are made, the local hospital now ranks as 5 star and the regional medical center as 4 stars. The investigators suggest that allowing patients to take command of their care, instead of basing their decisions on the governments' priorities, may be a better option.[29]

TOPPED-OUT MEASURES AND REMOVAL PROCESS: MEASURING IMPROVES AWARENESS

As mentioned earlier, in 2004, Epstein and colleagues'[16] "Paying Physicians for High-quality Care" suggested rotating measures and expanding performance indicators over time as a more successful long-term strategy to improve quality. MACRA has the goal of measuring, benchmarking, and shifting money from poor to good performers in a budget-neutral manner. One of the goals of CMS is to have a physician-compare Web site. The goal is to incentivize those that do a better job. For instance, if all physicians are doing the right thing, and thus scoring 100%, CMS would remove this measure because it has become ineffective at differentiating one physician's quality from another. However, what is the goal? To improve and maintain quality of care or to shift money from someone that documents poorly to someone that documents well? There are times when a topped-out measure should be maintained because the measure itself enhances outcomes, as is well shown by the perioperative patient handoff, which, although recently retired as a measure by

CMS, should be maintained as a clinical practice because the practice has been shown to improve outcomes.

The MIPS program does not detect preventable medical errors or the lack of evidence-based medicine, as long as they are being measured, because providers pay more attention to what is being measured. The Hawthorne effect states that outcomes tend to improve in response to the awareness of being observed or studied. Once clinicians stop measuring a specific measure, it is likely that performance on that measure would decrease as providers pay more attention to a new measure. Rotating measures can also create a clerical pitfall for the system. Because new measures for the following year are usually identified late in the current year, reporting may be difficult. Making changes to an anesthetic record or to a quality form is not a simple task and often requires approval by multiple committees, including the medical executive committee of a facility. This process could create a period in the year in which an action is being taken but not being recorded, or at least not recorded in a manner that can be easily captured by an EHR.

In 2004, the NHS implemented the Quality and Outcomes Framework (QOF), the largest pay-for-performance health care scheme. In 2014, a review of the QOF removed financial incentives for 40 of 121 quality-of-care indicators. The data continued to be collected and the documented quality of care decreased once financial incentives were removed for those specific indicators. This finding shows that paying providers to achieve a certain quality of care may not create a sustainable improvement in quality.[27,30,31]

THE FUTURE

The ASA Committee on Outcome and Performance Measures, in combination with the Committee of Ambulatory Surgical Care and the Society for Ambulatory Anesthesiology, has formed a Technical Expert Panel for the development of quality measures for ambulatory anesthesiology. The current focus is on developing measures relative to the assessment and management of dysglycemias, frailty, obstructive sleep apnea mitigation strategies, and discharge and follow-up care. Other efforts in progress include the development of multidisciplinary team shared measures, which encompass the surgeon, anesthesiologist and nurses.

Although substantial capital investment will be required, the development of a National Health Information Network is greatly anticipated and will be critical to quality improvement.[32]

The Medicare Payment Advisory Commission (MEDPAC) has analyzed the results of the first year of MIPS reporting and has become concerned about the direction the program has taken. MEDPAC suggests the reorientation of the MIPS program toward assessing the performance of groups of clinicians on population-based outcome measures. To increase financial incentives for APMs, MEDPAC has suggested elimination of the current MIPS program and replacing it with a claims-based program that CMS would calculate.[33] Making judgments about quality based on administrative data would bring significant errors to the system; administrative data are easy to obtain but have significant limitations, such as failing to distinguish a preexisting condition from complications that occur after an intervention. It would also require significant risk adjustment.[34]

The authors suggest creating a level of importance scale for quality measures in the MIPS program. Instead of just asking providers to report on 6 or 7 measures (depending on group size), measures should be reported by importance based on goals the government wants to achieve. For example, if a goal is to improve perioperative glycemic control in order to decrease complications, this should be a high-importance measure, representing (for example) 30% of the 100% quality score. Instead of retiring an old measure that has topped off, the measure should be labeled as a lower importance measure with a 10% quality score. Physicians or groups could report on a combination of high-importance and low-importance measures to achieve a minimal achievable score of 100%. They could, for example, choose to report on 3 high-importance and 1 low-importance measure to achieve 100% or 1 high-importance (30%) and 7 low-importance measures (10% each). This approach would prevent what happened in the United Kingdom once quality incentives were removed from certain indicators.[35]

SUMMARY

Health care professionals see measurement through their own eyes and biases. This article broadens the focal point to make the patient central to what is being measured. PREMs and PROMs are of the utmost importance. In addition, as clinicians continue to evolve how they measure what really matters, they need to be mindful of the time taken from direct patient care to achieve these activities. In addition, and most important, clinicians must ensure that all measures are designed to ensure that population health is improved, that patient experience and outcomes are enhanced, and that the cost of care is reduced.

REFERENCES

1. Institute of Medicine. Institute of Medicine. 2001. Available at: http://www. nationalacademies.org/hmd/Reports/2018/crossing-global-quality-chasm-improving-health-care-worldwide.aspx. Accessed February 22, 2015.
2. Appleby J, Devlin NJ. Getting the most out of PROMs - putting health outcomes at the heart of NHS decision-making. London: The Kings Fund; 2010.
3. Hostetter M, Klein S. Using patient-reported outcomes to improve health care quality. Quality matters. The Commonwealth Fund. 20 11/December 2011/January 2012. Available at: http://www.commonwealthfund.org/publications/newsletters/quality-matters/2011/december-january-2012/in-focus. Accessed February 22, 2015.
4. Keiningham T, Gupta S, Aksoy L, et al. The high price of customer satisfaction. Available at: https://sloanreview.mit.edu/article/the-high-price-of-customer-satisfaction/. Accessed February 28, 2019.
5. Black N, Varaganum M, Hutchings A. Relationship between patient reported experience (PREMs) and patient reported outcomes (PROMs) in elective surgery. BMJ Qual Saf 2014;23:534–42.
6. Kingsley C, Patel S. Patient-reported outcome measures and patient-reported experience measures. BJA Educ 2017;17(4):137–44. Available at: https://doi.org/10.1093/bjaed/mkw060.
7. Moro ET, Feitosa IMPSS, de Oliveira RG, et al. Ketamine does not enhance the quality of recovery following laparoscopic cholecystectomy: a randomized controlled trial. Acta Anaesthesiol Scand 2017;61(7):740–8.
8. Kohn LT, Corrigan JM, Donaldson MS. To err is human. Washington, DC: The National Academic Press; 1999. Available at: http://www.nap.edu/books/0309068371/html/. Accessed September 30, 2018.
9. Berwick DM, Calkins DR, McCannon CJ, et al. The 100,000 lives campaign: setting a goal and a deadline for improving health care quality. J Am Medical Assoc 2006;295(3):324–7.

10. Agency for Healthcare Research and Quality. Medical errors & patient safety. Rockville (MD): AHRQ. Available at: https://www.ahrq.gov/research/findings/factsheets/errors-safety/index.html. Accessed February 28, 2019.
11. McCannon CJ, Hackbarth AD, Griffin FA. Miles to go: an introduction to the 5 Million Lives Campaign. Jt Comm J Qual Patient Saf 2007;33:477–84.
12. A journey through the history of the Joint Commission. Oakbrook Terrace (IL): The Joint Commission. Available at: https://jntcm.ae-admin.com/assets/1/6/TJC_history_timeline_through_2018.pdf. Accessed February 28, 2019.
13. Guiding principles for the management of performance measures by the American Society of Anesthesiologists. Committee on performance and outcomes measures. Approved by the house of delegates on October 15, 2000, and last amended on October 19, 2011. Available at: http://www.asahq.org/~/media/Sites/ASAHQ/Files/Public/Resources/standards-guidelines/guiding-principles-for-management-of-performance-measures-by-asa.pdf. Accessed February 28, 2019.
14. Bloomstone J. Overcoming challenges–anesthesiologists in enhanced recovery in major abdominopelvic surgery. In: Gan TJ, Thacker J, Miller TE, et al, editors. American Society for Enhanced Recovery. West Islip (NY): Professional Communications, Inc; 2016. p. 207–24.
15. Institute of Medicine. Leadership by example: coordinating government roles in improving health care quality. Washington, DC: National Academies Press; 2002.
16. Epstein AM, Lee TL, Hamel MB. Paying physicians for high-quality care. N Engl J Med 2004;350:406–10.
17. Martin AB, Hartman M, Benson J, et al, National Health Expenditure Accounts Team. National health spending in 2014: faster growth driven by coverage expansion and prescription drug spending. Health Aff (Millwood) 2016;35(1):150–60.
18. Available at: https://www.healthaffairs.org/doi/10.1377/hlthaff.2015.1194.
19. Shen Y. Selection incentives in a performance-based contracting system. Health Serv Res 2003;38(2):535–52.
20. Petersen L, Woodard L, Urech T, et al. Does pay-for-performance improve the quality of health care? Ann Intern Med 2006;145:265–72.
21. Agency for Healthcare Research and Quality. Available at: https://www.ahrq.gov/professionals/quality-patient-safety/talkingquality/create/types.html]. Accessed September 30, 2018.
22. Dua A, Desai S, Seabrook GR, et al. The effect of Surgical Care Improvement Project measures on national trends on surgical site infections in open vascular procedures. J Vasc Surg 2014;60(6):1635–9.
23. Casalino LP, Gans D, Weber R, et al. US physician practices spend $15.4 billion annually to report quality measures. Health Aff (Millwood) 2016;35(3):401–6.
24. AHA/ACC Conference Proceedings. Measuring and improving quality of care: a report from the American Heart Association/American College of Cardiology first scientific forum on assessment of healthcare quality in cardiovascular disease and stroke. Circulation 2000;101:1483–93.
25. Walter L, Davidowitz N, Heineken P, et al. Pitfalls of converting practice guidelines into quality measures: lessons learned from a VA performance measure. JAMA 2004;291:2466–70.
26. Jha AK, Perlin JB, Kizer KW, et al. Effect of the transformation of the Veterans Affairs health care system on the quality of care. N Engl J Med 2003;348:2218–27.
27. Kontopantelis E, Springate D, Reeves D, et al. Withdrawing performance indicators: retrospective analysis of general practice performance under UK quality and outcomes framework. BMJ 2014;348:g330.

28. Ambulatory surgical center quality reporting specification manual listed by year of data collection. 2016. Available at: https://www.fsasc.org/assets/ASC%20Specification%20Manual.pdf. Accessed February 28, 2019.

29. Rumball-Smith J, Gurvey J, Friedberg MW. Personalized hospital ratings – transparency for the internet age. N Engl J Med 2018;379(9):806–7.

30. Lester H, Schmittdiel J, Selby J, et al. The impact of removing financial incentives from clinical quality indicators: longitudinal analysis of four Kaiser Permanente indicators. BMJ 2010;340:c1898.

31. Benzer JK, Young GJ, Burgess JF Jr, et al. Sustainability of quality improvement following removal of pay-for-performance incentives. J Gen Intern Med 2014;29: 127–32.

32. Kaushal R, Blumenthal D, Poon EG, et al, Cost of National Health Information Network Working Group. The costs of a national health information network. Ann Intern Med 2005;143:165–73.

33. Medicare Payment Advisory Commission (MEDPAC). Report to the Congress. Medicare and Health Care Delivery System. 2018. Available at: http://medpac.gov/docs/default-source/reports/jun18_medpacreporttocongress_sec.pdf. Accessed February 28, 2019.

34. Glance L, Neuman M, Martinez C, et al. Performance measurement at a "tipping point." Anesth Analg 2011;12(4):958–66.

35. Minchin M, Roland M, Richardson J, et al. Quality of care in the United Kingdom after removal of financial incentives. N Engl J Med 2018;379:948–57.

Value-Based Payment in Ambulatory Anesthesia
MACRA, MIPS, and More

Douglas G. Merrill, MD, MBA, MA

KEYWORDS

• MACRA • MIPS • CMS • Anesthesiology • Billing • Payment • Pay for performance

KEY POINTS

- The Medicare Access and CHIP Reauthorization Act of 2015 (MACRA) was passed in 2015 as a means to consolidate the many quality payment programs. MACRA combined all quality payment programs (Physician Quality Reporting System, Value-Based Payment Modifier, and Electronic Health Record [EHR] Incentive Programs) into 1 program, the Quality Payment Program (QPP). The QPP includes Merit-based Incentive Payment System (MIPS) and a potential for bonus payments for participation in eligible alternative payment models.
- Under MIPS, providers have their Medicare payments adjusted up or down based on their performance on 4 weighted metrics: quality, cost, clinical practice improvement activities, and meaningful use regarding EHR technology (Advancing Care Information).
- By 2022, a provider's Medicare payments will be adjusted up or down, ranging from a −9% to +27%, depending on the provider's or the group's performance on the 4 metrics. This is a budget-neutral process: the funding of bonuses to any will derive entirely from the reductions in payments to those who do not perform at or above benchmarks, as determined by the Centers for Medicare & Medicaid Services.
- Although ambulatory surgery center facilities are paid via the Ambulatory Surgical Center Payment System and not subject to MACRA, the anesthesiologists and other providers (eg, certified registered nurse anesthetists and anesthesia assistants) who work in them are subject to MACRA and its payment adjustments.

Disclosure: The author has no relationship with any entity that would constitute a conflict of interest in regard to the information provided in this article.

The material for this article was written in August 2018 as was necessary to meet the article deadline. The Centers for Medicare & Medicaid Services (CMS) announced potential changes to the program, open for public comment, on July 23, 2018. Readers should remain aware that substantive change in the programs may have come out since this material was published. Stay aware of CMS news releases.

Medicare Access and CHIP Reauthorization Act of 2015 and many other aspects of provider payment are subject to near constant tinkering (and interpretation) by CMS, so do not substitute the information in this article for professional advice from your practice manager and attorney.

Merrill Healthcare, Reno, NV 89511, USA

E-mail address: dougmd53@gmail.com

Anesthesiology Clin 37 (2019) 373–388
https://doi.org/10.1016/j.anclin.2019.01.011
1932-2275/19/© 2019 Elsevier Inc. All rights reserved.

anesthesiology.theclinics.com

INTRODUCTION

It might well be asked, "Why is this happening to our payment structure?" The short answer is that what is referred in the United States as *health care* is now so expensive that it is the focus of Congress rather than the work that would be more productive for that body to emphasize, which would be the more difficult (but more valuable approach) of improving the social networks for at-risk populations. As other nations have found, that effort would improve health and reduce the need for expensive rescue health care. For instance, making sure that the elderly have access to low-cost maintenance medication, social engagement, and adequate housing would greatly reduce their use of the nation's emergency rooms and the high cost of end-of-life care.[1]

US health care is so expensive because it is uncoordinated and provides low value (high cost but lesser outcomes) because most care is rescue care, which is highly reliant on technology and use of pharmaceuticals, the latter of which are expensive because Congress has eliminated most of the brakes on the ability of the drug manufacturing industry (Pharma) to overcharge for their products.

Other nations reduce the cost of health care by reducing the need for rescue care. They accomplish this by instead avidly investing in reducing the negative effects of the social determinants of health, such as available sources of nutritious food, safe neighborhoods that allow for regular exercise, education that leads to employment that allows for autonomy, and a reduction of the inherent racism that engenders stress, leading to early aging of minority and indigent populations.[2]

It is a reasonable question to ask why the government continues to push on the incomes of providers, when provider fees cost only 9% of US health care expenditures.[3] It might be answered, by health reimbursement policy experts, that physicians and allied health providers make most of the decisions around applications of the other 91% of expenditures, so their fees are tied to those costs, closely. One of the brightest of those experts, Uwe Reinhardt, however, recommended a different course more than a decade ago:

> Physicians are the central decision makers in health care. A superior strategy (to cutting physician income) might be to pay them very well for helping us reduce unwarranted health spending elsewhere.[4]

Unfortunately, the Centers for Medicare & Medicaid Services (CMS) and Congress each has failed to recognize Reinhardt's logic and instead constructed an arcane process in which unfocused goals (eg, use of electronic health records [EHRs]) are supposed to now be supported by both supplemented and reduced physician income.

Programs like MACRA and the QPP are nascent attempts to move payment for provider services from fee-for-service (FFS) bases to outcome-based and at-risk payments. These programs, along with the bundled care and value-based payments (VBPs), prospective risk payment policies, and other efforts on the facilities sides, should move the payment system away from an FFS model entirely. That would likely take, however, more than 2 decades, if the history of health care payment policy change is considered the harbinger of future rate of change.

Until the real direct causes of high health care costs are addressed, and if social networks are left uncreated, the costs of health care will continue to mount.

A good example is that pharmaceutical companies are currently allowed to set high prices on medication, generating nearly unlimited profits on sales of medication, purportedly because they require so much income for research and development. The industry, however, currently spends far more of those profits on direct-to-consumer advertising than it does on research, by more than 50% (**Fig. 1**). By statute (Medicare

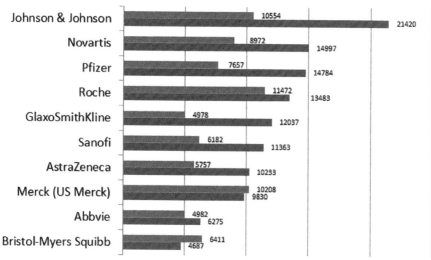

■ Research and Development (US$m)   ■ Sales and Marketing (US$m)

Fig. 1. The difference between spending by the 10 largest pharmaceutical companies on marketing versus research. These top companies spend 54% more on marketing than they do on research, belying their attempts to present themselves as scientific research organizations. Direct marketing to consumers drives overuse of expensive drugs. (*From* Intermede Investment Partners based on data taken from 2017 annual reports, 10-Ks and 20-Fs for each business. Figures have been converted to US$ at the average 2017 rate for direct comparability by Intermede. © Copyright Intermede Investment Partners Limited. All rights reserved; with permission.)

Part D), CMS is not allowed to negotiate lower prices for medications, cementing these high costs to the government and to patients. As to the latter cause, the cost of rescue care, what the United States calls health care will continue to climb if the social determinants of health, such as isolation, education, food deserts, unsafe transportation and neighborhoods, and inadequate housing, go ignored by the government.

WHAT IS THE MEDICARE ACCESS AND CHIP REAUTHORIZATION ACT OF 2015?

The Medicare Access and CHIP Reauthorization Act of 2015 (MACRA) was passed in 2015 to consolidate the many governmental quality (pay-for-performance) payment programs. It was also how Congress could eliminate the annually troublesome and euphemistically named Medicare Sustainable Growth Rate (SGR) process used to determine physician compensation, which proved both ineffective at reducing the rate of rise of health care costs and uniformly dissatisfying to policy makers and providers. SGR had been passed in 1997 to tie the rate of rise of health care provider costs to the gross domestic product growth, but it was arcane and repeatedly called for automatic and draconian cuts in provider pay each year, which were politically unsustainable. This required an annual override of the SGR calculation by Congress, which did not want to directly determine physician incomes if a means could be found instead for them managed by an algorithm that CMS bureaucrats would administer. In part because of everyone's exhaustion with the SGR, MACRA passed by remarkably wide margins (392–37 in the House of Representatives and 92–8 in the Senate), a reminding today that, just a few years ago, bipartisan action was still possible.

MACRA replaced the SGR and combined all quality payment programs (Physician Quality Reporting System [PQRS], Value-Based Payment Modifier, and the EHR

Incentive Programs) into 1 program, the Quality Payment Program (QPP). The QPP includes the Merit-based Incentive Payment System (MIPS), and a potential for bonus payments for participation in eligible alternative payment models (APMs).

The MIPS is now intended to determine all Medicare payment adjustments, increasingly supplanting more and more of the FFS methodology. Providers (not just physicians) will have their Medicare payments adjusted up or down based on their performance on 4 weighted metrics:

1. Quality
2. Cost
3. Clinical practice improvement activities (IAs)
4. Meaningful use regarding EHR technology (Advancing Care Information [ACI]—note this name was changed in the summer of 2018 to Promoting Interoperability, with no changes to the nature of the program itself).

By 2022, a provider's Medicare payment will be adjusted up or down, ranging from −9% to +27%, depending on the provider's or the group's performance on these 4 metrics. This is a budget neutral process: the funding of bonuses will derive entirely from the reductions in payments to those who do not perform at or above benchmarks, as determined by CMS.

The Advanced APM (AAPM) in the QPP for 2018 consists of programs that meet the following 3 criteria:

1. Require participants to use certified EHR technology (CEHRT)
2. Provide payment for covered professional services based on quality measures comparable to those used in the quality performance category of the MIPS
3. Either
   • Is a medical home model expanded under CMS Innovation (CMMI) authority
   • Requires participating APM eligible clinicians (ECs) to bear more than a nominal amount of financial risk for monetary losses.

As discussed previously, AAPMs are inherently risky (more than a nominal amount of financial risk) but have potential high value to the participants under the new system.[5]

APMs are of 2 types: MIPS APMs and AAPMs. So, there are 3 value-based options for providers:

1. MIPS adjustments only
2. MIPS APMs that will provide additional, APM-specific rewards plus MIPS adjustments
3. AAPMs

In brief, AAPM-specific rewards provide their qualifying participants (QPs) protection from certain MIPS requirements and eligibility to receive a 5% lump sum bonus payment each year for up to 6 years, 2019 to 2024. Furthermore, QPs would receive a consistently higher annual fee schedule update from 2026 onward.

Recent and Proposed Changes in Medicare Access and CHIP Reauthorization Act of 2015 (Mostly Good)

No surprise, as with any CMS program, tinkering began early. Changes include:

1. Exclusion of Medicare Part B drug costs from MIPS payment adjustments.
2. Elimination of improvement scoring for the cost performance category for the third through fifth years of MIPS.

3. Elimination of the requirement that CMS increase the weighting of the cost category from 10% to 30% in 2019 (year 3). That weighting, however, likely will still increase. The proposed changes open for public comment as of submission of this article are to increase cost to 15% with quality dropping to 45% and all else staying the same. The proposed rule also recommends that the weighting of cost will rise to 30% by 2024 (ie, 5% per year) (see https://qpp.cms.gov/about/resource-library).
4. Increased flexibility for CMS in setting the performance threshold for years 2 through 5 to ensure a gradual and incremental transition to the performance threshold set at the mean or median for the sixth year.
5. There is allowance for the Physician-Focused Payment Model Technical Advisory Committee (PTAC) to provide initial feedback and guidance to stakeholders developing APMs on their own. Anyone can propose an APM to the Health and Human Services (HHS) Secretary. Such proposals will be reviewed (and now advice given) by PTAC, prior to presentation to the Secretary.
6. New: a cost evaluation will be added to the quality, informatics, and improvement metrics.
7. In 2017, the cost metric was weighted at zero, but it is increased to 10% in 2018, with the quality metric dropping from 60% to 50%, pending involvement in AIC or AI metrics. 2018 data impact providers' Medicare payments in 2020.
8. Finally, the weighting assigned to the cost metric will increase to 30% next year (2019) unless a legislative fix can be created.

How are the Merit-based Incentive Payment System and Physicians Doing?

Overall, the MIPS and physicians are doing well, according to some media reports. *Modern Healthcare* reported in May 2018 that "90% of clinicians required to report under MIPS submitted data this year, but thousands of physicians will still face penalties for not complying with the program, according to CMS Administrator Seema Verma."[6] CMS had set a goal of 90% of physicians reporting and that was surpassed, with 91% submitting. Verma went on to note that only 39% (just over 621,000) of physicians are eligible to report under the MIPS program and 55,000 of those did not report. CMS admitted that the barriers of the program itself were likely responsible for many or most of those reporting failures, and Verma noted that CMS hopes to reduce those in the future.

Verma noted that submission rates for rural ACOs and clinicians were remarkably high, at 98% and 94%, respectively.[7] She went on to aver that part of the reason these numbers were so high was a CMS emphasis on support of small practice access to bonuses and easier reporting methodologies.

The Ambulatory Anesthesiologist and the Medicare Access and CHIP Reauthorization Act of 2015

Eligibility

A common question for those who work in an ambulatory surgery center (ASC) is whether MACRA applies to them. The short answer is "yes," but the long answer gets more complicated. Although ASC facilities are paid via the Ambulatory Surgical Center Payment System and not subject to MACRA, the physicians and other providers (eg, CRNAs and anesthesia assistants) who work in them are subject to MACRA and its payment adjustments.

How to check potential participation capability

First, log on to https://qpp.cms.gov and enter your National Provider Identifier (NPI) number into the system. This indicates if CMS has already determined that you are or are not an MIPS EC.

It is likely that you are a MIPS EC if:

1. You reported more than $90,000 in allowed Medicare Part B FFS charges AND
2. You have cared for more than 200 Medicare Part B beneficiaries (not 200 episodes, actual patients).

Another question is whether the provider would create reports based solely on Medicare patients or all patients. Providers and groups must report on 50% of all patients for the quality category, unless they are reporting via claims, in which case they only need to report on 50% of Medicare Part B patients. Physicians must also report on all patients for the ACI category.

Here is a quick run-down of who and what are covered by QPP:

1. Included payments: all services billed under the Medicare Physician Fee Schedule (MPFS) will be impacted
2. Excluded payments
   a. Inpatient Prospective Payment System
   b. Outpatient Prospective Payment System
   c. Ambulatory Surgical Center Payment System
3. Included clinicians
   Physicians, physician assistants, nurse practitioners, clinical nurse specialists, CRNAs, and groups that include any of these clinicians
4. Excluded clinicians
   a. Groups with fewer than 15 ECs
   b. Clinicians or groups that fall under the low-volume threshold, which CMS defines as clinicians or groups with $90,000 or less in annual Medicare charges OR with 100 or fewer Medicare patients
   c. Clinicians in their first-year billing Medicare
   d. Clinicians in an APM (either receiving 25% of their Medicare payments or seeing 20% of their Medicare patients through an AAPM)
   e. Place of Service (POS) exclusions: if 75% of services to patients were provided in these POS settings, you will automatically be excluded from some metrics:
      - Modifier 19: Off- Campus–Outpatient Hospital[a]
      - Modifier 21: Inpatient Hospital
      - Modifier 22: On Campus–Outpatient Hospital[b]
      - Modifier 23: Emergency Room

Bottom line: check, using your NPI, to see what CMS has designated you as at this point. Go to https://qpp.cms.gov and enter your NPI number to find out.

SCORING AND MEASURES

MIPS scoring: you are scored this year (2018) for payment in 2020.

The MIPS quality component will make up at least 50% of the MIPS score.

To succeed maximally, an EC must report 6 measures for 60% of the patients for whom the measure applies. ECs must report on 50% of all patients for the quality

---

[a] Effective January 1, 2016, a new POS code (19) for services provided in outpatient settings outside of the main hospital campus.

[b] POS code 19, Off Campus–Outpatient Hospital, was created and the description of POS code 22 was revised to On Campus–Outpatient Hospital (originally Outpatient Hospital). Providers must know which code the facility uses for billing.

category, unless reporting via claims, in which case they need to report on only 50% of Medicare Part B patients.

To report, most anesthesiologists use either a qualified registry or a qualified clinical data registry (QCDR) (less often, an EHR). A good example of a QCDR is the American Society of Anesthesiologists (ASA) National Anesthesia Clinical Outcomes Registry (NACOR) or another that is proprietary (eg, a MEDNAX provider would use the company's reporting system). Some may be covered by an accountable care organization (ACO) that provides this service.

Measures: 1 of 6 measures must be an outcome measure or, if 1 is not available, it should be a high-priority measure. A high-priority measure measures appropriate use, patient safety, efficiency, patient experience, or care coordination. There can also be a population health measure used if the group is large enough. There are 9 measures that may be useful for anesthesiologists, supplied by CMS for 2018 (https://qpp. cms.gov/about/resource-library). Sixteen measures can be reported via the Anesthesia Quality Institute (AQI) NACOR (a QCDR) that are approved by CMS. If you participate in AQI NACOR, you can use this approach[8]:

For outpatient anesthesiologists, there are 9 metrics that can be used:

1. Assessment of sleep apnea patients
2. Documentation of anticoagulation prior to neuraxial or interventional pain procedures
3. Infection control for interventional pain procedures
4. Multimodal pain management
5. New corneal injury avoided
6. Patient experience scores
7. Safe opioid prescribing
8. Peripheral nerve blocks or neuraxial anesthesia for total knee arthroplasty
9. Use of pencil-point needles for spinal anesthesia

CMS has identified benchmarks for each measure and the measures that are topped out (eg, temperature monitoring and preventative postoperative nausea and vomiting medication) are weighted as less valuable (3.0 points maximum). Benchmarks may change during the year.

Here are some tips:

1. Reporting on 6 is minimum; try for more.
2. If fewer than 6 are reported on, CMS will find the ones that could have been reported and potentially give zero points for those.
3. If working in a practice of 16 or more providers, a population-based measure may be able to be used, possibly achieving more points.

The Merit-based Incentive Payment System Advancing Care Information Metric

The MIPS ACI metric category has a weight of 25% in the component scoring. Physicians must report on all patients for the ACI category. There are exemptions. If qualifying for an exemption from ACI, then all that weight (25%) moves to the quality component. Check https://qpp.cms.gov.[9]

Exemptions that are automatic:

1. Non–patient-facing clinicians.
2. Hospital-based MIPS clinicians (who do 75% of their care in the hospital).
3. ASC-based clinicians—those who provide 75% or more of their work in site-of-service 24 locations.

4. These MIPS ECs can still choose to report if they would like, and if data are submitted, CMS will score their performance and weight their ACI performance accordingly.

Other exemptions that had to have been applied for by December 31, 2018:

1. If practicing in a location with no Internet access
2. If experiencing uncontrollable circumstances (hospital closure or natural disaster) during the reporting period
3. If you or your group lack of control over the availability of a CEHRT in more than 50% of patient encounters
4. If solo or group has fewer than 16 fewer ECs
5. ACI score is calculated such that you must get more than 100 percentage points to get full ACI credit.

A common question is around the meaning of a non–patient-facing clinician. CMS recognizes that hospital-based doctors do not have long-term patient relationships, so they created the non–patient-facing category:

1. Individual who bills for fewer than 100 Medicare patients
2. A group so qualifies if more than 75% of the individual ECs in the group meet the individual criteria (fewer than 100 patients billed for)
3. Most anesthesiologists (not ICU or pain doctors) may well qualify as non–patient-facing clinicians

Even if qualifying as a non–patient-facing provider, 6 quality measures or a specialty measure set (like ASA has created) must still be reported, but CMS will reweight categories if there are not enough to report on.

A hospital-based provider will be excluded entirely from ACI reporting. For more information, see www.asahq.org/macra.

The Merit-based Incentive Payment System Improvement Activities Component

The improvement activities (IAs) measures can be reviewed at https://qpp.cms.gov; to earn the highest score, 40 points are needed, reached by reporting medium activities (10 points) or by reporting high-weighted activities (20 points each). Small or rural groups may be eligible for doubling of the scores. There are 112 different activities available. See https://www.aqihq.org/MACRAOverview.aspx and https://www.aqihq.org/files/MIPS/2018/2018_MIPS_Measures_Available_for_Reporting_through_AQI.pdf for a list of 23 that should work for anesthesiologists. You will attest that you did the activity for a minimum of 90 days and maintain the supporting documentation for 6 years (do not send it in).

CMS will audit and validate what it considers "consistent and meaningful engagement."

A special note about the MIPS IA component and the perioperative surgical home (PSH) is in order. If you either have not started a PSH or are doing the work without declaring it, this is a good reason to consider doing those. For CY 2018 MIPs reporting, CMS has recognized 2 sets of PSH activities as IAs:

1. PSH care coordination: allows for reporting of strategies and processes related to care coordination of patients receiving surgical or procedural care within a PSH:
   a. Coordinate with care managers/navigators in preoperative clinic to plan and implementation comprehensive postdischarge plan of care.
   b. Deploy perioperative clinic and care processes to reduce postoperative visits to emergency rooms.

    c. Implement evidence-informed practices and standardize care across the entire spectrum of surgical patients.

    d. Implement processes to ensure effective communications and education of patients' postdischarge instructions.

2. Use of patient safety tools: use of tools that assist specialty practices in tracking specific measures that are meaningful to their practice, such as a surgical risk calculator; evidence-based protocols, such as enhanced recovery after surgery (ERAS) protocols; the Centers for Disease Control and Prevention Guide to Infection Prevention for Outpatient Settings (https://www.cdc.gov/hai/settings/outpatient/outpatient-care-guidelines.html); predictive algorithms; and other such tools.

Each of these activities has been assigned a weight of medium, which means that reporting of these PSH activities constitutes 50% of all the reporting requirements for the IAs category under MIPS.

Additionally, most clinicians designated as non–patient-facing (which most anesthesiologists are designated) can receive 100% of their requirements through participating with just these 2 activities.

If all 40 points are scored on the IA, not getting a negative MIPS adjustment for 2020 is assured.

The Fourth Merit-based Incentive Payment System Metric is Cost

This component is considered by CMS from claims data and, therefore, will not include any reporting by the provider. In 2019, the cost score is to be weighted at 10% but will increase to 30% after 2020, assuming no changes in the plans for MACRA. If CMS cannot determine an EC cost score, then that weight will roll to quality. Most anesthesiologists will not have a qualifying cost score (discussed later), although CMS is working on an alternate methodology to capture cost for anesthesiologists.

ECs will be scored on 2 cost measures for 2018:

1. Medicare Spending per Beneficiary (MSPB)—this is the cost of the services provided during a patient's hospital care episode (begins 3 days preadmission and 30 days after discharge). In 2018, they are not including Medicare Part D (prescription costs).

2. Total Per Capita Costs (TPCCs) for all attributed beneficiaries—this should not apply to any anesthesiologists unless they are providing primary care services.

ASA recommends reading Quality and Resource Use Reports (QRURs) from the Enterprise Identity Management system on the CMS portal twice a year. This allows checking to see if any patients are attributed to a practice.

In Summary, Things to Remember About Scoring

In 2018, 50% is apportioned to quality, 25% for ACI, 10% for cost, and 15% for clinical practice improvement.

You could be measured only for quality (85%) and IAs (15%), however, if you do not have enough attributable patients such that your group is exempt from the ACI requirement.

Once a score is calculated by CMS, if above its 2018 15-point score (threshold), you will get a positive adjustment.

To avoid a negative adjustment, here are 4 things that can be done in 2019:

1. Submit 6 quality measures that meet data completeness criteria (at least 60% of the patients to whom they would apply).

2. Attest to 40 points of IAs.

3. Earn the ACI base score AND submit just 1 quality measure that meets data completeness criteria.
4. Earn the ACI base score AND attest to 1 medium-weighted IA.

For more specific information, see the ASA module at www.asahq.org/macra/solutionsresources/macramodules.

REPORTING

Most anesthesiologists will likely report via a QCDR.

Other options are via other qualified registries, the EHR vendor, the CMS Web interface, by attestation (only usable for ACI and IA metrics), and via claims data (only usable for quality metrics).

You can participate and report as an individual, or, if 2 or more providers share the same tax ID number, then they can report their performance as a group.

Alternative Payment Models

AAPMs can lead to an annual 5% bonus through 2026 and an exemption from MIPS. To do this, the APMs must:

1. Be designated (approved) by CMS
2. Meet a patient volume threshold of 25% of patients or 20% of payments for the individual or group must run through the APM
3. Include "more than nominal" downside risk

Most of the physicians in the APM must use a certified EHR. Again, check to see if you are a qualified participant in an APM at https://qpp.cms.gov.

APMs consist of MIPS APMs and non-MIPS APMs. If you think you might be in a MIPS APM, check to see if your group has a contract with CMS under one of these models. If you are, then you must also make sure that you meet threshold requirements (eg, you do not if fewer than 20% of your patients fit into the APM), and, if you do not, then you may have to report under MIPS after all.

Here is what you should do next:
1. Review your eligibility at https://qpp.cms.gov.
2. Review the resources at www.asahq.org and review your options with your group members and practice manager.
3. Consider starting a PSH program if you do not already do that.
4. Join the AQI NACOR both to benchmark your work and to make MIPS reporting easy.

At-risk Contracting

Finally, if you are thinking about joining an ACO or with another entity to negotiate an at-risk contract, either within an APM or with a private payer, there are several factors to consider.

You must be sure to evaluate what is included (eg, preoperative in-depth consults in person vs phone preoperative consultations?), how many days postoperative, other costs you do not control (eg, skilled nursing facility [SNF] costs for postoperative total joints?):

1. Know where the data are coming from that determine the payment. Be sure they are from a certified actuary (or CMS).
2. You must also be sure that there is reasonable risk adjustment (eg, you should get credit for an ASA III vs an ASA I, age, socioeconomic status, and so forth).

3. How difficult is the documentation going to be?
4. When do you get paid?
5. How do you obtain relief for dispute or how do you exit the contract?
6. Know your practice—if you are considering joining a bundle:
   a. Your demographics—how many of the patients in the plan do you care for?
   b. Your surgeons' complication rate—how many of them end up in the hospital after outpatient surgery?
   c. Your surgeons' use of ancillary services (SNF, home health, and durable medical equipment) that will cut into your income, that is, where are your costs controllable?
   d. What have you not been able to control?
   e. Do you know your outcomes over a longer period time than 24 hours?
   f. Who in the community can you align with? Surgeons only or do you have a potential network regarding primary care docs?
7. When you are negotiating when entering an at-risk contract, planning is critical:
   a. First, know what you want (the best you could ask for).
   b. Second, know what you will not do ("we will stay engaged but I can't do that…")?
   c. Third, know what you will accept (not what you wanted but will not hurt you fatally).
   d. Fourth, know what would make you walk away (it would injure your core integrity to stay at the table)?
   e. Finally, recognize your actual power—what options does your "opponent" have rather than you? Do not overstep your power.
   f. Definitions count: know the specific definition of the bundle and when the episode starts and stops.
   g. Downside risk control: write in reasons to bail out without penalty (eg, a new expensive drug or procedure or a natural catastrophe).

SUMMARY

As discussed, MACRA is an attempt by CMS and Congress to reduce health care costs but primarily, errantly, focuses on the smallest of causes of those costs: provider income. Most providers find that the opportunities to report and succeed under MACRA are in the MIPS. The first step that every provider should take is to go to the QPP performance program Web site to determine eligibility and how CMS has characterized the provider, as an individual or a group member.

After that step, every provider should report data if required to. There is no reason to accept a negative impact on 2020 payments because you simply ignored this program in 2018. Finally, stay tuned: this program and its "opportunities" for participation will likely change as the months go by.

A GLOSSARY OF RELEVANT TERMS

ACA – The Affordable Care Act, which is a shortening of the term, Patient Protection and Affordable Care Act (PPACA), which is law enacted in 2010 (see **PPACA**).

ACI – Advancing Care Information was the name applied to the effort to pay providers to implement EHRs, with the presumption that this would lead to higher-quality care. In the last year, this metric has been renamed Promoting Interoperability (PI) but there has been no change in the specifics of the metric itself.

ACOs – Accountable care organizations are groups of providers who typically accept some form of risk (payment decreases) for the opportunity to earn incentives by successfully managing care for large groups of patients, including goals of reduced cost, reduced medical error, and improved clinical and process outcomes.

AHRQ – The Agency for Healthcare Research and Quality is 1 of the 12 agencies of HHS (CMS being another), originally created in 1989 as the Agency for Health Care Policy and Research as part of the Public Health Service. It was rechartered in its current state in 1999 and is charged with developing evidence bases for the delivery of high-quality, efficient, and effective health care.

ASA – The American Society of Anesthesiologists is the largest professional organization of anesthesia providers and sponsors the AQI and, therefore, NACOR.

APM – An Alternative Payment Model provides incentive payments to those providers whom CMS determines provide high-quality and cost-efficient care (see **MIPS APM**).

AAPM – The Advanced APM track of the QPP gives providers access to an additional 5% incentive (as of now) for achieving certain metrics within the AAPM. If achieved, the added benefit for the provider is that he or she or they can opt out of the MIPS reporting requirements and payment adjustments.

AQI – The Anesthesia Quality Institute was created by the ASA in 2008 as a PSO to channel the quality-improvement efforts supported by the ASA. AQI manages the NACOR database.

ASC – Ambulatory surgery center

BCPI – A Bundled Payment for Care Improvement Initiative payments was authorized under PPACA, under which the CMMI is charged with sponsoring innovation in payment methodology. In a BCPI model, health care organizations can participate in 1 of 4 different payment models, all of which combined the payments from CMS to 1 entity for the entire episode of care. Elective total joint replacement has been a frequent focus of BCPI participation as those procedures lend themselves to the standardization of care needed to improve outcomes while reducing costs.

CEHRT – Certified EHR technology is the term given by CMS to qualified EHRs that meet certain standards, which will allow providers to qualify for incentive payments if they choose to implement CEHRT under MACRA.

CMMI – The Center for Medicare and Medicaid Innovation was established under the PPACA to create experimental models of payment for health care. Such models can be proposed by either CMMI or by outside parties for consideration as BPCIs.

CMS – The Centers for Medicare & Medicaid Services is the branch of HHS that oversees the management of the Medicare and Medicaid Trust and payment and certification programs.

EC – An eligible clinician under an APM.

EHR – Electronic health record

ERAS – Enhanced recovery after surgery is an evidenced-based guideline set that includes various aspects of preoperative-, intraoperative, and postoperative care that improve the outcomes of patients who undergo certain surgical interventions. Appropriate use of ERAS may be reported as a patient safety tool, which will in turn qualify as an IA for reporting under MIPS.

FFS – Fee for service is the traditional means by which physicians and other providers have been paid, either by patients, insurance companies, or the government. The provider is paid by doing things, irrespective of outcomes (clinical or process). This contrasts with the QPPs or at-risk payment programs now increasingly used by insurance companies and governmental payers.

HIPAA – The Health Insurance Portability and Accountability Act was passed in 1996 and was intended to strengthen safeguards on data privacy regarding medical information. It also protects the health insurance coverage for people who change or lose their jobs, established national standards for electronic transactions regarding health care, and bolstered protections for patients with preexisting conditions.

HHS – Health and Human Services is the cabinet-level department that oversees all health care services for the federal government. CMS is a department within HHS.

IAs – Improvement activities is a component of the metrics chosen to measure for MIPS. The IA measures are listed at https://qpp.cms.gov.

MACRA – Medicare Access and CHIP Reauthorization Act of 2015

Medicare Part D – This program was passed in 2003 and is how self-administered prescription medications are paid for under Medicare. The program is widely recognized as a boondoggle and windfall for Pharma, who heavily lobbied for its passage. The legislators most involved and many of the administrators in CMS who championed its passage were rewarded Pharma jobs soon thereafter. More than 1 economist has put the cost of the program above and beyond the reasonable cost of the drugs at $50 billion or more per year, due to overpayment to drug companies. Under the bill, CMS is not allowed to negotiate reduced prices with the companies, in contrast to remarkable savings achieved by the Veterans Administration, which can negotiate. As many as 25% of Medicare "beneficiaries" (patients) pay more than $2500 per year extra out of their own pockets because of the high charges allowed by the program.

MIPS – The Merit-based Incentive Payment System replaced SGR and is part of MACRA; it determines most of the provider payment with Medicare and includes incentives and penalties resulting from provider success or failure, respectively, to meet its metric targets. It will lead over time to much reduced FFS and more VBP payments for care.

MIPS APM – An MIPS APM requires scoring on metrics that are determined by the APM and the providers will be held to those requirements instead of MIPS (ie, no duplicate reporting is required). Most AAPMs are also MIPS APMs so if an EC participating in the AAPM fails to achieve the metrics of the AAPM and, therefore, is not able to be a APM QP, thereby achieving exclusion from MIPS, that clinician will be scored under normal MIPS standards.

MSPB – The Medicare Spending per Beneficiary metric is the cost of Medicare Part A and Part B services provided during a patient's hospital care episode, beginning 72 hours prior to admission and extending 30 days after discharge. It does not currently include Medicare Part D costs (for prescription drug costs incurred in the outpatient arena) and is one of the cost methodologies (the other is TPCC) used to calculate the cost of care for MIPS reporting.

NACOR – The National Anesthesia Clinical Outcomes Registry is managed by the AQI, an arm of the ASA and is a database that collects and reports on quality clinical and process outcomes for participating anesthesiologists or their groups. It qualifies under MACRA as a QCDR and the AQI can manage MACRA reporting for any participating anesthesiologist or group.

NPI – The National Provider Identifier is the unique 10-digit code assigned to each provider of Medicare services by CMS. It is used for billing and for assigning eligibility for MACRA programs, and is often used by nongovernmental insurers now as well. If inputting NPI into the database query system at https://qpp.cms.gov, then it will identify status regarding eligibility for MIPS (ie, a MIPS EC).

PCMHM – The patient-centered medical home model is the term given to care entities that provide team-based care and care management to help integrate care delivery for any given patient. The PSH is an example of such a model.

Pharma – This is a collective term used to refer to the highly profitable drug manufacturing industry.

PI – Promoting Interoperability is the new name of the payment metric formerly known as ACI. No change has been made in the metric, which is designed to incentivize providers to purchase and deploy "qualified" EHR systems.

Population health – Population health is an approach to health that aims to improve the health of an entire human population, consisting of 4 components:

- Outcomes of clinical health care delivery
- Outcomes and patterns of personal health and disease
- Social determinants of health
- Health care policies

PPACA – The Patient Protection and Affordable Care Act (often shortened to ACA) was passed by Congress and enacted in 2010 as an attempt at an omnibus overhaul of the federal government's various administrative rules and guidelines regarding health care policy and provision. It is popularly known as Obamacare in response to President Obama's championing of its creation and passage.

PQRS – Physician Quality Reporting System

PSH – The perioperative surgical home is a team-based care model developed by members of the ASA and recognized by MACRA as an effective means of improved perioperative (preoperative, postoperative, and intraoperative) care via coordination of the many care services that will improve clinical outcomes of surgical intervention.

PSO – Patient Safety Organization is the name given to organizations certified by the Agency for Healthcare Research and Quality, allowing them certain confidentiality and privilege protections regarding sharing of patient data in the effort to improve patient safety.

PTAC – The Physician-Focused Payment Model Technical Advisory Committee is a group of providers and other stakeholders who assess potential APM programs for recommendation to the HHS Secretary for inclusion in future MACRA payment models.

QCDR – A qualified clinical data registry is the means for most providers to report required metric performance under MACRA. These may include an EHR or may be a proprietary entity, such as the AQI NACOR.

QPs – APM qualifying participants are those APM participants who achieve the metric requirements of an APM and thereby avoid MIPS scoring requirements.

QPP – Quality Payment Program—this program is a product of the MACRA legislation and ties all the former VBP programs into 1. It includes MIPS and the APM programs.

QRURs – Quality and Resource Use Reports are available on the CMS portal to all providers and groups of providers and portray which patients have been attributed to a given provider or provider group and the data on cost and quality that are thereby also attributed to a provider.

SDHs – Social determinants of health (eg, access to education, higher socioeconomic status, safe neighborhoods, autonomy in the workplace, and freedom from discrimination) are the progenitors of approximately 60% to 70% of health, with genetics forming another 20%, and only 10% due to health care delivery.

SGR – The Medicare Sustainable Growth Rate was a methodology created in the Balanced Budget Act of 1997 to reduce the annual increase in expense of Medicare beneficiary coverage to no more than the increase in the gross domestic product. It, however, failed to recognize the increasing cost of care delivery, such that it would have required most providers to lose money by participating in Medicare. As a result,

Congress overrode the price inhibitions resulting from the SGR calculation annually but with great amounts of lobbying and difficult negotiations. As a result, it was finally replaced by the MACRA program in 2015 and is no longer active.

SNF – A skilled nursing facility is a licensed sites that provide care to patients who need longer-term, nonacute care. SNFs are often important in the schema of BCPIs and ACOs, which may be at risk for the cost of care provided in these sites. A good example is the often routine use by orthopedic surgeons of such sites to deliver care after discharge from an acute care hospital after elective total joint replacement.

Telehealth – Telehealth is a site-to-site service where a patient presents at an originating site with a presenter and a cart or device capable of some level of biometric measurement. As well, such care may take the form of provider-to-provider interactions, such as with consultation with specialists.

Telemedicine – Telemedicine (also referred to as telehealth or e-health) allows health care professionals to evaluate, diagnose, and treat patients in remote locations using telecommunications technology. Telemedicine allows patients in remote locations to access medical expertise quickly, efficiently, and without travel. Telemedicine provides more efficient use of limited expert resources who can "see" patients in multiple locations wherever they are needed without leaving their facility.

Telephonic visit – A telephonic visit is real-time care provided using a telephone.

TPCCs – Total Per Capita Costs for all attributed beneficiaries refers to the total Parts A and B costs of care for all Medicare beneficiaries who are attributed to a provider or group of providers through the year. Again, Part D costs are not included. This is 1 of the 2 cost measures (the other is the MSPB) used by CMS to calculate the cost metric success or failure under MIPS. Unlike MSPB, the TPCC is not connected to a single hospitalization episode but instead is for the cost of care for a beneficiary through an entire year.

VBPs – Value-based payment programs are payment programs that do not simply pay for performance of activities (FFS), but which instead include incentives or penalties for good or bad outcomes, such as clinical quality, cost, or other process outcomes.

Virtual Care – Virtual care is device-agnostic, direct-to-consumer service that does not require a presenter or biometric monitoring, for example: using an iPhone to FaceTime with a provider.

REFERENCES

1. Shaw JG, Farid M, Noel-Miller C, et al. September 17). Social Isolation and Medicare Spending: among older adults, objective isolation increases expenditures while loneliness does not. J Aging Health 2017;29(7):1119–43.

2. Barr DA. Health disparities in the United States: social class, race, ethnicity, and health. 2nd edition. Baltimore (MD): The Johns Hopkins University Press; 2014.

3. Jackson Healthcare. Physician compensation eight percent of healthcare costs 2011. Jackson Healthcare. Available at: https://jacksonhealthcare.com/media-room/news/md-salaries-as-percent-of-costs/. Accessed March 30, 2019.

4. Rampell C. Doctor's salaries and the cost of health care 2008. N.Y. Times. Available at: https://economix.blogs.nytimes.com/2008/11/14/do-doctors-salaries-drive-up-health-care-costs/. Accessed March 30, 2019.

5. CMS. Alternative payment models in the quality payment program as of February 2018. 2018. CMS Quality payment program. Available at: https://www.cms.

gov/Medicare/Quality-Payment-Program/Resource-Library/Comprehensive-List-of-APMs.pdf. Accessed March 30, 2019.

6. Dickson V. CMS meets MIPS reporting goals, but thousands of doctors still face penalties 2018. Modern Healthcare. Available at: http://www.modernhealthcare.com/article/20180531/NEWS/180539986/cms-meets-mips-reporting-goals-but-thousands-of-doctors-still-face. Accessed March 30, 2019.

7. John Commons. CMS says quality payment program exceeds year 1 participation goal 2018. HealthLeaders. Available at: https://www.healthleadersmedia.com/strategy/cms-says-quality-payment-program-exceeds-year-1-participation-goal.

8. ASA. 2017 MIPS Overview. 2017. ASA AQI. Available at: https://www.aqihq.org/files/2017%20MIPS/MIPS%20at%20a%20Glance%202017.pdf.

9. CMS. CMS quality payment program 2018. QPP. Available at: https://qpp.cms.gov/.

Ambulatory Surgery Center Medical Director

Visionary Leader

Michael Guertin, MD, MBA, CPE[a],*, Jarrett Heard, MD, MBA[b],
Timothy Del Rosario, MD[b]

KEYWORDS

- Physician leadership • Organizational culture • Organizational behavior
- Patient selection • Patient safety • Patient satisfaction • Innovation
- Ambulatory surgery center (ASC)

KEY POINTS

- The ambulatory surgery center (ASC) medical director should be a visionary physician leader who helps create an effective organizational culture by fostering collaboration and empowering people.
- The 3S of ASC patient care—selection, safety, and satisfaction—require policies and procedures that safeguard patients to be developed and enforced.
- Innovation and sustainability present additional opportunities for the medical director to establish meaningful changes that further the success, credibility, and impact of the ASC.

On March 2, 2018, *USA Today* published an article entitled "How a Push to Cut Costs and Boost Profits at Surgery Centers Led to a Trail of Death."[1] Autopsy records, Medicare inspection records, and other data were used, and revealed that more than 260 patients have died after outpatient procedures at surgery centers from 2013 to 2018. The report stated that most surgery center procedures do not result in any complications, especially if the ambulatory surgery center (ASC) possesses the appropriate equipment and highly trained staff to deal with emergencies. The investigators found more than 12 instances, however, in which ASCs were not compliant.[2] The article presented a negative view of the ASC industry and might be easily dismissed by industry

Disclosure: There are no disclosures for any of the authors.
[a] Department of Anesthesiology, The Ohio State University Wexner Medical Center, Jameson Crane Sports Medicine Institute, 2835 Fred Taylor Drive, Office 2214, Columbus, OH 43202, USA; [b] Department of Anesthesiology, The Ohio State University Wexner Medical Center, 410 W. 10th Avenue, N410 Doan Hall, Columbus, OH 43210, USA
* Corresponding author.
E-mail address: Michael.Guertin@osumc.edu

Anesthesiology Clin 37 (2019) 389–400
https://doi.org/10.1016/j.anclin.2019.01.009
1932-2275/19/© 2019 Elsevier Inc. All rights reserved.

representatives as an example of fake news. The Ambulatory Surgery Center Association (ASCA) sharply rebuked the article and stated in its press release that "By not putting the number of adverse events into context, this article misleads readers into thinking that ASCs have more adverse events than other sites of service, when they actually have fewer." [3] The ASCA further pointed out that the article did not mention that more than 200 million procedures were safely performed at ASCs in that same 5-year timeframe. As is the case in most point-counterpoint arguments, there is some validity on each side; however, this article and the rebuttal statement provide several examples of opportunities for effective medical leadership to improve safeguards for patients and increase the credibility of the tremendous care that is delivered at most ASCs. The goal of this article is to discuss some of the opportunities for improvement that were presented in the USA Today article and to describe how, among other things, an engaged and effective ASC medical director can guide and set the foundation for

- Organizational behavior and culture of the ASC
- The 3S of ASC patient care: selection, safety, and satisfaction
- Innovation in the ASC.

The position of ASC medical director requires a mix of managerial and leadership skills. A manager is an individual who oversees a certain group of tasks or a certain subset of a company, and often has a staff of people who report to him or her.[4] Some of the management duties of an ASC medical director are developing and overseeing policies and procedures that optimize

- Quality of perioperative medical care
- Surgeon access and appropriate utilization of valuable time
- Patient access to timely surgical and procedural services
- Efficiency of perioperative workflow
- Cost-effectiveness of treatments, medications, instruments, and implants.

Like a good administrator, the medical director can make the difference between a good facility and a great facility.[5] The ability, along with the ASCs administrator, to articulate and implement the policies set forth by a board of directors is a critical function that helps drive the center's success. Although strong management skills are essential for this role, it is the capability and credibility as a leader that transforms the effective medical director into one who can truly guide the organization in a meaningful way.

LEADERSHIP, ORGANIZATIONAL BEHAVIOR, AND CULTURE

Leadership involves establishing a clear vision and sharing that vision with others by providing the information, knowledge, and methods to realize that vision. Coordinating and balancing the conflicting interests of all members and stakeholders is also essential. An effective leader steps up in times of crisis and can think and act creatively in difficult situations.[6] In their book, Inspired Physician Leadership, Charles Stoner and Jason Stoner[7] cite 3 reasons why "physician leadership has never been more critical":

1. As health care reform continues to evolve, physician leaders help preserve patient wellbeing despite pressures to contain costs and reform payment models.
2. Physician leaders, due to their expertise and credibility, are uniquely capable of facilitating discussions between practicing physicians and nonclinical leadership.
3. When doctors are more involved in improving organizational performance, "better financial and clinical outcomes occur."

Although there is a school of thought that leaders are born with the ability to lead, it is becoming increasingly accepted that leadership skills are learned as much as they are innate. In their book, *The Extraordinary Leader*, John Zenger and Joseph Folkman[8] use the example of the 234 years that the US Marine Corps has been developing leaders to make the statement "Leaders are made, not born." If leadership skills are indeed acquired, then an essential step in this acquisition is to develop a personal leadership philosophy. Dr Dale Benson,[9] a prominent figure in the American Association for Physician Leadership, wrote that "you should be able to clearly and concisely articulate your philosophy of leadership. Your leadership philosophy gives you consistency." He further opined that if one is guided by one's philosophy, then others have less to fear because they know what to expect in the way that one acts and reacts. Dr Benson described empowerment as "the understanding that no organization will be as effective as it could be if all the decisions are left to management. It is letting the decisions be made at the level where they are most relevant." Taking that further, enlightened empowerment is the empowerment of people who clearly understand the goals and direction of the organization. An effective leader who is guided by a personal leadership philosophy will clearly communicate that organizational vision by what he or she says and the way in which he or she acts. Benson concludes by stating, "Enlightened empowerment means first aligning my people, then unleashing their talents."[9]

Legendary Ohio State football coach Woody Hayes titled his autobiography *You Win with People*.[10] Hayes understood the importance of surrounding oneself with good people and giving them a goal-directed culture; he won 5 national collegiate football championships by creating a culture of success and giving young men the direction and motivation to succeed. Following a similar theme, Benson[9] wrote, "I have one final perspective to share with you now. This perspective is that it all has to do with people." These leaders, from very different occupations, understood the fundamental reality that supporting, directing, and motivating people is the key to success in any business.

If people are the life-blood of the enterprise, then the organizational culture is what motivates them. In an ASC, the medical director, together with a board of directors and administrator, determines the specific culture of the organization, selecting a balance of business, academic, and altruistic priorities. It is, therefore, incumbent on the true physician leader to clearly communicate that culture and to guide the employees so that each person understands the organization's objectives and strategies, can determine how they can optimize their own personal potential within that culture, and can work together to achieve the common goals. Although getting the people in an organization to work together as a team is a challenge, the payoff can be significant. In a large analysis of patient satisfaction survey scores by the consulting firm Press-Ganey, developing effective teamwork has been shown to be 1 of the 3 key drivers of patient satisfaction.[11,12] Furthermore, one of the findings of a recent study[13] was that effective communication is among the key elements for developing the teamwork that is essential to safe patient care in the perioperative setting: "You have anesthesiologists working with a variety of surgeons and different OR [operating room] staff ... So, communication becomes especially important."[14] An effective ASC medical director understands this link between teamwork and communication and helps foster that communication through her or his words and actions and by developing clinical pathways that create an environment that is conducive to effective patient safety practices and leads to high patient satisfaction.

In summary, the ASC physician leader must remember that the people on the frontline are critical to success and among her or his most important roles is to encourage effective communication practices and to provide employees with the resources and direction that they need to be successful. A successful leader engages people to share a common organizational vision in ultimately giving patients what they need and want.

A final note about leadership is the mantra to always do the right thing. Because the ultimate effect of the decisions and actions of a medical director is to take care of patients, this cannot be overemphasized. While learning the skill set necessary to be a leader, it is possible to lose sight of this vision. General Norman Schwarzkopf is credited with the quote that should summarize the essence of a physician leader: "Leadership is a potent combination of strategy and character. But if you must be without one, be without strategy."[15]

THE 3S OF AMBULATORY SURGERY CENTER PATIENT CARE: SELECTION, SAFETY, AND SATISFACTION

There are now more than 5600 surgery centers in the United States, outnumbering hospitals. These centers are performing increasingly complex procedures on sicker patients owing to advances in surgical and anesthesia techniques and capabilities. Excerpts from the March 2018 *USA Today* article (**Box 1**) highlight the opportunities for ASC medical directors to establish clinical pathways, as well as policies and procedures, that address and alleviate concerns related to the 3S of ASC patient care: selection, safety, and satisfaction.

PATIENT SELECTION

In a recent review of anesthesia closed claims from ASCs, among the key findings was the need to improve preoperative assessment of patients in advance of the day of surgery (DOS).[14] The investigators found that the most critical opportunities included "improving strategies for thorough screening, preoperative assessment, and risk stratifying of patients." The ASC medical director is in a unique position to design and implement these processes in the interest of patient safety, as well as operational efficiency. In the authors' institutional experience at The Ohio State University Wexner Medical Center, implementation of a comprehensive preanesthesia center (ComPAC) allowed ASC nurses to meet with patients on the day that they see their surgeon and decide to have surgery. This provides the time needed to adequately evaluate and

---

Box 1
Excerpts from the March 2018 *USA Today* article

Medicare asks surgery centers to assess each patient's risk, but inspectors flagged 122 surgery centers in 2015 and 2016 alone for lapses in risk assessments. Some centers failed to gauge risk at all.

Surgery centers have steadily expanded their business by taking on increasingly risky surgeries.

Because surgery centers have less safety equipment and staffing than hospitals, industry leaders stress the importance of selecting patients healthy enough to fare well.

Some surgery centers risk patient lives by skimping on training or lifesaving equipment. Others have sent patients home before they were fully recovered.

Some patients have been sent home to grapple with complications on their own.

From Jewett C, Alesia M. How a push to cut costs and boost profits at surgery centers led to a trail of death. USA Today. Available at: https://www.usatoday.com/story/news/2018/03/02/medicare-certified-surgery-centers-safety-deaths/363172002/. Accessed January 9, 2019; with permission.

optimize patients before the DOS. The comprehensive component refers to the patient education that is to delivered to educate patients for the DOS and to set realistic expectations for the perioperative experience. At the same time, preventable DOS delays and cancellations were reduced to less than 1% despite a patient population with moderately high acuity. Patient safety is indirectly improved because it is much more problematic to cancel surgery on the DOS. This pressure to avoid cancelations can lead to caring for patients who are not optimized or appropriate for ambulatory surgery. The ComPAC allows those decisions to be made days or weeks before surgery and avoid last-minute changes for the patient and surgeon. Moreover, it leads to caring for more patients because it allows time to optimize comorbid factors that may facilitate ambulatory surgery in patients who might not otherwise be considered appropriate for an ASC without preoptimization. Finally, it can have an overall positive effect on patient satisfaction for several reasons (see later discussion).

When the preoperative assessment and optimization are complete, risk stratification and determining which patients are appropriate for an outpatient surgery center can be accomplished in a more efficient manner. This is not to imply that determining who should have surgery in an outpatient center is clear-cut or straightforward. As surgical techniques and anesthetic care have expanded the possibilities for outpatient surgery,[16] more patients with significant comorbidities are being considered. To date, there is no validated algorithm for patient selection that gives appropriate attention to the type of surgery, type of anesthesia, and patient factors. A 2013 retrospective study of more than 200,000 cases found ambulatory surgery to have a low rate of perioperative morbidity and mortality but it did identify 7 risk factors for perioperative adverse events: overweight body mass index, obese body mass index, chronic obstructive pulmonary disease, history of transient ischemic attack or stroke, hypertension, previous cardiac surgical intervention, and prolonged operative time.[17] However, depending on the type of surgery and the anesthetic needed, these patients are often cared for in ASCs. There have been several studies that looked at frailty scores to predict morbidity and mortality in elderly patients undergoing surgery.[18,19] Currently, there are other ongoing initiatives to use frailty scales or other indices for risk stratification in ambulatory surgery but, to date, no clinically useful method has been described.

Clearly, patient selection is an area in which an effective physician leader can have a significant impact on patient safety and satisfaction, as well as on the financial performance of the ASC. It is vital to develop a good process for evaluation and optimization, and to provide guidance for selecting appropriate patients. By communicating a vision to the center's surgeons and anesthesiologists, the medical director can build consensus and have a profound impact on the ultimate success of an ASC. Effective leadership skills, particularly communication and consensus-building proficiency, are critical in this endeavor.

PATIENT SAFETY

Although patients enjoy the convenience and low costs associated with ASCs, the continued growth has led to more scrutiny regarding patient safety. The *USA Today* article concluded that some ASCs are expanding business by taking on increasingly risky surgeries and overlooking high-risk health problems. The article also suggested that some surgery centers have looked to reduce costs by skimping on training or life-saving equipment, and that patients have been discharged home before being fully recovered. Recent data suggest that more than twice as many inpatient surgical patients have high severity outcomes compared with patients in ASC settings.[20] Despite this, there is growing concern that the changing nature of ambulatory surgery in which sicker patients are requiring more complex surgeries on an outpatient basis may ultimately change this balance.[21] Additionally, the various accrediting bodies and state agencies have different standards and different reporting requirements, which lead to confusion for consumers and potential patient safety issues. To improve safety, the ASC Quality Collaboration was created to collect outcome data at ASCs, including number and causes of hospital transfers from ASCs, incidence of falls, wrong site–wrong side surgery, and emergency department visits within 1 day of discharge. For example, in the second quarter of 2018, 0.945 out of 1000 surgeries at ASCs resulted in hospital transfers or admissions.[22] The ASC Quality Collaboration asked Medicare to collect additional reports on every patient transferred to a hospital to improve transparency and accountability. However, Medicare is proposing to no longer collect hospital transfer and other quality measures, saying the differences between different surgery centers is too small to be meaningful.[23] This represents an example of how medical leaders can improve ASC credibility by advocating for improved transparency through timely and complete reporting of outcomes.

The ASC medical director must be familiar with the standards of care and guidelines consistent with the Centers for Medicare & Medicaid Services (CMS), state laws, and the ASC's accrediting bodies to provide continual quality improvement and the safest possible environment for patients and staff. A medical director can have a major impact on patient safety by developing a well-defined scope of care that is agreed on by physician leadership and staff, is well-enforced, and is refined on a routine basis to match the agreed-on cases to be performed at the center. This also allows for some adaptability given the continued growth of ambulatory surgeries, even permitting those patients and procedures that were previously considered less than ideal for the outpatient setting.

It is the responsibility of the ASC medical director to ensure that the center avoids many of the shortfalls previously listed and identified in the USA Today article. The medical director should ensure that the ASC has the necessary emergency equipment (eg, crash cart) and highly trained staff, including those certified in basic life support and advanced cardiac life support. Despite the associated cost, an adequate supply of dantrolene, as determined by the Malignant Hyperthermia Association of the United States, should be kept onsite whenever volatile anesthetic gases or succinylcholine are administered.[24] To maintain staff competency, there should be regular in-service trainings that include code blue and malignant hyperthermia drills, at a minimum. It should be written in the center's policies and considered mandatory that an anesthesiologist remain in the center until all patients who have received anesthesia services have recovered sufficiently to be ready for discharge. By developing patient-centered policies, and ensuring compliance with them, the ASC medical director can be the ultimate patient-safety advocate.

PATIENT SATISFACTION

With a move toward a model of value-based care, it is important to remember that "value in healthcare is the balance between outcomes that matter to patients and the cost to achieve those outcomes."[25] Because patients have come to expect convenience and quality, it is paramount that the medical director embraces and develops continuous changes that provide excellent patient satisfaction to ensure continued success of the ASC. Very satisfied customers provide the greatest profitability due to excellent customer retention because the cost of acquiring a new customer is

5 to 10 times costlier than retaining one.[26] Very satisfied customers are more likely to create additional business via loyalty and by recommending services to others.

The medical director should recognize that much of what shapes patient satisfaction is subjective and is based on the preoperative and postoperative experience of both the patient and family members. Companies such as Press-Ganey administer and benchmark patient satisfaction surveys that provide ASCs with insights into their patients' perceptions of the care that they received. The Outpatient and Ambulatory Surgery Consumer Assessment of Healthcare Providers and Systems survey (OAS CAHPS) is currently a voluntary national reporting system initiated by the CMS in January 2016. It "is designed to measure the experiences of care for patients who visited Medicare-certified hospital outpatient departments (HOPDs) and ambulatory surgery centers (ASCs) for a surgery or procedure."[27] Public reporting of OAS CAHPS scores commenced in 2018 and CMS has proposed to continue voluntary participation in the survey through 2019. By 2020, it is very possible that reporting will be linked to reimbursement, probably by penalizing poor scores and/or nonreporting. In addition to raw percentages of satisfied patients and percentile benchmarking against ASCs across the country, surveys often contain patient comments that span the entirety of patient experiences. The ASC medical director can use this information to make operational improvements and to develop care pathways that enhance patient care.

In a quality improvement project at the authors' ASC, patient satisfaction survey comments were examined over a 6-month period and all negative comments grouped into broad classifications. After evaluating the negative comment classifications, it was found that communication, facility, and intravenous (IV) catheter needle placement were the top recurring themes for patient dissatisfaction. It was not fiscally practical to renovate the facility, so improvement projects were focused on improving communication and the process of starting the IV therapy preoperatively.

To improve the communication element, the ComPAC was developed (see previous discussion) to evaluate patients on the same day as the preoperative surgeon appointment. In addition to getting information from the patient, an emphasis was also placed on giving information to the patient. Face-to-face interaction, videos, and printed material were used to prepare the patient and family for the DOS. This allowed the providers to set reasonable and appropriate expectations for the postoperative recovery period.

On the DOS, among the identified issues of concern was that the family and the patient were separated very early in the process. A process change brought the family into the preoperative area, which not only reduced patient anxiety but also allowed the family to observe the care and interventions, and to listen to the instructions that physicians and nursing staff provided. This was a major contributor to increased patient satisfaction in the communication metric. By including the staff in the development of this new process, buy-in was much easier because they were part of the change management from the beginning.[28]

A protocol for IV catheter needle placement was established that defined the appropriate catheter size and number of attempts allowed, and thus decreased the variability that was seen between individual nurses at the surgery center. Perhaps most importantly, the surgery center now uses buffered lidocaine infiltration before IV catheter needle insertion. Not only did placement of local anesthetic reduce the discomfort associated with the IV catheter needle but it also demonstrated to the patient that every attempt is being made to make this part of the process less threatening. The positive psychological and physiologic effects of this simple procedure cannot be overestimated.[29,30] This change reduced the number of negative comments about

IV catheter needle placement. More significant, after implementation of this process there were 35 positive comments about IV catheter needle placement in a 12-month period. This was in stark contrast to prior surveys when there were no positive comments about IV catheter needle placement.

Largely due to these changes, the surgery center improved its overall rating on Press-Ganey surveys from the 73rd percentile to the 98th percentile. Increasing patient readiness and optimization also contributed to a 16% decrease in OR turnover time and a 20% increase in case volume during the same OR hours of 7 AM to 3 PM.[31] This allowed for increased accuracy in case scheduling times, which improved patient satisfaction because entry into the OR more closely mirrored the time that the patient and family were expecting. The reduction in turnover time also increased surgeon satisfaction.

Finally, the proliferation of Perioperative Surgical Home (PSH) and Enhanced Recovery After Surgery (ERAS) protocols seen in the last few years offers the ASC medical director yet another opportunity to improve patient outcomes and satisfaction.[32–34] Use of evidence-based techniques, such as multimodal analgesia and postoperative nausea and vomitting prevention, as well as opioid-sparing anesthetics, are examples of methods that can be operationalized by a physician leader interested in providing patients with the best perioperative experience.

INNOVATION

If visionary is a desirable characteristic for a physician leader as the ASC medical director, then innovation should be a by-product of that vision. In today's complex health care setting, the concept of innovation can take on various forms. Innovation can be understood as "the intentional introduction and application within a role, group, or organization, of ideas, processes, products or procedures, new to the relevant unit of adoption, designed to significantly benefit the individual, the group, or wider society."[35] Translated into the realm of health care, innovation can refer to any method by which a health system can function faster, more efficiently, and at a reduced cost, all while improving patient outcomes. Novel technologies, policies, workflows, and organizational structures all have the potential to significantly affect various aspects of patient care, thus belonging within a medical director's purview.

Thakur and colleagues[36] broadly described the typical process by which innovative ideas arise and are subsequently executed within a health system. The phases of this process include

1. The generation of ideas
2. Decision-making
3. Rolling out
4. Evaluation
5. Modification

Both internal, as well as external, factors contribute to the generation of ideas, which are then reviewed by those in management and leadership positions. A decision on whether to adopt the idea is made and is usually based on its overall compatibility with the culture that is present within a health system. The next step, referred to as rolling out, involves multiple stakeholders and is typically the phase wherein most challenges are encountered as the idea is executed. Further fine-tuning (or conversely, cancellation) of the innovation is performed throughout the subsequent evaluation and modification phases. Of note, the final 2 phases might also loop back to the initial phase because novel innovative ideas may be generated from the preceding steps.

Furthermore, in the setting of today's fast-paced technological advancements, innovative ideas may likely be replaced with innovative products, including software and devices. After a procurement decision is made, such products are similarly rolled out, evaluated, and modified to fit the needs of the system in varying ways.

A prevailing aspect of health care innovation involves the widespread utilization of information technology (IT). In this context, IT describes a wide array of products that, among other functions, use networks and computerized algorithms to obtain, process, organize, and present data. From electronic health record software to devices such as infusion pumps, surgical robotic systems, and automated drug and equipment dispensing systems, IT has reshaped the overall delivery of patient care. Computerized coding and billing systems have likewise been developed to optimize costs and efficiency. Furthermore, information databases have allowed for rapid access to the latest medical knowledge. From the medical director's standpoint, IT represents a powerful tool in the delivery of safe and efficient patient care. However, as with any other innovative idea, each product should undergo a rigorous process of evaluation, examining not only its perceived merits but also its compatibility with existing structures within a health system. Bhattacherjee and Hikmet[37] investigated the phenomenon of clinician resistance toward the introduction of new IT, citing "perceived usefulness" and "perceived ease of use" as contributing factors. As IT related products and systems are rolled out, evaluation in terms of feedback from clinicians and other users are paramount to optimization. Continuous improvements regarding the efficient use of IT necessitates a close working relationship between administrative teams (led by the medical director), clinicians, and IT personnel. Furthermore, and most especially during implementation (rolling out) and modification phases, it is important to consider the resistance to change that is inherent in most organizations. Within a health system, resistance is usually a result of the perceived and actual disruptions in patient care that accompany such changes.[38] It is apparent that innovation, regardless of sector, requires top-down as well as bottom-to-top approaches in management. However, the health care setting is unique in that the overall goal in innovation not only involves improving operational efficiency and costs but also patient outcomes. As IT continues to evolve, especially with the recent developments in artificial intelligence, it will increasingly become engrained within the fabric of health care. The medical director occupies a unique position to facilitate faster and more impactful innovations.

In line with this, a popular trend found in many sectors today is the increased awareness of the concept of environmental sustainability. It has been estimated that the US health care industry is responsible for 9.8% of the country's total greenhouse gas emissions.[39] As society (and regulatory agencies) becomes more cognizant of these data, measures to improve sustainability in a health system will likely become part of a medical director's area of responsibility. Decisions regarding the use of disposable versus reusable equipment, methods to reduce environmentally detrimental gas emissions, waste disposal, and energy efficient facility designs, are a few examples of sustainability-related opportunities available to ASC medical directors. A recently addressed issue in anesthesiology is the global warming effect of waste anesthesia gasses (WAGs). Nitrous oxide, a commonly used anesthetic with an atmospheric lifetime of 114 years, not only has the ability to absorb and emit ultraviolet radiation in the form of heat, it also causes direct degradation of the ozone layer. Global warming potential (GWP) is a measure of a substance's ability to warm the atmosphere relative to an equivalent mass of carbon dioxide (CO_2). Sevoflurane has a GWP value of 130, whereas nitrous oxide and isoflurane have GWPs of 298 and 510, respectively. The volatile anesthetic desflurane, however, weighs in at a GWP of 2540. Furthermore, it has been demonstrated that use of desflurane for 1 hour has the CO_2 equivalent of driving 400 miles.[40] Measures to reduce this impact have been identified and require propagation. Using lower fresh gas flows (FGFs), turning off gas flows (as opposed to the vaporizer) during intubation and any other time the circuit is disconnected, and turning the vaporizer dial to a higher setting than intended (instead of using high FGFs) to increase gas concentrations, are a few practical methods to avoid expelling WAGs into the atmosphere. Innovations in volatile anesthetic recapturing technology have also been developed. Perhaps a more complex challenge will lie in convincing staff of the merits of such efforts. As with any innovation that may temporarily disrupt usual workflows, such measures may be met with resistance. However, as benefits are realized, consistent with what has been observed in the energy and automotive sectors, environmentally sustainable health care delivery will likely become incorporated into standard practice. ASC medical directors are in a unique position to be at the forefront of this change by communicating the methods and the benefits of integrating sustainable practices into their centers, and by ensuring that these practices are accepted and adopted.

SUMMARY

The visionary ASC medical director is a physician leader who recognizes the need to develop a culture in the ASC that encourages communication and empowerment of employees and professional staff, leading to engagement that sustains the mission of the organization. Development and execution of operational processes that optimize the 3S of ASC patient care—selection, safety, and satisfaction—requires vision and guidance from the medical director and is central to the success of the ASC. Innovative thinking presents the chance to further improve patient care and long-term success by leveraging advances in technology and sustainable practices.

REFERENCES

1. Jewett C, Alesia M, Kaiser Health News. How a push to cut costs and boost profits at surgery centers led to a trail of death. USA Today 2018. Available at: https://www.usatoday.com/story/news/2018/03/02/medicare-certified-surgery-centers-safety-deaths/363172002/. Accessed August, 2018.
2. Wood M. Ambulatory Surgery Center Association 'sharply rebukes' Kaiser Health News, USA Today for report on surgery centers: 6 things to know. In: Becker's spine review. 2018. Available at: https://www.beckersspine.com/orthopedic-spine-practices-improving-profits/item/40140-ambulatory-surgery-center-association-sharply-rebukes-kaiser-health-news-usa-today-for-report-on-surgery-centers-6-things-to-know.html. Accessed August, 2018.
3. ASCA. Ambulatory Surgery Center Association faults Kaiser Health News and USA Today for sensationalism and misrepresentation of safety and quality in Ambulatory Surgery Centers. In: Ambulatory Surgery Center Association news. 2018. Available at: https://www.ascassociation.org/asca/aboutus/pressroom/press2018/2018-03-khn-usa-today-misrepresentation-ascs. Accessed August, 2018.
4. Business dictionary definition of manager. In: Business Dictionary.com. 2018. Available at: http://www.businessdictionary.com/definition/manager.html. Accessed August, 2018.
5. Earnhart S. The Medical Director's role in same day surgery. Relias Media 2018. Available at: https://www.ahcmedia.com/articles/42729-the-medical-director-8217-s-role-in-same-day-surgery. Accessed August, 2018.

6. Business dictionary definition of leadership. In: Business Dictionary.com. 2018. Available at: http://www.businessdictionary.com/definition/leadership.html. Accessed August, 2018.
7. Stoner C, Stoner J. Inspired physician leadership. Tampa (FL): American Association for Physician Leadership; 2015.
8. Zenger J, Folkman J. The extraordinary leader, turning good managers into great leaders. United States: McGraw-Hill; 2009. p. 25.
9. Benson D. Pursuit of increased leadership effectiveness. Physician Leadersh J 2016;3:54–7.
10. Hayes W. You win with people. Columbus (OH): Woody Hayes; 1973.
11. Heath S. Nurse communication, teamwork to boost care experience scores. In: Patient engagement HIT. 2017. Available at: https://patientengagementhit.com/news/nurse-communication-teamwork-to-boost-care-experience-scores. Accessed August, 2018.
12. Heath S. 3 tips for nurses to improve patient satisfaction, experience. In: Patient engagement HIT. 2017. Available at: https://patientengagementhit.com/news/3-tips-for-nurses-to-improve-patient-satisfaction-experience. Accessed August, 2018.
13. Ranum D, Beverly A, Shapiro FE, et al. Leading causes of anesthesia-related liability claims in Ambulatory Surgery Centers. J Patient Saf 2017. https://doi.org/10.1097/PTS.0000000000000431.
14. Anesthesiology News. Analysis of anesthesia closed claims compares ambulatory surgery centers with hospital based operating rooms. In: Policy and management. 2018. Available at: http://www.anesthesiologynews.com/Policy-and-Management/Article/01-18/Analysis-of-Anesthesia-Closed-Claims-Compares-Ambulatory-Surgery-Centers-With-Hospital-Based-Operating-Rooms/46569/ses=ogst?enl=true. Accessed August 2018.
15. Kruse K. 100 best quotes on leadership. 2012. Available at: Forbes.com; https://www.forbes.com/sites/kevinkruse/2012/10/16/quotes-on-leadership/#75c61c742feb. Accessed August, 2018.
16. Ambulatory Surgery Center Association. Ambulatory surgery centers: a positive trend in healthcare 2011. Available at: https://www.ascassociation.org/advancingsurgicalcare/aboutascs/industryoverview/apositivetrendinhealthcare. Accessed August, 2018.
17. Mathis M, Naughton N, Shanks A, et al. Patient selection for day case-eligible surgery, identifying those at high risk for major complications. Anesthesiology 2013;119(No 6):1310–21.
18. Kim S, Han HS, Jung HW, et al. Multidimensional frailty score for the prediction of postoperative mortality risk. JAMA Surg 2014;149(7):633–40.
19. Makary M, Segev D, Pronovost PJ, et al. Frailty as a predictor of surgical outcomes in older patients. J Am Coll Surg 2010;210(6):901–8.
20. Jensen T. Ambulatory Surgery Center malpractice risk overview 2017. Available at: https://cdn.ymaws.com/www.pldf.org/resource/collection/370BDA06-7DC5-4667-B278-EFB8FEB482C1/ASC_Malpractice_Materials.pdf. Accessed October, 2018.
21. Metzner J. Ambulatory surgery: is the liability risk lower? Ambul Anesth 2012;25(6):654–8.
22. ASC Quality Collaboration. ASC quality collaboration quality report 2nd quarter 2018. In ASC quality collaboration, partners in ASC quality 2018. Available at: http://www.ascquality.org/qualityreport.cfm#Transfer. Accessed August, 2018.

23. Advisory Board. 17 states don't require surgery centers to disclose patient deaths, USA Today investigation finds. 2018. Available at: Advisory.com; https://www.advisory.com/daily-briefing/2018/08/14/surgery-centers. Accessed August, 2018.

24. Malignant Hyperthermia Association of the United States. Available at: https://www.mhaus.org/. Accessed August, 2018.

25. Porter ME, Lee TH. The strategy that will fix health care. Harv Bus Rev 2013;91: 50–70.

26. Best RJ. Market based management. 6th Edition. Upper Saddle River (NJ): Pearson Education, Inc; 2013. p. 12.

27. Outpatient and ambulatory surgery CAHPS Survey. Available at: https://oascahps.org/. Accessed August, 2018.

28. Bowers B. Managing change by empowering staff. Nurs Times 2011;107(32–33): 19–21.

29. Harris T, Cameron PA, Ugoni A. The use of pre-cannulation local anaesthetic and factors affecting pain perception in the emergency department setting. Emerg Med J 2001;18(3):175–7.

30. Burke SD, Vercler SJ, Bye RO, et al. Local anesthesia before IV catheterization. Am J Nurs 2011;111(2):40–5.

31. Aggarwal N, Stoicea N, Shabsigh M, et al. Improving OR turnover time: a better process starts with the patient. Int J Adv Res (Indore) 2017;5(8):102–8.

32. Lungqvist O, Scott M, Fearon K. Enhanced recovery after surgery-a review. JAMA Surg 2017;152(3):202–8.

33. Lyass S, Link D, Grace B, et al. Enhanced recovery after surgery (ERAS) protocol for out-patient Laparoscopic Sleeve Gastrectomy in Ambulatory Surgery Center – safe and effective. Surg Obes Relat Dis 2015;11(6):198.

34. Gapinski K. The guidelines that are changing surgical patient's care. Outpatient Surgery Magazine 2016. Available at: https://www.outpatientsurgery.net/surgical-facility-administration/patient-management/the-guidelines-that-are-changing-surgical-patients-care–08-04-16. Accessed August, 2018.

35. West M. The social psychology of innovation in groups. In: West MA, Farr JL, editors. Innovation and creativity at work: psychological and organizational strategies. Chichester: John Wiley & Sons, Ltd; 1990. p. 309–33.

36. Thakur R, Hsu S, Fontenot G. Innovation in healthcare: issues and future trends. J Bus Res 2012;65(4):562–9.

37. Bhattacherjee A, Hikmet N. Physicians' resistance toward healthcare information technology: a theoretical model and empirical test. Eur J Inf Syst 2007;16(6): 725–37.

38. Landaeta RE, Mun JH, Rabadi G, et al. Identifying sources of resistance to change in healthcare. Int J Healthc Tech Manag 2008;9(1):74–96.

39. Eckelman MJ, Sherman J. Environmental impacts of the US health care system and effects on public health. PLoS One 2016;11(6):1–2.

40. ASA Task Force on Environmental Sustainability Committee on Equipment and Facilities. Greening the operating room and perioperative arena: environmental sustainability for anesthesia practice, Revised 2017. Available at: https://www.asahq.org/about-asa/governance-and-committees/asa-committees/committee-on-equipment-and-facilities/environmental-sustainability/greening-the-operating-room. Accessed August 2018.

Moving?

Make sure your subscription moves with you!

To notify us of your new address, find your **Clinics Account Number** (located on your mailing label above your name), and contact customer service at:

Email: journalscustomerservice-usa@elsevier.com

800-654-2452 (subscribers in the U.S. & Canada)
314-447-8871 (subscribers outside of the U.S. & Canada)

Fax number: 314-447-8029

Elsevier Health Sciences Division
Subscription Customer Service
3251 Riverport Lane
Maryland Heights, MO 63043

*To ensure uninterrupted delivery of your subscription, please notify us at least 4 weeks in advance of move.

Printed and bound by CPI Group (UK) Ltd, Croydon, CR0 4YY

08/05/2025

01864746-0001